Renal Pathology Express

An Essential Companion for a Nephrologist

Renal Pathology Express
An Essential Companion for a Nephrologist

Dr. Radhika Krishna Patil

M.D (Pathology), D.P.B, FISN-ANIO, PDCC (Renal & Transplant Pathology)

Director and Consultant Nephropathologist,
Shri Balaji Kidney Care Private Limited,
Madhapur, Hyderabad, Telangana, India.

Vice-President, Basic Sciences, Indian Society of Organ Transplantation (ISOT)

Renal Pathology Express: An Essential Companion for a Nephrologist
by Dr. Radhika Krishna Patil

Disclaimer: This book has been published with all efforts to ensure error-free material after the author's consent. However, the author and publisher disclaim any liability for any damage caused as a result of use of this book. The respective user must check the accuracy from other sources too. The drug selections and doses given in this book are for illustration only. The authors and publishers take no responsibility for any actions consequent upon following the contents of this book without first checking current sources of reference.

Published with arrangement by

Shri Balaji Kidney Care Pvt. Ltd.
First Floor, Door No. 1-99/14,
Hitech City Road, Megha Hills,
Hyderabad, Telangana 500081, India.

e-mail: sbhcindia2021@gmail.com

International ISBN: 978-93-340-8546-4

ISBN: 978-93-341-3075-1 (e-book)

Foreword

Renal Pathology Express is amongst the latest in the textbooks devoted solely to non-neoplastic Renal Pathology. It is unusual in that it is composed entirely of well-curated case records from the author's practice. The entire spectrum of glomerular, tubular, interstitial, and vascular lesions has been organized into separate chapters, along with an introductory chapter outlining clinical and pathology definitions.

The book is an atlas of light and immunofluorescence microscopy images of all the common conditions encountered in day-to-day practice interspersed with minimal text pertaining to relevant clinical, diagnostic, and management details, making it easy to read. A special mention must be made of the electron microscopy images hand drawn by the author, bringing out the details very accurately.

The book will be a valuable resource for pathologists and nephrologists in training and for those in practice as a ready reference.

Swarnalata G.

DR SWARNALATA GOWRISHANKAR

Senior Consultant Pathologist and Head,
Department of Histopathology
Apollo Hospitals, Jubilee Hills
Hyderabad, India

Foreword

With immense enthusiasm and a profound sense of duty, I present the first edition of the 'Renal Pathology Express' by Dr. Radhika Krishna Patil. This atlas transcends a mere collection of histological images; it forms a pivotal link between the intricate domain of renal pathology and the pragmatic demands of newcomers in nephrology. The genesis of this atlas was motivated by a clear gap in the existing literature - a need for a concise yet comprehensive guide that distills the essence of renal pathology into an accessible format. Amidst the vast sea of detailed textbooks and extensive atlases, the unique aim here was to sculpt a resource that stands out for its clarity, relevance, and ease of use. This atlas, crafted by Dr. Radhika, serves as a tool for learning and a companion for quick reference, tailored to the hectic schedules of practicing nephrologists and resident doctors alike. In creating this atlas, Dr. Radhika has strived to forge a resource that sparks learning enthusiasm, encouraging users to engage with the content actively through clinical case presentations. Each case is structured to cultivate a diagnostic thought process reflective of real-world challenges, promoting a hands-on learning approach. Integrating high-quality histopathology images, immunofluorescence, and immunohistochemistry studies provides a thorough insight into the microscopic worlds foundational to renal diseases. It is crafted with the hope that it will stand as a reliable guide for nephrology residents during their exam preparations and serve as a swift, effective refresher for experienced practitioners revisiting renal pathology fundamentals.

Having reviewed the book, I recognize that assembling this atlas has been an immensely fulfilling endeavour, propelled by a commitment to deepening our understanding of renal diseases.

I wholeheartedly endorse her work, acknowledging the dedication and perseverance required to create such an exemplary educational resource. As you explore this atlas, I hope you will find it informative and motivating, stirring a curiosity that drives you deeper into the study of renal pathology, enriching your clinical practice, and ultimately enhancing patient care.

Welcome to a journey of discovery, learning, and professional advancement through the 'Renal Pathology Express.'

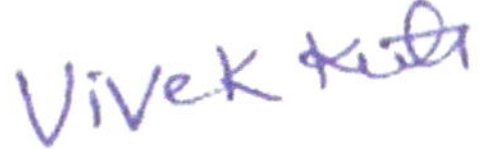

DR VIVEK KUTE

MBBS, MD, FCPS, DM Nephrology (Gold Medalist), FASN, FISOT, FISN, FRCP (London)

Professor, Nephrology and Transplantation
Institute of Kidney Diseases and Research Center, Ahmedabad, India.

Member of Apex Technical Committee NOTTO, Treasurer Indian Society of Organ Transplantation (ISOT), The Transplantation Society (TTS): Councillor (Asia), Asian Society of Transplantation: Councilor (India), Member TTS Data Harmonization committee, Editor, Indian Journal of Transplantation, Former Secretary, ISOT (2018-2023), Member TTS 2024 Finance committee

Testimonials

Absolutely thrilled with this Atlas! It's the perfect companion for anyone diving into the world of nephrology. Its engaging presentation and focused content make learning complex renal pathologies surprisingly accessible and enjoyable. A game-changer for both residents and seasoned practitioners looking to refresh their knowledge efficiently. Highly recommended for its practical approach and ease of use!

Dr. Manjusha Yadla
Professor and HOD Nephrology,
Gandhi Medical Collage/Hospital, Hyderabad

This Atlas emerges as a quintessential beacon for those traversing the intricate landscapes of nephrology. It adeptly demystifies complex renal pathologies with an elegance and precision that is both engaging and enlightening. Its meticulously curated content, designed for both novices and experts, makes it an unparalleled resource for enriching one's practice and study. This work is not merely informative; it is a testament to the art of medical education. An indispensable treasure for the discerning practitioner.

Dr. Rajsekhar Chakravarthy
Senior Consultant Nephrologist,
Yashoda Hospitals, Hi-tech city, Hyderabad, India.

The Renal Pathology Express stands out as a concise, yet thorough guide for those entering nephrology. Its practical case scenarios and clear histopathology images make it an indispensable tool for residents and busy practitioners alike, offering a straightforward way to navigate the complexities of renal pathology. A must-have for efficient learning and quick reference."

Dr. Kamal Kiran
Senior Consultant Nephrologist,
Medicover Hospitals, Hyderabad, India.

For students and budding nephrologists, I highly recommend The Renal Pathology Express. With detailed case scenarios and histopathology pictures to go along with, studying this book, students are going to understand the concepts of renal pathology by the impeccable presentation the author has displayed.

Dr. Sree Bhushan Raju
Senior Professor Nephrology,
Nizam's Institute of Medical Sciences, Hyderabad, India.

For those seeking to deepen their understanding of renal pathology, "Renal Pathology Express" stands out as an exceptional resource. This comprehensive compilation offers a wealth of cases, complete with histopathology images, fundamental studies, and advanced diagnostic insights. Its thorough approach to correlating clinical findings with differential diagnoses makes it an invaluable reference for both students and professionals in the field of Nephrology.

Dr. Krishna V Patil
Senior Consultant Nephrologist,
KIMS Hospitals, Gachibowli, Hyderabad, India.

"Renal Pathology Express - As the first of its kind from an Indian author, this book stands out for its innovative approach and unique style of presentation. I highly recommend it for: Nephrologists seeking to deepen their understanding of renal pathology and trainee pathologists looking for a comprehensive and concise guide.
Renal Pathology Express is a must-have resource that will revolutionize your learning experience!"

Dr. Manisha Sahay
Professor and HOD Dept. Nephrology,
Osmania Medical College, Hyderabad, India.

There has been an imperative need for a book on practical points of Nephropathology, especially from India. This book fulfills the void with Illustrative and comprehensive clinical pathology on both native and allograft biopsies. A must-read for all nephrologists.

Dr. P N Jikki,
Retired Principal Kurnool Medical College & Additional Director of Medical Education Andhra Pradesh, Retired Professor and Head of Dept. of Nephrology Kurnool Medical College Kurnool, India.

"Renal Pathology Express" is an invaluable resource for both Nephrologists and Pathologists. As a Nephrologist, I appreciate the clarity and depth it provides in correlating clinical presentations with microscopic findings. The case-based approach not only facilitates student learning but also allows busy clinicians to refer to key pathological entities quickly. This book significantly enhances our understanding of renal pathology and bridges the communication gap with pathologists during biopsy interpretation. It's not just a reference guide, but an essential tool for improving diagnostic precision and patient care in nephrology. My sincere appreciation to Dr. Radhika Krishna Patil for her remarkable work on this book, and I extend my best wishes for her future endeavors.

Dr. Swarnalatha Guditi,
Professor and HOD, Department of Nephrology,
NIMS, Hyderabad, India.

Preface

Welcome to the first edition of my Renal Pathology Express. This atlas, enriched with clinical case scenarios, has been carefully crafted to introduce the intricacies of renal pathology to newcomers in the field of nephrology in a precise and engaging manner. In a landscape abundant with elaborate textbooks and atlases, my goal was to create a streamlined refresher- a compact yet comprehensive resource filled with focused, relevant information. Designed to be both easy to access and navigate, this atlas aims to be a convenient reference for busy practitioners, ready to be consulted during brief moments of downtime without the risk of information overload. This atlas is intended as a quick, efficient tool for pathology review, especially useful for resident doctors preparing for their nephrology examinations. It compiles a range of common and some less frequent clinical cases, presenting them in a manner that encourages clinicians to engage in differential diagnosis. This is followed by histopathology images featuring various stains, along with immunofluorescence and immunohistochemistry studies, guiding clinicians toward identifying the underlying pathology and reaching a diagnosis. This approach mirrors real-life clinical practice, making the atlas a unique and practical learning/ guiding tool. I hope, befitting its name, 'Renal Pathology Express,' that it shall meet the needs of nephrology residents and busy practitioners alike, providing a straightforward means to refresh their knowledge of renal pathology with minimal effort.

I would like to acknowledge all the nephrologists who have contributed with their kidney biopsy samples.

Dr. Radhika Krishna Patil

Contents

CHAPTER 1

Journey of the Renal Tissue from Needle to Slide

I. NEPHROLOGIST'S CONTRIBUTION IN OPTIMIZING THE DIAGNOSTIC YIELD

Role of Kidney biopsy:

Invariably, the kidney diseases in which a nephrologist considers doing a biopsy are those with impending or ongoing kidney or graft failure. These situations can frequently be compared to a building on fire, and the earlier you douse the fire, the more damage is prevented. Similarly, the earlier you identify the cause and degree of damage in the kidney, the better you stand. You can salvage kidney function and decide how aggressive or observant you need to be when choosing your therapeutic options. Kidney biopsy is, therefore, the gold standard diagnostic test to find out what's happening inside the kidney.

Kidney biopsy specimen undergoes microscopic evaluation (Shown in the Fig. 1.1).

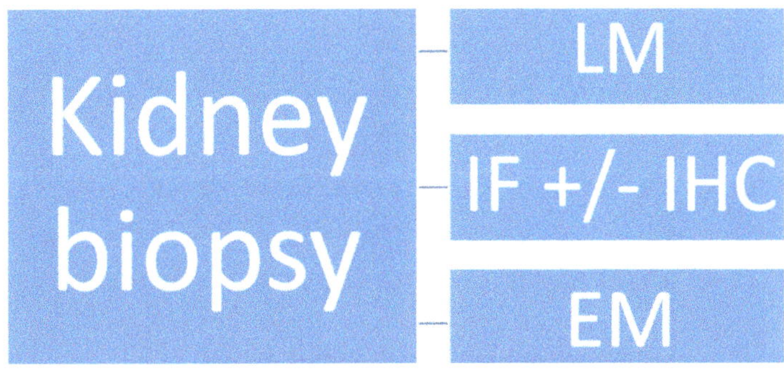

Figure 1.1: LM: Light microscopy, IF: Immunofluorescence, IHC: Immunohistochemistry, EM: Electron microscopy.

For an accurate diagnosis, the indispensable requirements are:

1. **Relevant Clinical History**: Detailed information the nephrologist provides is crucial for accurate diagnosis.
2. **Adequate Sample/Core Size**: The biopsy core must contain both cortex and medulla. It should be placed in an appropriately labeled and tightly sealed container.
3. **Proper Transportation:** The sample should be sent in appropriate transport media.
4. **Trained histopathology technician**: A skilled technician must appropriately handle and process the biopsy sample.
5. **Dedicated Renal Pathologist**: A renal pathologist who can discuss the case with the nephrologist before finalizing the report ensures a thorough and accurate diagnosis.

Optimizing the diagnostic yield of the biopsy:

It is an invasive procedure that cannot be repeated casually due to the risk involved, the expenses associated, and the patient's apprehension. Hence, when the procedure is planned, it is paramount to perform it with utmost care to obtain a core with maximum diagnostic yield.

A) Choosing the appropriate needle gauge (G):

The sample size is related to the gauge of the needle. The average glomerular diameter ranges from 200 to 350 microns for individuals above eight years of age. The internal diameter of an 18G biopsy needle is 300 to 400 microns, while that of a 16G biopsy needle is 600 to 700 microns. Therefore, a 16G biopsy needle is appropriate for individuals above eight years of age, and an 18G biopsy needle is adequate for those under eight.

Serial sections taken from a core obtained with a 16G needle:

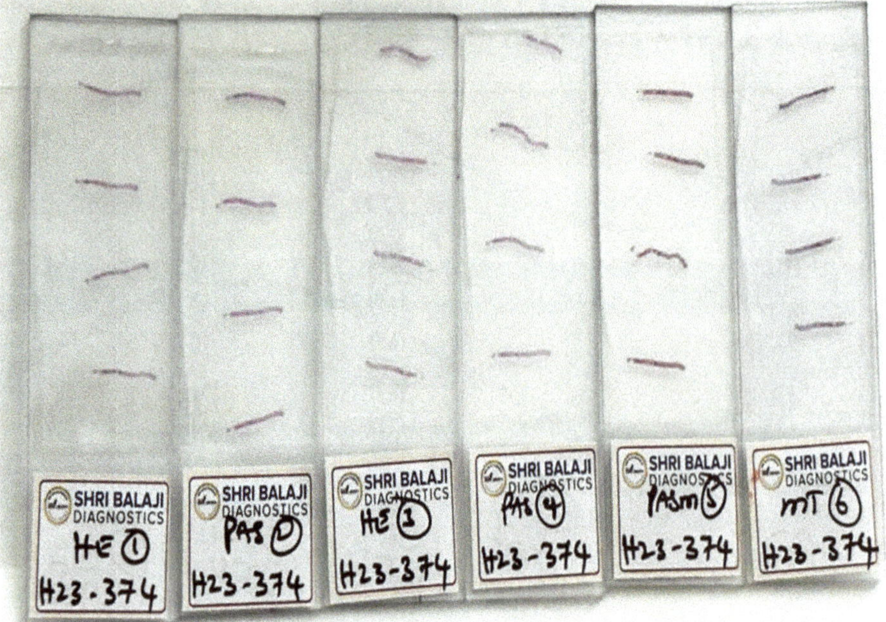

Figure 1.2: Serial sections: 16G needle: The thickness of the tissue is maintained till the last 24th section.

The core obtained with a 16G needle doesn't usually get exhausted even after sections are taken for light microscopy. It is available for further studies like Immunohistochemistry/Electron Microscopy when a separate core is unavailable. Also, if an inadequate sample was obtained for an IF study, this core taken with a 16G needle can suffice for the Paraffin IF procedure.

Serial sections were taken from a core obtained with an 18G needle:

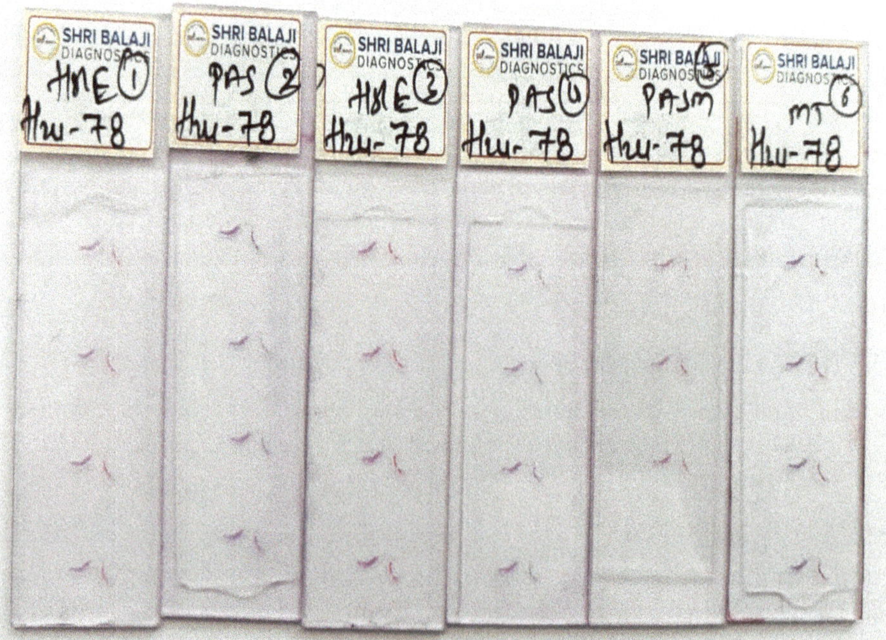

Figure 1.3: Serial sections: 18G needle: the tissue volume is less and likely to get exhausted.

Comparing the microscopic view of the samples obtained through 16G versus 18G needles:

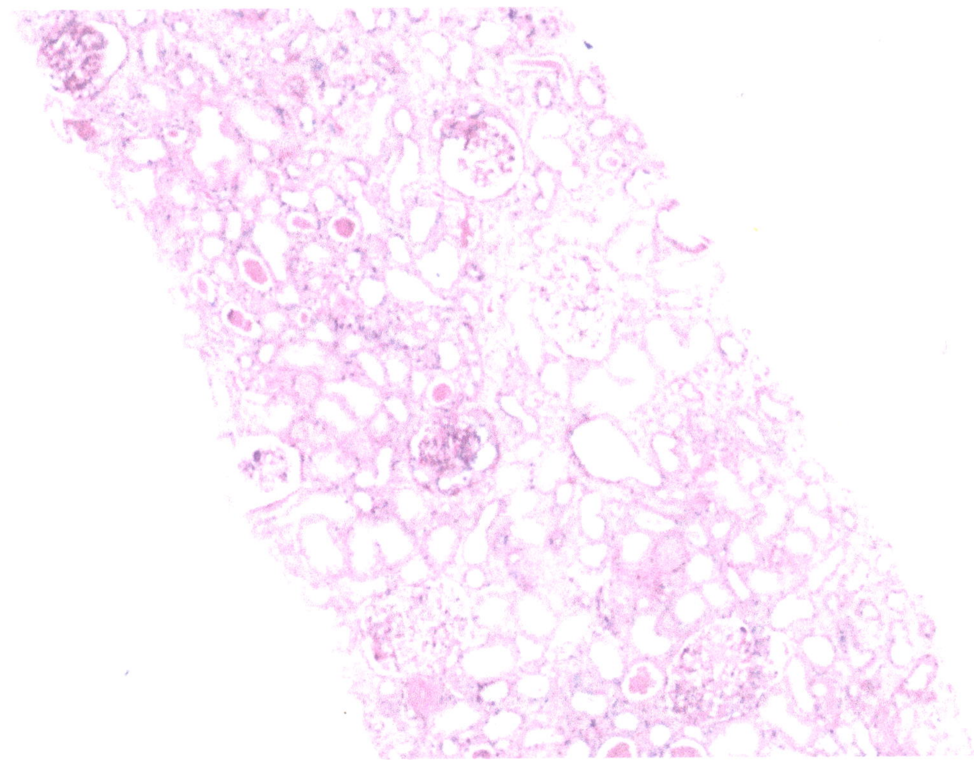

Figure 1.4: H&E (Haematoxylin & Eosin) Stain: Scanner view 4x: With a 16-gauge needle, a broader view with a more significant number of glomeruli, so there is a lesser chance of missing focal pathologic changes.

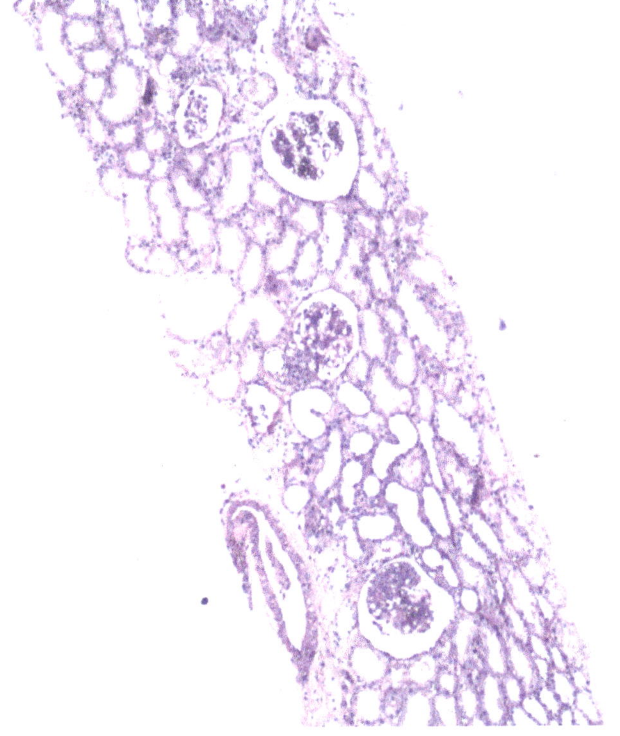

Figure 1.5: PAS (Periodic Acid Schiff) Stain: Scanner view 4x: With an 18-gauge needle, a narrower view with fewer glomeruli, a greater chance of missing focal pathologic changes.

B) Obtaining the Core from the appropriate location:

The core should contain the cortex and medulla.

Diagnostic pitfalls related to the location of the sample:

(i) Renal cortex:

(a) Subcapsular: subcapsular-scarred glomeruli may give an overrepresentation of global sclerosis related to aging/hypertension.

Age-related glomerulosclerosis appears to be an ischemic process more evident in the superficial (subcapsular) region. Diabetes-related glomerulosclerosis is more evident in the deeper(juxtamedullary) region. Obesity is more strongly associated with larger glomeruli in the superficial region.

When a biopsy is obtained with the needle entering only the superficial subcapsular region of the kidney, we get only the subcapsular cortex with more features of chronicity. The needle should enter perpendicularly so that the cortex and medulla are proportionately obtained.

Reference: Glomerular Volume and Glomerulosclerosis at Different Depths within the Human Kidney: Aleksandar Denic et al. J Am Soc Nephrol. 2019 Aug; 30(8): 1471–1480

(b) Juxtramedullary: Glomeruli in this region are involved early in FSGS and Alport syndrome. So, if the obtained core lacks the medulla, the diagnosis of FSGS can be missed.

Reference: Juxtramedullary glomeruli appear to be more vulnerable to developing FSGS than superficial glomeruli, likely because of their greater single-nephron glomerular filtration rate (GFR) and higher glomerular capillary pressures and flow rates: Newbold KM, et.al: Comparison of size of juxtramedullary and outer cortical glomeruli in normal adult kidney: Virchows Arch A Pathol Anat Histopathol 1992;420(2):127-129.

(ii) Renal medulla:

If only the medulla is obtained with no cortex, most glomerular diseases cannot be diagnosed, but the following diseases can still be diagnosed:

1. Acute pyelonephritis.

2. Light chain cast Nephropathy

3. Medullary interstitial amyloid.

4. Medullary angiitis.

5. Polyoma Virus Nephropathy.

C) Looking for glomeruli before placing in fixative:

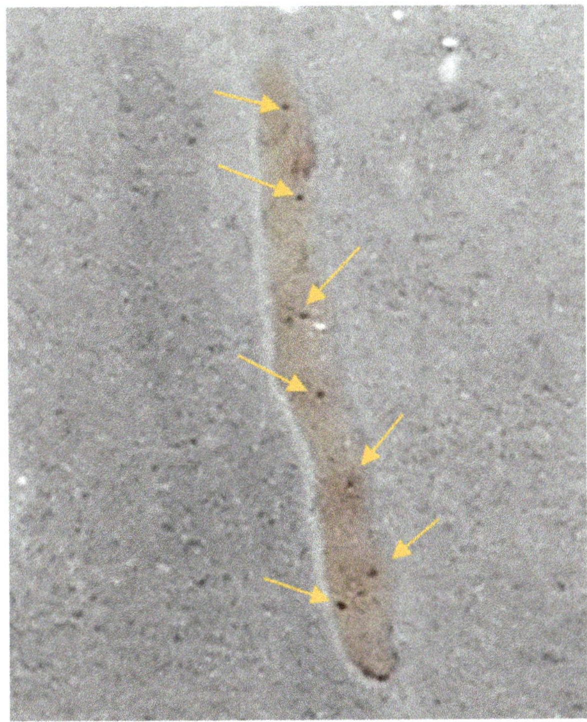

The handheld magnifying lens or zoomed view of a smartphone camera may not always show the presence of glomeruli as in this picture. Sclerosed glomeruli or glomeruli with diminished capillary blood due to proliferative glomerulonephritis, may not be visible as red dots.

Figure 1.6: Renal (needle) biopsy core: Smart phone camera view: glomeruli seen as red dots pointed by orange arrows.

D) Transporting the sample to the laboratory:

Ideally, three cores should be obtained, and each core should be placed in the following mentioned fixatives for different studies:

Core one: In 10% NBF- Neutral buffered Formalin – For Light Microscopy

Core two: In Michel's medium or Normal Saline – For Immunofluorescence study.

Core three: In 2% to 3% Glutaraldehyde – For Electron microscopy.

If only a single core is obtained, then place in 10% NBF so that after the light microscopy, the same tissue can be processed for Paraffin Immunofluorescence.

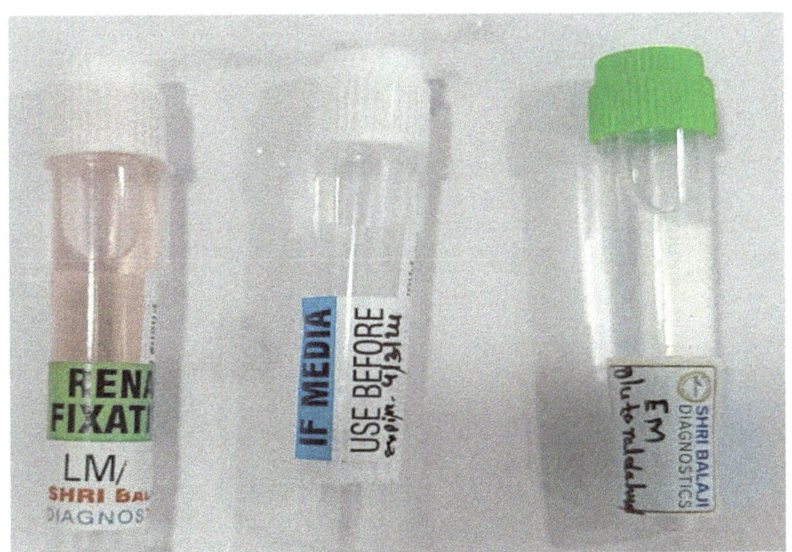

Renal biopsy vials: Eosin stain drops are placed in 10% Neutral Buffered Formalin to differentiate the LM vial from other vials.

Figure 1.7: Vials from left to right: LM vial (10% Neutral Buffered Formalin), IF media vial (Michel's media) and EM vial (3% Glutaraldehyde).

E) Fixation:

When live tissue is kept open in the air, it will dry up within minutes, and autolysis begins. To avoid drying and autolysis and preserve the structures as they are in living condition, the tissue needs to be fixed using a fixative that prevents the structure from crumbling.

***10%NBF:** neutral buffered formalin is the most common fixative used in laboratories. It is made up of:

1. Formalin: 100ml: 37% to 40% Formaldehyde solution, called Formalin. Pure Formaldehyde is a vapor that is dissolved in water, forming an aqueous solution called Formalin.

2. Tap water: 900ml

3. Sodium phosphate monobasic monohydrate: 4g

4. Sodium phosphate dibasic, anhydrous: 6.5gm

5. The Ph: 7 to 7.2.

   ***Reference:** Theory and Practice of Histological Techniques: John D Bancroft, Sixth edition: Chapter 4: Fixation of tissues: page no. 68.

Advantages of using 10% NBF:

1. Formalin is stable at room temperature for months.
2. It preserves morphology by the formation of protein cross-linkage.
3. It allows IHC to be performed.
4. The tissue can be used for EM and Paraffin Immunofluorescence if separate tissue is unavailable.

A minimum fixation time of 4 hours is required before tissue processing.

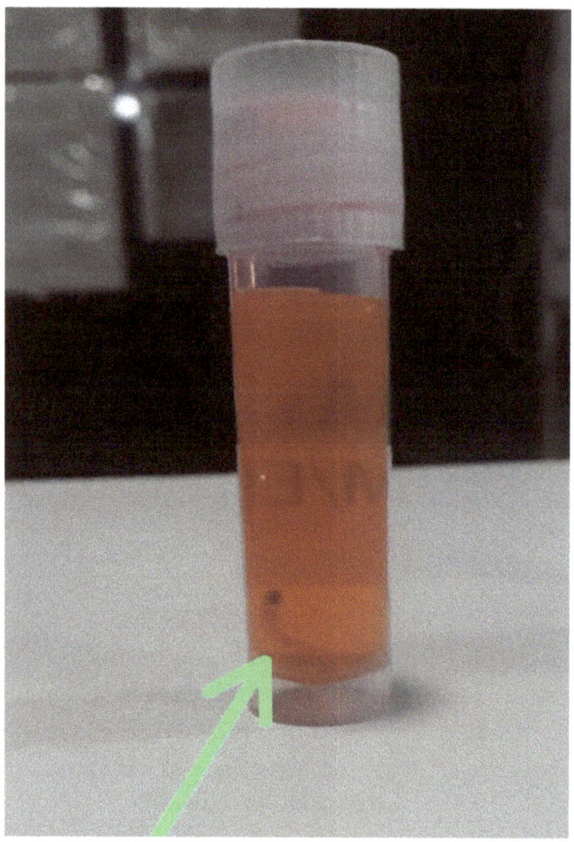

10% Neutral-Buffered Formalin: Renal tissue (green arrow) sinks to the bottom, whereas fatty tissue floats on the surface.

Figure 1.8: LM vial:10% NBF containing vial with renal tissue.

II. PATHOLOGIST'S CONTRIBUTION IN OPTIMIZING DIAGNOSTIC ACCURACY

Procedure for Light Microscopy:

For accurate results with high-quality images, grossing and processing must be performed according to Standard operating procedures (SOPs) with attention and without haste, giving appropriate time for each step.

1. Steps in Grossing:

a) **Labelling the sample:** The requisition form should consist of proper clinical history and relevant details, along with correctly labeled vials with the patient's name, age, and gender (Fig. 1.7 (a)).

b) **Measurement of the core:** Pour the respective LM vial sample core/s into a clean Petri dish/cap of a Coplin jar. Remove the sample core/s with blunt forceps and place them on pre-labeled 10% NBF-soaked Whatman filter paper number zero. Document the number of core/s and measure it with a measuring scale (Fig. 1.7 (b)).

c) **Staining the core:** Place a drop of Eosin stain on the tissue core so that the core stands out (Fig. 1.7 (c)).

d) **Placing in Tissue Cassette:** The carefully folded filter paper containing the stained tissue is placed into the labeled cassette (Fig. 1.7 (d)).

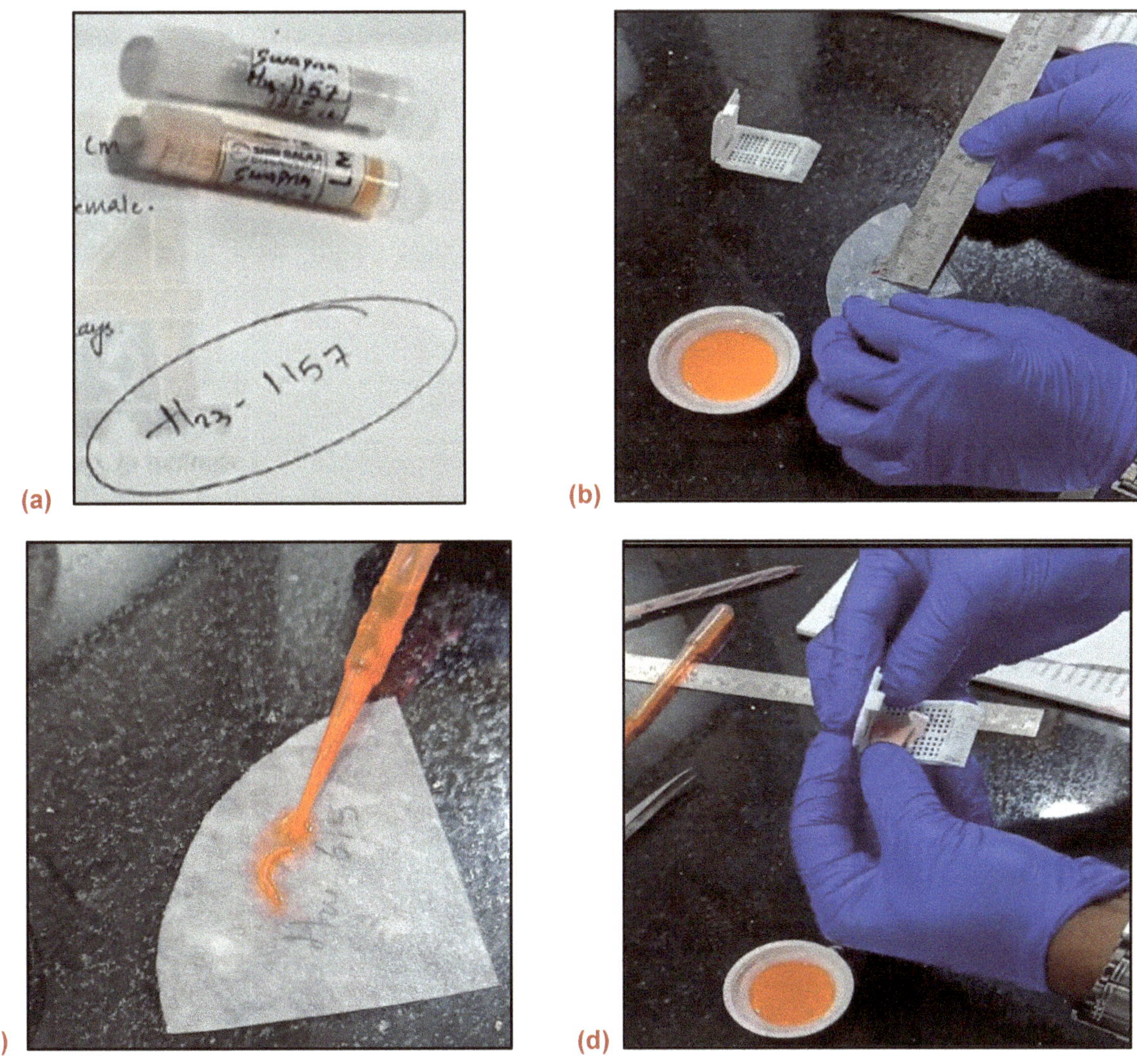

Figure 1.9: Steps in Grossing (a), (b), (c), and (d).

Steps of Tissue Processing

The labeled tissue cassette is placed into the Automatic Tissue Processor's first jar (10% NBF). (Figure 1.13).

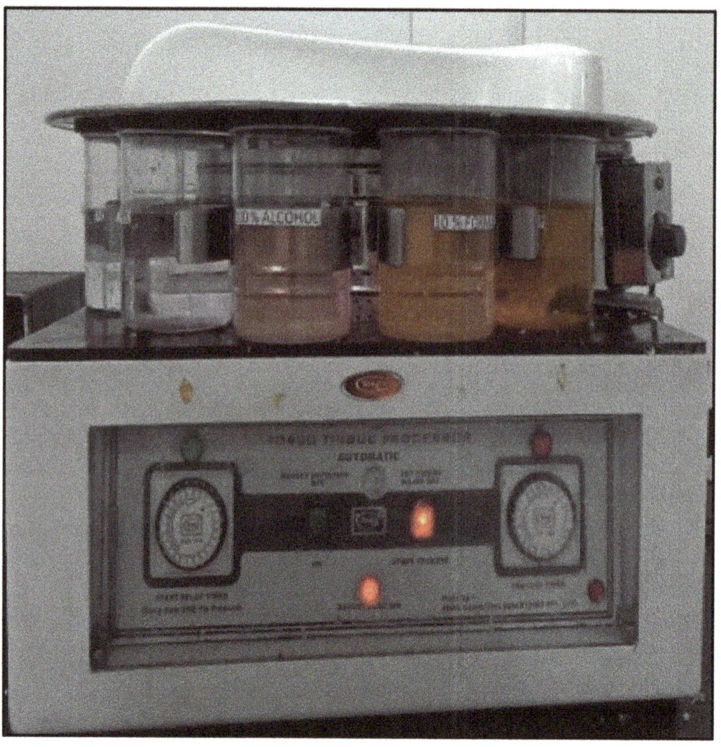

Figure 1.10: Automatic tissue Processor: Glass jars containing different solutions.

Time required for processing:

The processing time can be set based on the urgency of reporting, the sample size, and staff availability on weekends and holidays.

1. Short processing: 6 hours
2. Overnight processing: 12 hours
3. Delayed Processing: 24 hours

The sample size is small for kidney (needle) biopsy, so short processing for 6 hours would be sufficient if the tissue is fixed in 10% NBF for a minimum of 4 hours.

A. Fixation:

First jar: 10% NBF
Second jar: 10% NBF

B. Dehydration:

It is the removal of unbound water and aqueous fixatives from the tissue by serially increasing the percentage of alcohol (alcohol diluted with distilled water).

Third jar: 70% alcohol
Fourth jar: 80% alcohol
Fifth jar: 90% alcohol
Sixth jar: 100% alcohol
Seventh jar:100% alcohol

C. Clearing:

Xylene removes the dehydrating agent(alcohol) from the tissue.

> Eighth jar: Xylene I
> Ninth jar: Xylene II
> Tenth jar: Xylene III

D. Impregnation:

By Paraffin wax

> Eleventh jar: Paraffin wax I
> Twelfth jar: paraffin wax -II

After that, the Automatic tissue processor stops, and the processed tissue core is removed for Embedding.

E. Embedding:

Manual embedding: with Liquid Paraffin at 60 to 65 degrees Celsius. The tissue core is placed into a steel Mold filled completely with Hot Paraffin from the paraffin dispenser (Figure 1.14).

F. Paraffin block:

The plastic cassette is placed on the Mold and kept in an ice tray for cooling. After some time (30 min.), the block is ready, with the orange-pink tissue standing out in white Paraffin (Figure 1:1.15). The paraffin block can easily pop out of the mold; the wax block should not stick. Figure 1.15: A paraffin block is prepared, and the tissue stands out in the white paraffin block.

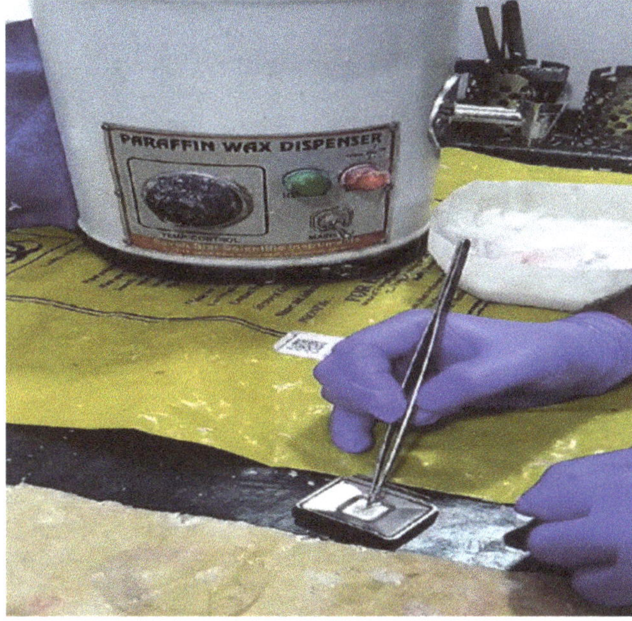

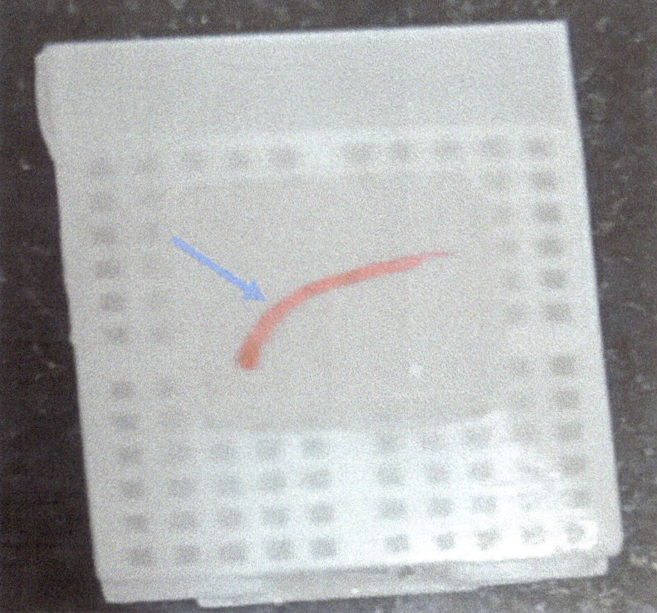

Figure 1.11: Manual Embedding in steel Mold filled with Liquid Paraffin Wax.

Figure 1.12: Paraffin block is prepared, and the tissue stands out in the white paraffin block.

PREPARING THE SLIDES

1. Cutting: Cool the paraffin-embedded tissue blocks on ice before sectioning. The small amount of moisture penetrating the block from the melting ice makes the tissue easier to cut. A Rotary Microtome is used for cutting serial sections of 2 to 3 microns thickness (Figure 1:1.15).

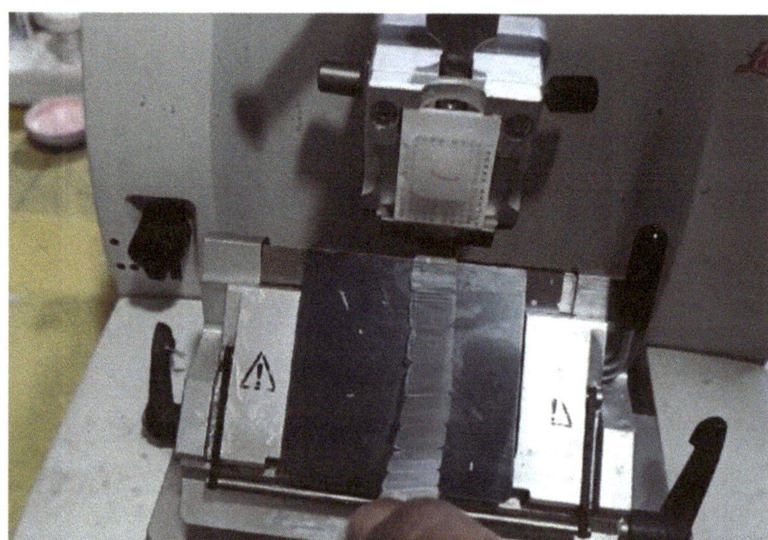

Figure 1.13: Cutting the serial sections from the Paraffin block. It should be like a tissue ribbon.

2. Sections in Distilled water(D/W): Placing the serial sections in distilled water to correct folding artifacts if any.

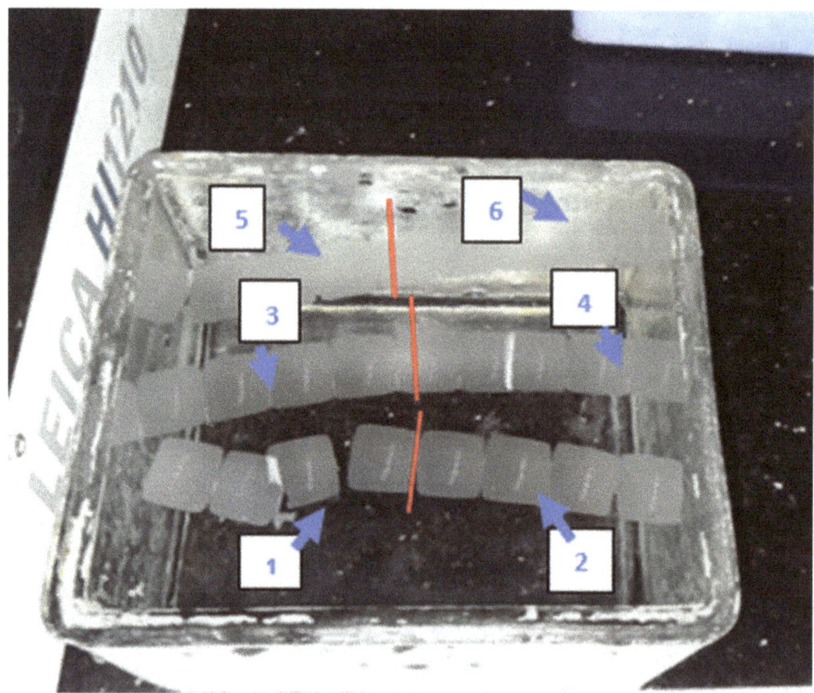

Figure 1.14: Serial sections in distilled water(D/W): numbers and arrows in blue colour are the slide numbers. At least 4 serial sections are to be taken on each slide; in total, 6 slides and a minimum of 24 sections are to be viewed under the microscope after staining.

3. Sections in Hot Water Bath: The serial sections taken on the slide from the D/W bath are then placed in a Hot water bath (temperature:50 to 55 degrees Celsius) in which a pinch of Gelatine powder is already added so that the sections remain stuck to the slide.

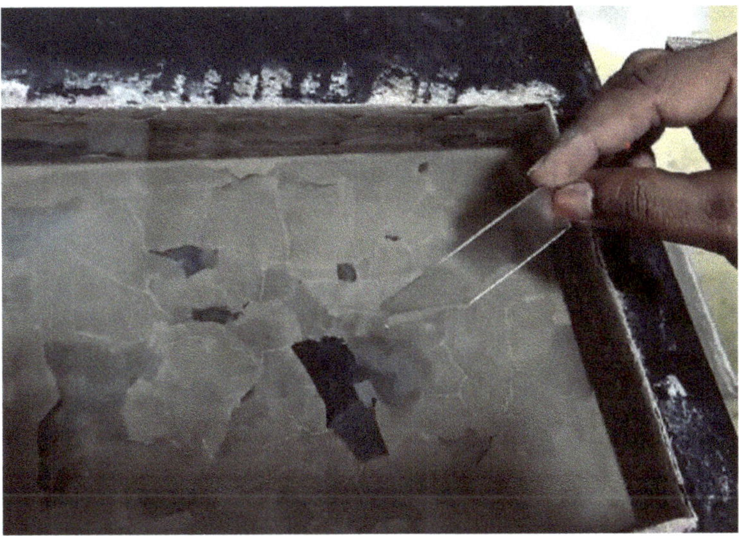

Figure 1.15: Hot water bath containing Gelatine: Sections are taken on a glass slide.

4. Slide Warming: The slides are then placed on a warming table until the wax melts (60 degrees Celsius for 10 min).

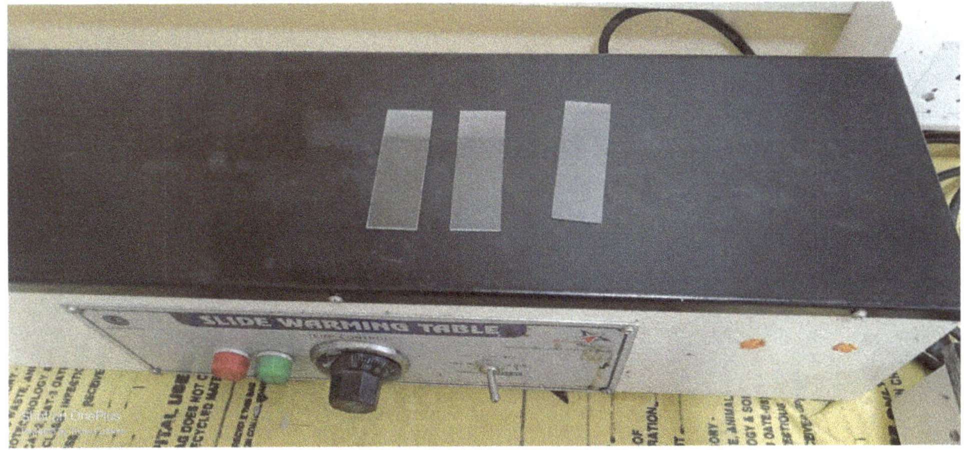

Figure 1.16: Slide warming table for melting the wax. Finally, only tissue core is visible.

5. Deparaffinization:

It is removing of Paraffin from the tissue before staining the section. The following steps are performed for it:

> Xylene: I: 5 min.
> Xylene: II:5min.
> 80%Alcohol:2 min.
> 90% Alcohol:2min.
> 100% Alcohol:2 min.
> Water Wash: under running Tap water: 5 min.

6. Staining station:

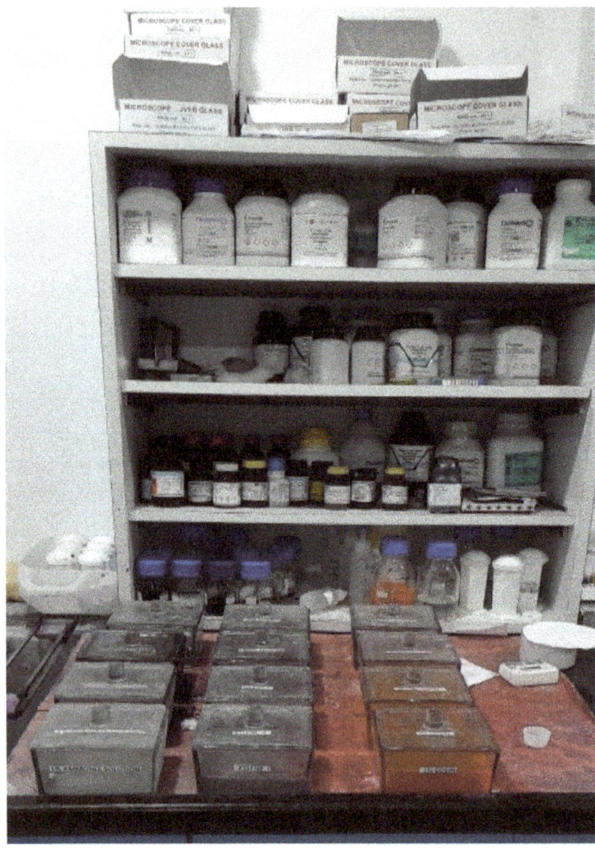

Figure 1.17: The following stains are done according to their standard operating staining procedures.

1. Hematoxylin & Eosin (H&E)
2. Periodic Acid Schiff (PAS)
3. Periodic acid Schiff Jones Methenamine Silver (PASM)
4. Masson Trichrome (MT)

*Congo red and Prussian Blue stains are done whenever needed.

The total time required for sample fixation, processing, and staining for Light microscopy is about 12 hours /18 hours.

7. Observing the slide under the Light microscope:

4. Compartments

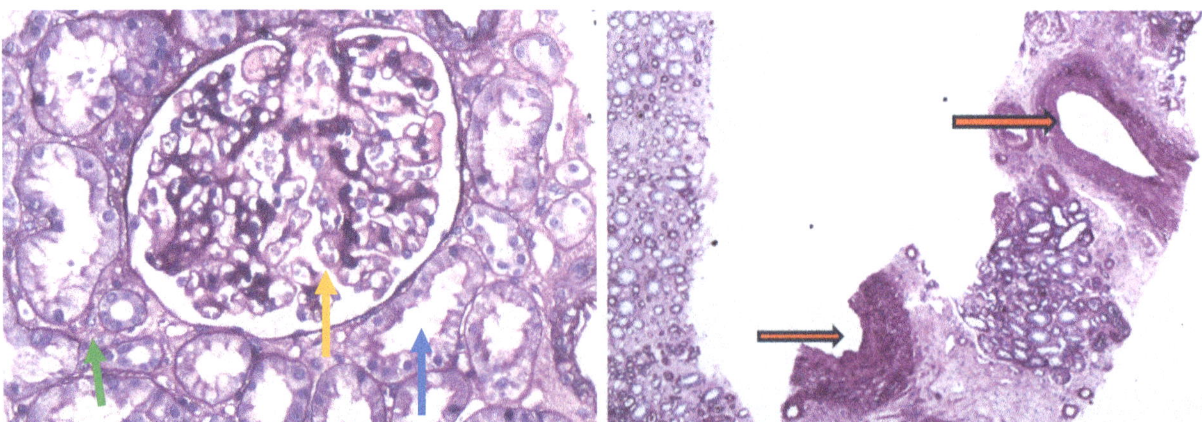

Figure 1.18: The following 4 compartments are to be viewed under the microscope:

1. Glomerulus: orange arrow   **2.** Tubules: blue arrow
3. Interstitium: green arrow (space in between the tubules) **4.** Vessels: red arrow

Assessing sample adequacy under the microscope:

1. In most cases, a minimum of 10 glomeruli are needed to assess the severity and distribution of lesions.

2. For FSGS, a sample of at least 20 glomeruli is required to confidently exclude the presence of FSGS affecting 10% of glomeruli: Corwin HL, et al. The importance of sample size in the interpretation of the renal biopsy. Am J. Nephrol 1988;8(2):85-89.

3. Membranous glomerulonephritis can be diagnosed from a single glomerulus on light microscopy.

4. For IgA Nephropathy, a single glomerulus for Immunofluorescence study is sufficient to make the diagnosis.

Table: 1.1: Mandatory Stains in Renal biopsy.

Renal structures	Hematoxylin & Eosin (H&E)	Periodic acid-schiff (PAS)	Silver/ PASM	Masson Trichrome (MT)
Types of inflammatory cells	To be seen in H&E	-	-	-
Mesangial cellularity	-	To be seen in PAS	-	-
Mesangial matrix appearance	Pink	Magenta	Black	Dark Blue
Extracapillary cellularity	-	To be seen in PAS stain	To be seen in PASM stain	
Glomerular Basement membrane (GBM)	Pink	Magenta	Black : 1. Breach in Bowman capsule: Crescent 2. Rupture of GBM: necrosis of the tuft	Dark blue
Tubular Basement membrane	Pink	Magenta. To assess tubular atrophy	Black	Dark blue
Hyaline	Homogeneous -smooth pink	Homogeneous -smooth magenta	Homogeneous - smooth Silver negative	Homogeneous - smooth Fuchsinophilic (reddish)
Fibrin	Fibrillar - pink	Granular- magenta	Silver negative- orange- fibrillar	Fuchsinophilic (reddish) - fibrillar
Immune complex deposits	-	-	-	Can be seen in MT stain -reddish

Immunofluorescence (IF) study:

Tissue is transported in:

1. **Michel's medium**: It is a transport medium, and the tissue is stable at room temperature for 5 to 7 days. It is used to transport the sample to other cities.
2. **Normal saline**: For samples expected to reach the laboratory within two hours, vials containing Normal saline can be used, or the tissue can be placed in saline-moistened Whatman filter paper number zero, wrapped with a Saline-soaked gauze piece, and transported with an ice pack.

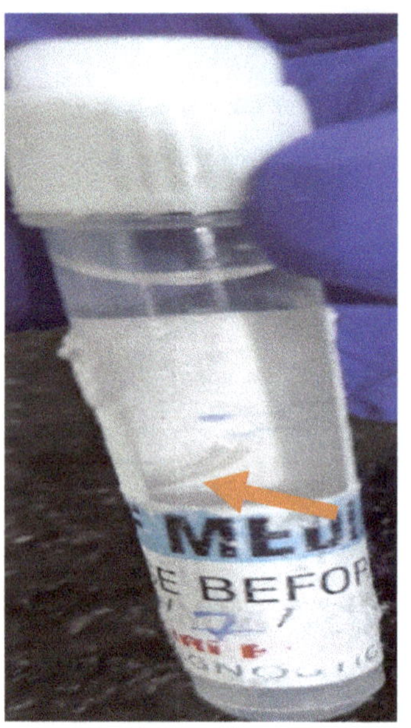

Michel's media: It inhibits proteolytic enzymes thus prevents autolysis. It preserves immuno-antigenicity by its ability to precipitate macromolecules hence it is useful for detection of Immunoglobulins and complements by Immunofluorescence technique.

The tissue may float /sink in it.

Tissue is preserved for 5-7 days at room temperature in Michel's medium.

This solution is stable at room temperature for about one month.

Figure 1.19: Michel's medium vial: orange arrow is pointing towards the renal biopsy core.

Cryostat : A Cryostat is required to prepare frozen sections from the saline /Michel's medium specimen.

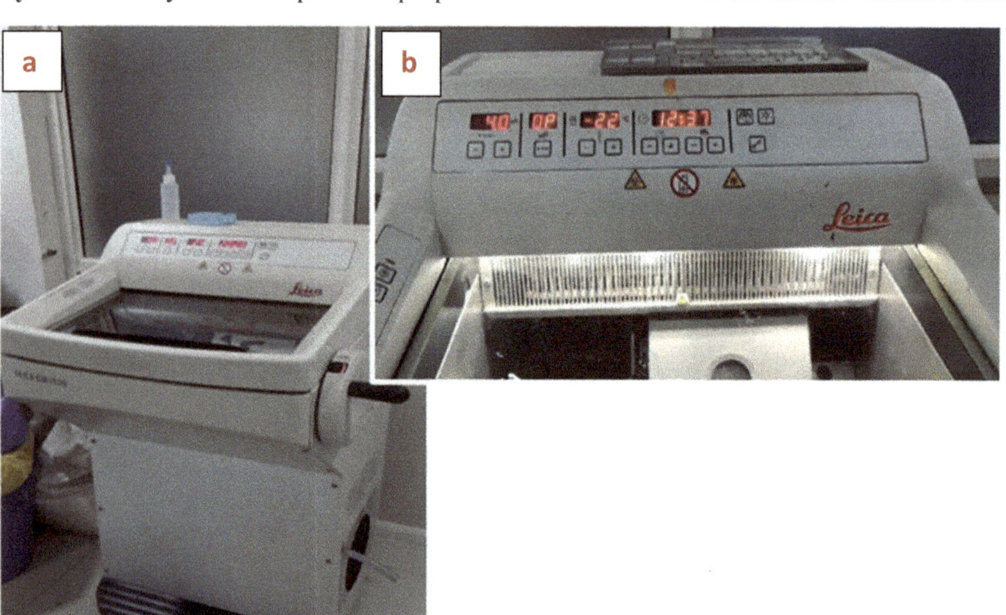

Figure 1.20: (a) Cryostat: Freezing Rotary microtome. **(b)** Temperature at cryostat is minus 22 to minus 24 degree celcius for kidney Immunofluorescence studies.

1. Label the sample with the appropriate laboratory number.
2. If sample is received in normal saline; then sample can be taken directly for cryostat cutting.
3. If sample is received in Michel's medium, it has to be washed three times with 10% Sucrose solution before cutting.
4. Measurement of the sample is done.
5. Label the cryostat chuck with the appropriate number
6. Mount the tissue with freezing medium for section cutting on the prelabeled cryostat chuck, place the chuck in the cryostat freezing chamber. Within a minute it gets frozen and ice block (orange arrows) is ready for cutting.

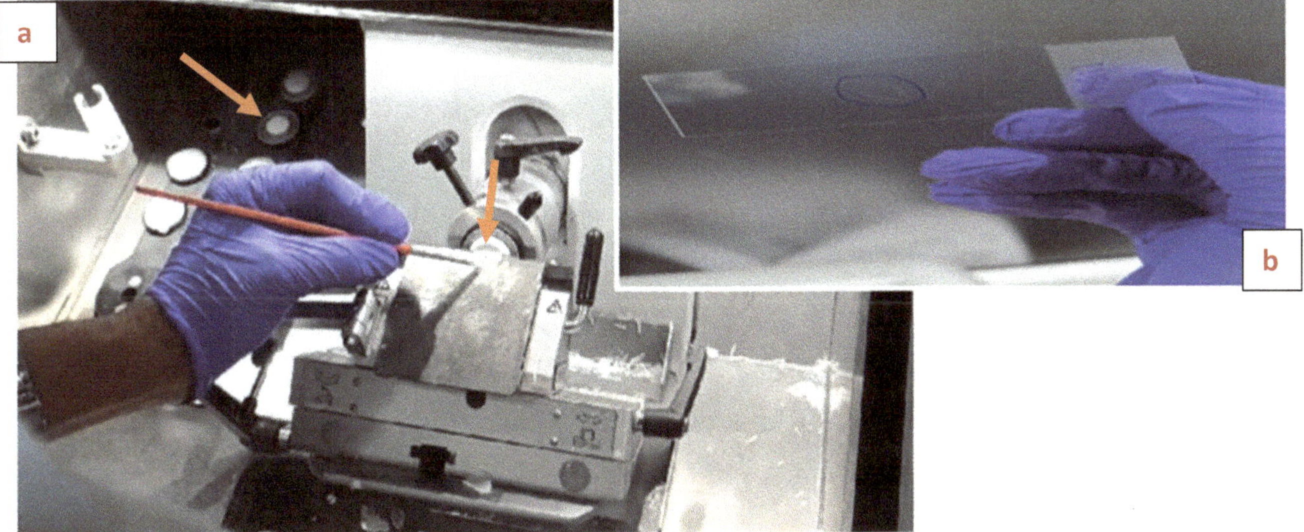

Figure 1.21: (a) Cryostat: 3-4 microns thickness sections are taken. **(b)** Cryostat: Sections are placed on the pre-labeled and clean glass slide and marked with blue circle on the back side of the section to indicate the sample.

7. **Staining:** Sections are stained with pre-made FITC-labeled antibodies targeting IgG, IgM, IgA, C3c, C1q, and light chains Kappa and Lambda. The entire sectioning and staining process takes 2 hours.

8. **Microscopy:** A fluorescent microscope is necessary for examining the IF slides. Fluorescent stains can fade with repeated exposure to light during microscopy, hence it should be examined in a dark room. Interpretation: Positive results are indicated by bright green fluorescence against a dark background.

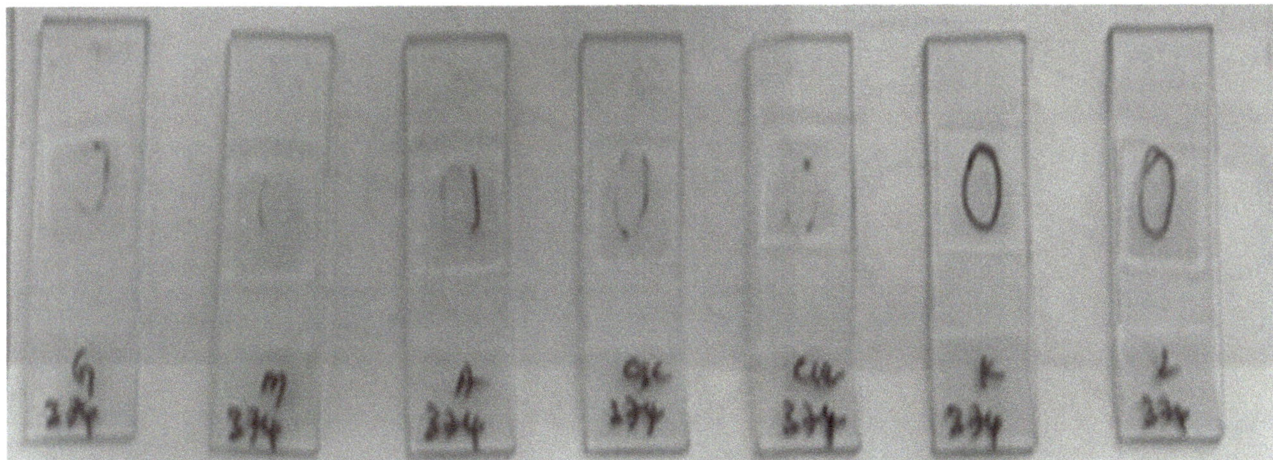

Figure 1.22: For each case these 7 slides need to be viewed under fluorescent microscope in a dark room.

Internal controls: To ensure that the process has worked and the negative IF result is not due to error in processing, internal control helps.

1.   **IgG:** The tubular epithelial cells often take up IgG fluorescence in all cases, hence the IgG in tubular epithelial cells work as positive internal control for the glomerulus.

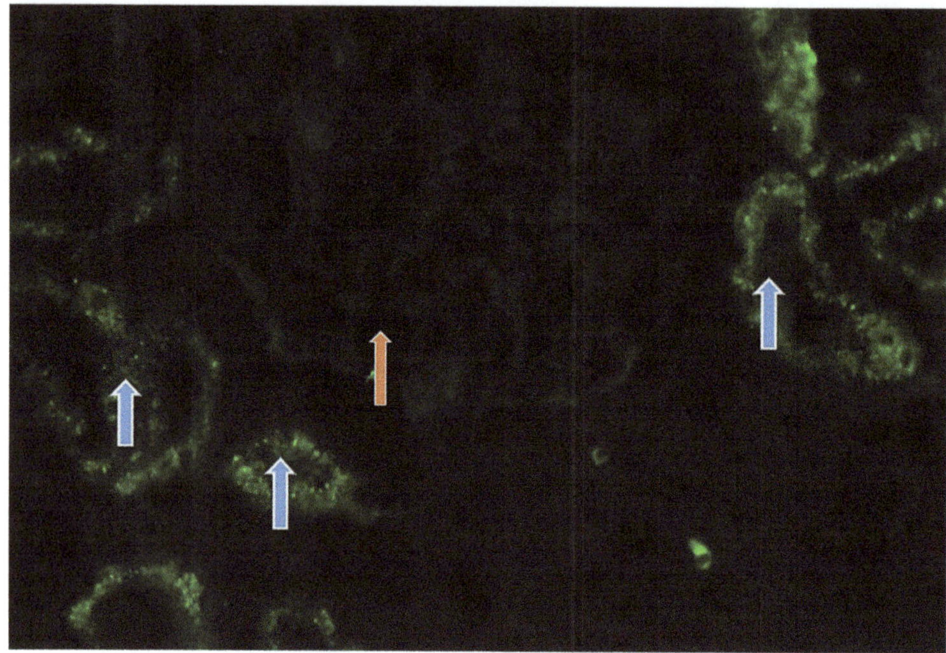

Figure 1.23: IgG :20x: is negative in the glomerulus **(orange arrow)** as there is no granular bright green positivity in it. The tubular epithelial cells are positive for IgG, which acts as internal control for that antibody.

2.   **IgA:** Tubular casts always take up IgA Flourescence hence these IgA positive tubular casts serve as positive internal control for the IgA in the glomeruli.

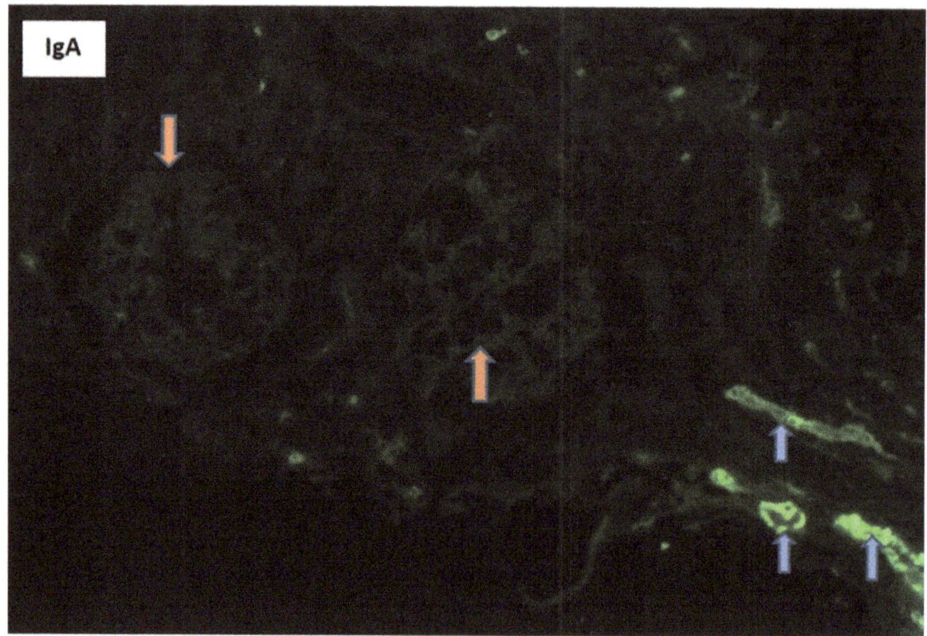

Figure 1.24: IgA :20x: Tubular casts **(blue arrow):** internal control for IgA,
glomeruli **(orange arrow):** negative for IgA

3.   **C3c:** Vessels are always lit up with C3c hence C3c in the vessels serve as positive internal control for C3c in the glomeruli.

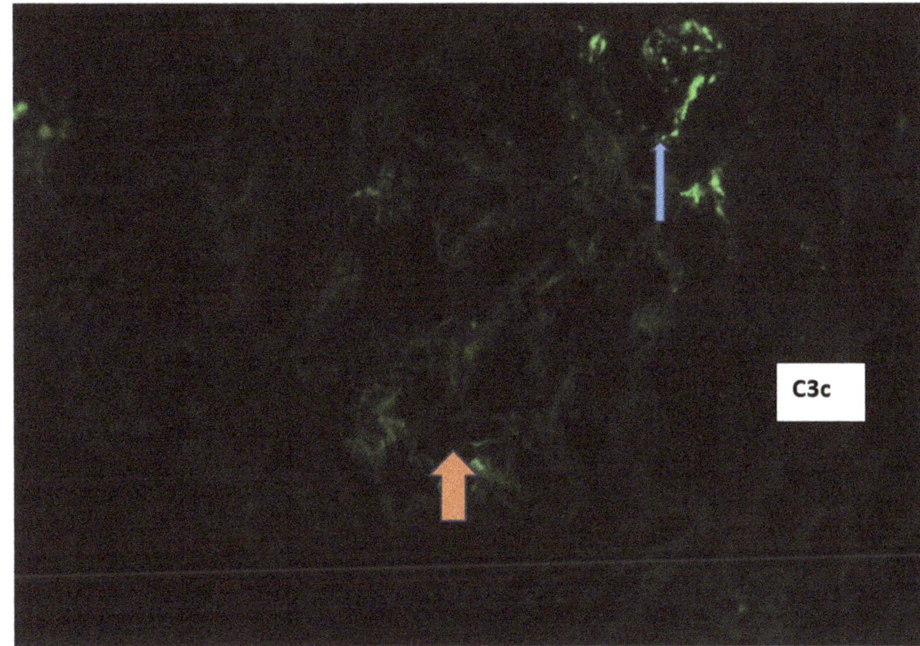

Figure 1.25: C3c:20x: Hilar arteriole is positive (blue arrow) and glomerulus (orange arrow) is negative for C3c.

***Paraffin Immunofluorescence: Pronase Immunofluorescence:** When a single core is received in formalin and no separate core available for IF study then we can perform IF using Pronase digestion (paraffin immunofluorescence). It is also useful in unmasking the false negative immune deposits on routine immunofluorescence study.

Formalin induces protein cross linking; this blocks the antigenicity & reduces the ability of antibodies to bind with these antigens giving false negative IF results. Pronase digestion is the process of breaking these cross linkages allowing the antibody to attach to the antigen.

Diagnostic insights about Paraffin Immunofluorescence:

1.   Non-specific trapping of serum within capillary loops of glomeruli should not be mistaken for immune complex deposition.

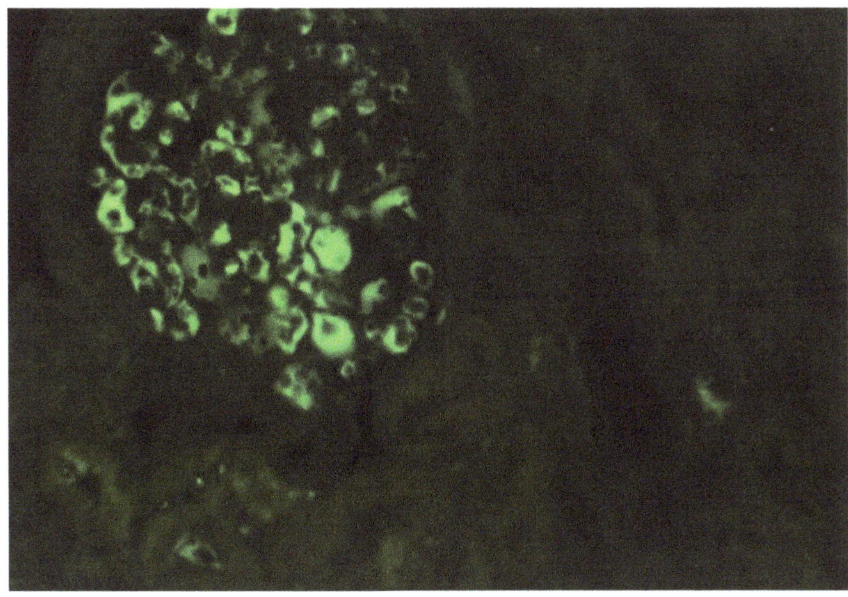

Figure 1.26: Paraffin Immunofluorescence: IgA: 20x: There is non-specific trapping of serum in the capillary lumina and not in mesangium.

2. C3c often stains weaker by paraffin immunofluorescence than by routine immunofluorescence done on saline/Michel's medium fixed tissue.

3. In conditions where you suspect a false negative IF (due to masked antigens), Paraffin IF unmasks these masked antigens and helps in confirming true negative from false negative result. For e.g. When only C3c is positive and IgG is negative, before reporting it as C3 GN we suggest doing Paraffin IF study. If with paraffin IF the IgG turns out positive, it suggests Immune complex mediated GN rather than C3 GN. This way paraffin IF helps in unmasking of false negative IF results.

***Reference:**

Paraffin immunofluorescence in the renal pathology laboratory: more than a salvage technique: Nidia C Messias, et.al, Modern Pathology (2015) 28, 854–860

Immunohistochemistry (IHC):

Utility of IHC in native kidney biopsy:

IHC is useful in detection of following entities:

1. AA Amyloid : For AA Amyloidosis

2. Myoglobin : For Myoglobin cast nephropathy

3. Kappa/ Lambda light chain: In light chain restricted diseases- Paraproteinemias

4. IgG4: In IgG 4 related tubulointerstitial disease

5. PLA2R / NELL 1 / THSP7A / Semaphorin 3B / EXT-1 – In Membranous Nephropathy

6. DNAJB9 : In Fibrillary Glomerulonephritis.

Utility of IHC in Allograft biopsies:

IHC is useful in identifying following entities :

1. C4d : In Antibody mediated rejection.

2. SV 40 : In Polyomavirus nephropathy

3. CMV : In Cytomegalovirus nephritis

4. Adenovirus: In Adenovirus nephritis.

***Suggested reading:**

*Approach to Renal Biopsy: AB Fogo: AJKD:2003: Core curriculum in Nephrology
*Basics of Kidney biopsy: A nephrologist's perspective: S. K. Agarwal, et.al, Indian J Nephrol.2013 Jul-Aug; 23(4): 243–252.

III. WRITING A NATIVE KIDNEY BIOPSY REPORT

A. Light Microscopy:
1. Mention Number of cores
2. Mention the presence of Cortex/medulla/corticomedullary tissue.
3. Note the total number of glomeruli & presence of an artery /not.
4. **Glomeruli:**
   a. Mention the number of globally sclerosed glomeruli if any.
   b. Viable glomeruli –
      Cellularity: Normocellular /Hypercellular: mesangial/ endocapillary/ extracapillary-crescents: segmental/circumferential.
      Basement membrane: thickening/duplication/spikes/holes.
      Mesangial matrix: Expansion with PAS/Silver – Stain Positive/Negative.
      Capillary lumina: Patent / Obliteration: Hyaline/ Fibrin thrombi
      Segmental lesions: sclerosis/necrosis.
5. **Tubules:**
   a. Acute Tubular Injury/Acute tubular necrosis/Tubulitis /Tubular casts /Tubular atrophy
   b. Tubular epithelial cells: Cytoplasmic Vacuolizations / viral inclusion bodies/ pigmented epithelial cells
6. **Interstitium:**
   Interstitial fibrosis: Percentage
   Interstitial Inflammation: in fibrosed /non – fibrosed areas, degree of inflammation, patchy or diffuse, type of inflammatory cells and any granulomas or hemorrhage if present.
7. **Vessels:**
   Arteriolar hyalinosis/arteriosclerosis/vasculitis/mucoid intimal hyperplasia (onion skinning), fibrinoid deposits.

B. Immunofluorescence findings:

Number of glomeruli

A. Location of immune deposits:
   a. Glomerular: Capillary wall/Paramesangial/mesangial
   b. Extraglomerular: Tubular Basement membranes/tubular casts/Interstitium (in case of amyloidosis)/vessel walls
B. Pattern of deposits: linear smooth/linear continuous/linear interrupted/fine granular/coarse granular/smudgy
C. Intensity: Insignificant (Grade: 0 / Trace / 1+) , minimal (Grade : 2+), significant (Grade 3+/4+).

Diagnosis/Comments:

The kidney (needle) biopsy shows features of………

IV. SOME CLINICAL DEFINITIONS

1. **Acute Kidney Injury (AKI):** Increase in Serum Creatinine by 0.3 mg/dl within 48 hours; or Increase in Serum Creatinine by >1.5 times baseline, which is known or presumed to have occurred within the prior 7 days; or Urine volume <0.5 ml/kg/hour ≥ for 6 hours.

2. **Simple definition of AKI:** Renal dysfunction evolving over hours to days.

3. **Rapidly progressing renal failure (RPRF):** Renal dysfunction evolving over days to weeks.

4. **Chronic Kidney Disease (CKD):** CKD is defined as abnormalities of kidney structure or function, present for a minimum of 3 months, with implications for health.

5. **Nephrotic range Proteinuria:** In Children: First morning urine sample or 24 hour Urine Protein to creatinine ratio of ≥ 2 g/ g, or Urine dipstick protein 3+ or more.

   In adults: 24 hour urine protein ≥3.5 gm per day or UPCR ≥3 g/g. With no edema, no or mild dyslipidemia, with serum albumin >3 g/dl.

6. **Nephrotic syndrome:** Nephrotic range proteinuria and Serum albumin level of < 3 g/dl, (or with edema when serum albumin level is not available), with dyslipidemia.

CHAPTER 2

Glomerular Diseases

DEFINITIONS

Basic Definitions in Glomerular Histology

Focal: Involving < 50% of glomeruli.

Diffuse: Involving ≥ 50% of glomeruli.

Segmental: Involving part of a glomerular tuft.

Global: Involving all of the glomerular tufts.

Sclerosis: Increased collagenous extracellular matrix, expanding the mesangium and forming adhesions to the Bowman capsule.

Endocapillary Hypercellularity: Increased cellularity internal to the GBM composed of leukocytes, endothelial cells, and /or mesangial cells.

Extracapillary Hypercellularity: Increased cellularity in Bowman space.

Crescent: Extracapillary hypercellularity, composed of at least 2 layers of parietal epithelial cells, involving 10% or more of the circumference of Bowman's capsule with/ without fibrin and fibrous matrix.

Circumferential Crescent: ≥ 50% circumference of Bowman capsule.

Cellular Crescent: > 75% cells and fibrin and < 25% fibrous matrix.

Fibrocellular Crescent: 25% – 75% cells and fibrin and the remainder fibrous matrix.

Fibrous Crescent: > 75% fibrous matrix and < 25% cells and fibrin.

Fibrinoid Necrosis: Fibrin + glomerular basement membrane disruption + lysis of the mesangial matrix ± karyorrhexis.

Nodule: Mesangial matrix expansion without cellularity, giving a nodular appearance.

Enlarged glomerulus: The normal glomerulus is approximately 2.5 times the size of the proximal tubules and also when it exceeds the field of vision under the high power 40x lens.

PATTERNS

Patterns of Glomerular Injury

A.   No Abnormality in Light Microscopy (LM).

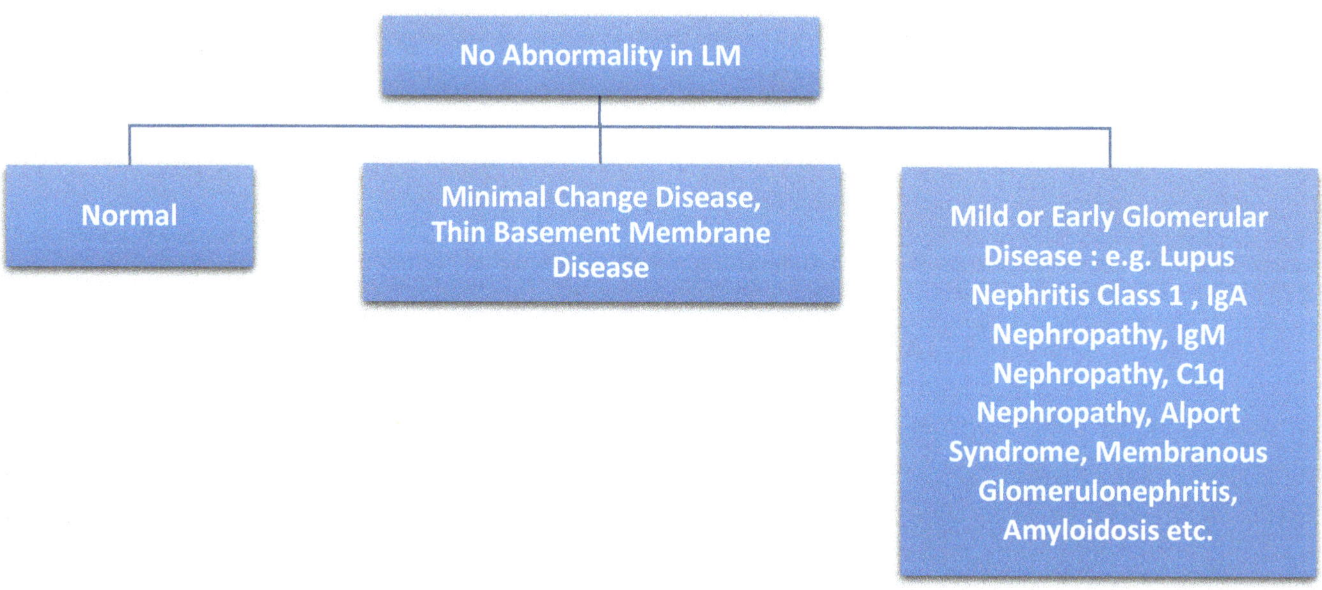

B.   Focal Segmental Glomerulosclerosis with no Increase in Cellularity on LM.

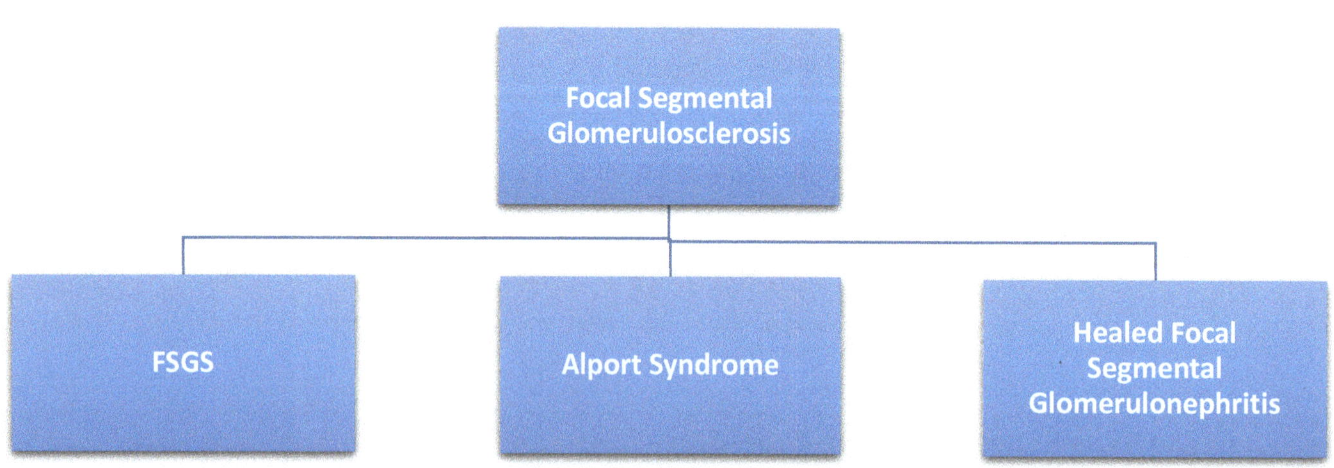

C.　Mesangial Hypercellularity on LM with and Non-IgA Deposits on the Immunofluorescence (IF) Study.

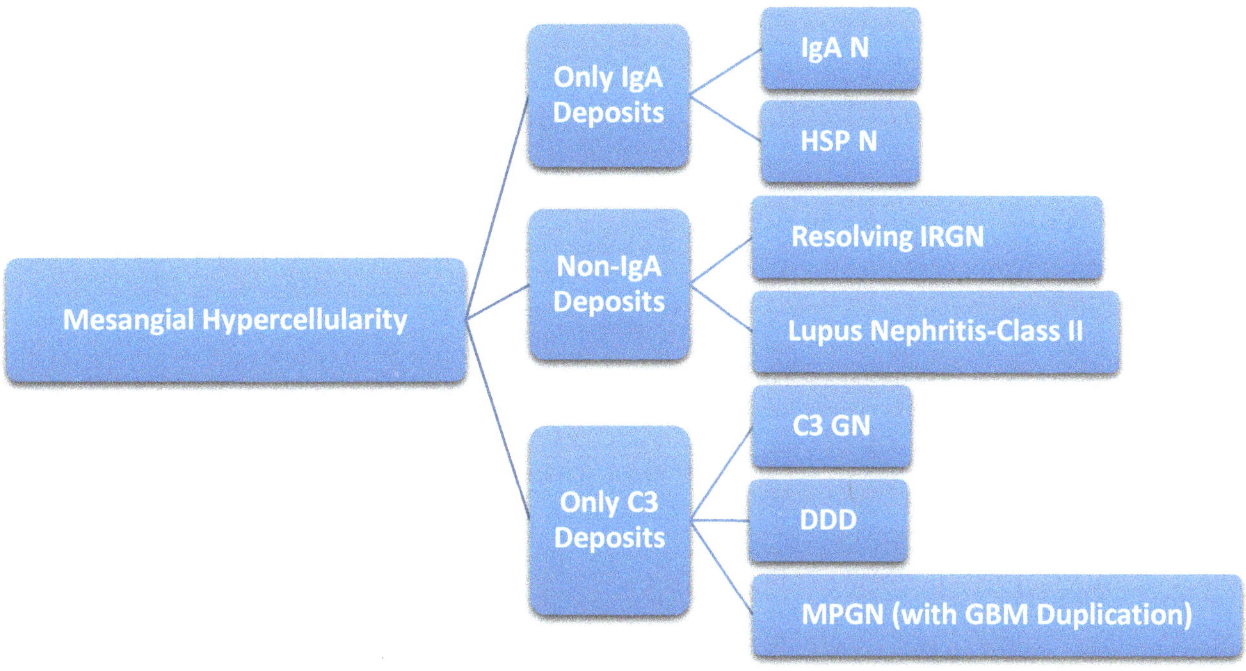

GN: Glomerulonephritis, IgA N: IgA Nephropathy, HSP N: Henoch Schonlein Purpura Nephritis, C3GN: C3 Glomerulonephritis, DDD: Dense Deposit Disease, IRGN: Infection related Glomerulonephritis.

D.　Endocapillary Hypercellularity on LM.

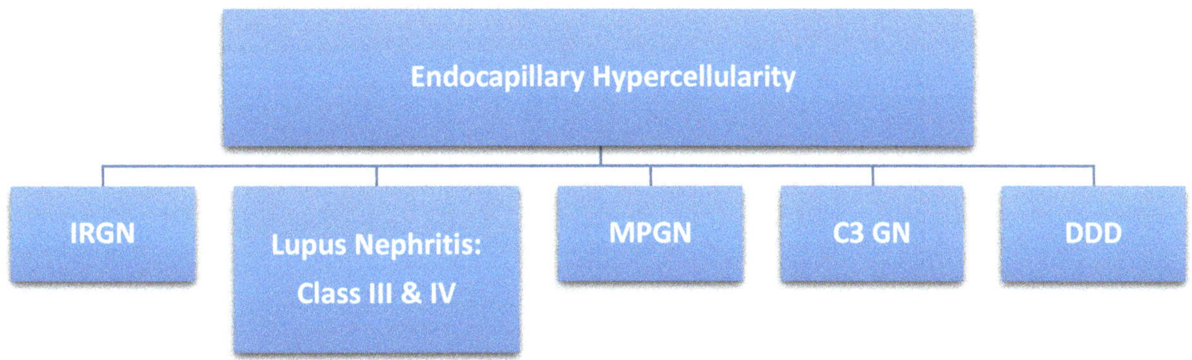

E. Nodular pattern

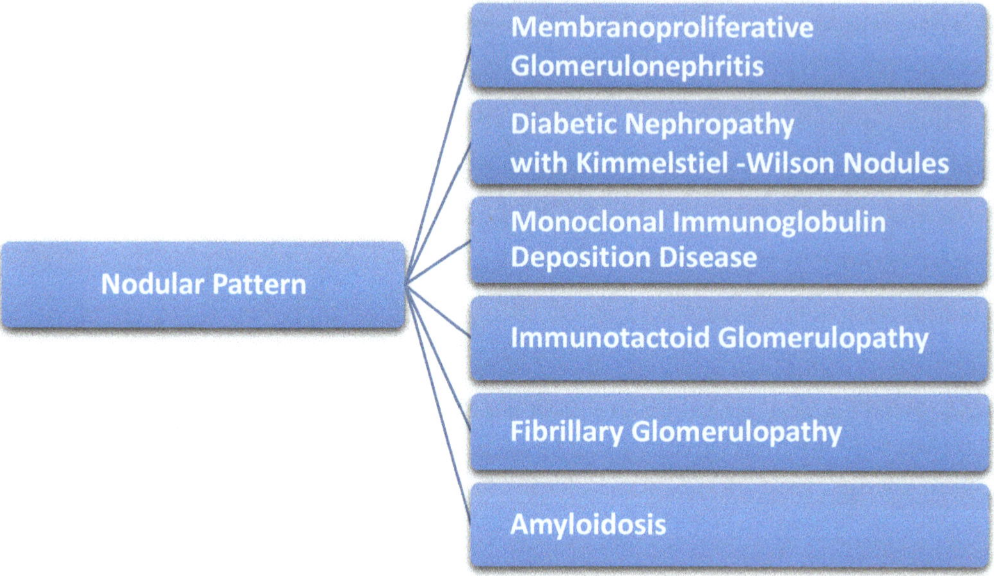

E. Extracapillary Hypercellularity.

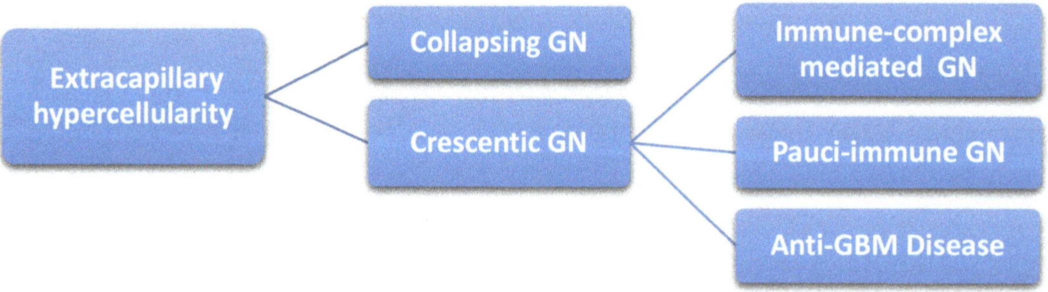

F. Normocellular Glomerulus with Thick GBM without Mesangial Matrix Expansion.

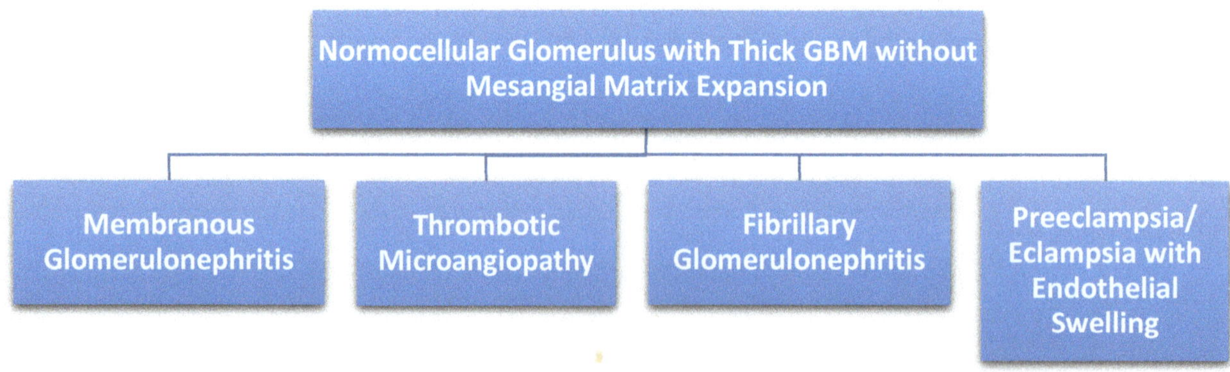

G. Normocellular glomerulus with Thick GBM with mesangial matrix expansion:

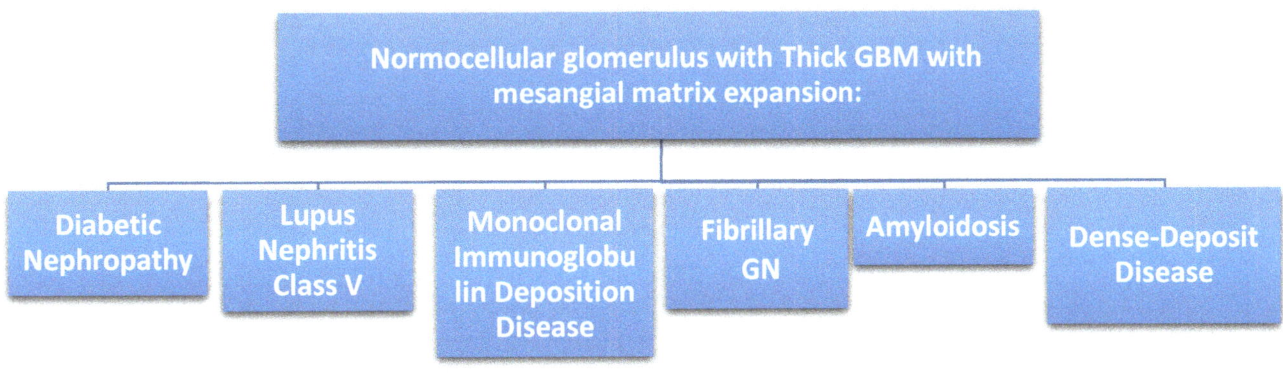

Reference

Heptinstall's Pathology of Kidney, Seventh Edition, Chapter 3, Primer on the Pathologic Classification and Diagnosis of Kidney Disease: Page no. 100.

Patterns of Glomerular Immunofluorescence (IF)

Direct Immunofluorescence: A readymade FITC-labelled antibody is added to the tissue antigen, and the antigen-antibody complex is visualised under a fluorescent microscope.

A. No/significant immune deposits:

 MCD, FSGS, Pauci-immune crescentic GN

B. Capillary wall: Linear deposits of IgG:

 Diabetic nephropathy

 Anti-GBM Disease

C. Capillary wall: Fine granular immune deposits: IgG:

 Membranous Nephropathy

D. Mesangial coarse granular immune deposits:

 Immune-complex mediated GN, IgA Nephropathy

E. Mesangial smudgy immune deposits:

 Amyloidosis, Fibrillary GN, Immunotactoid GN

CASE 1

History: An 11-year-old boy presented with pedal edema and facial puffiness with no history of preceding vaccination/infection in the last one month. No family history of kidney disease. No h/o skin rash/abdominal pain/hematuria. BP:100/60mm of Hg.

Investigations: Urine protein to creatinine ratio (UPCR): 3g/g, Urine analysis: protein: 3+, RBCs: 2 to 3/HPF, Pus cells: 1to2/HPF, serum albumin: 1.9 gm/dl, serum cholesterol: 260 mg/dl, serum TG: 280mg/dl, HDL: 50mg/dl, LDL: 140 mg/dl.

Clinical Diagnosis: Childhood-onset Nephrotic syndrome.

Differential Diagnoses: Minimal Change disease (Most likely) / FSGS / Membranous Nephropathy.

Light microscopy:

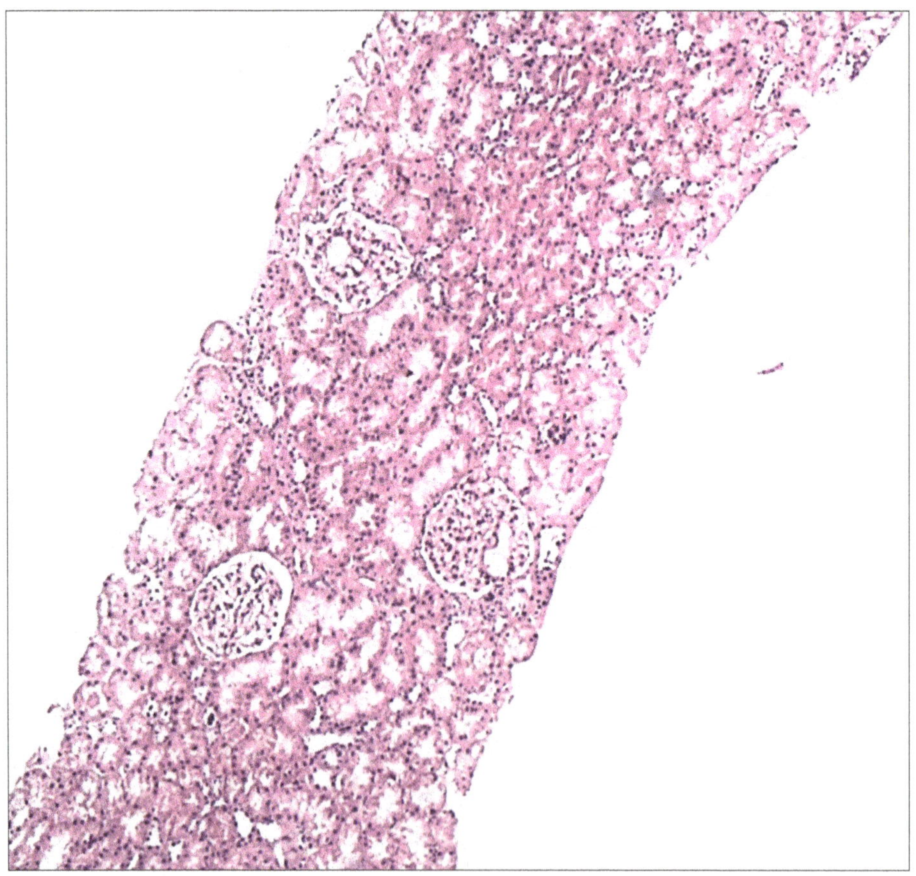

Figure 2:1.1: H&E Stain 4x: Renal cortex: normal glomeruli, tubules are closely apposed to each other.

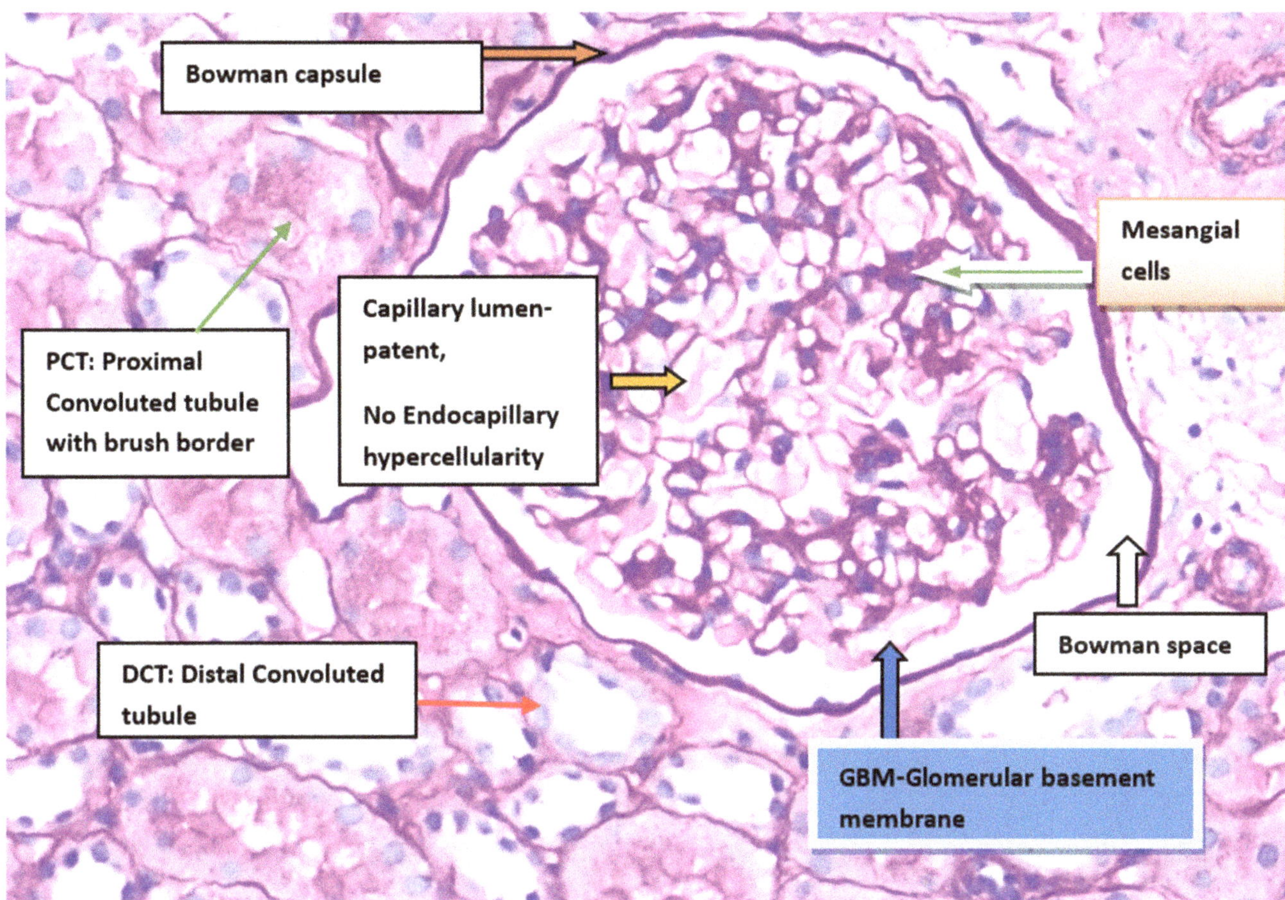

Figure 2:1.2: PAS Stain 20x: Glomerulus - normal histology.

Glomeruli:

Cellularity: Normal

Basement membrane thickening: Absent

Segment of sclerosis: Absent

Crescents: Absent

Tubules & Interstitium: IF/TA: The tubules are closely apposed to each other, and there is no evidence of Tubular atrophy, Interstitial Fibrosis, or inflammation.

Blood vessels: Normal.

Immunofluorescence:

IgG, IgM, IgA, C3c, C1q, Kappa & Lambda: Negative.

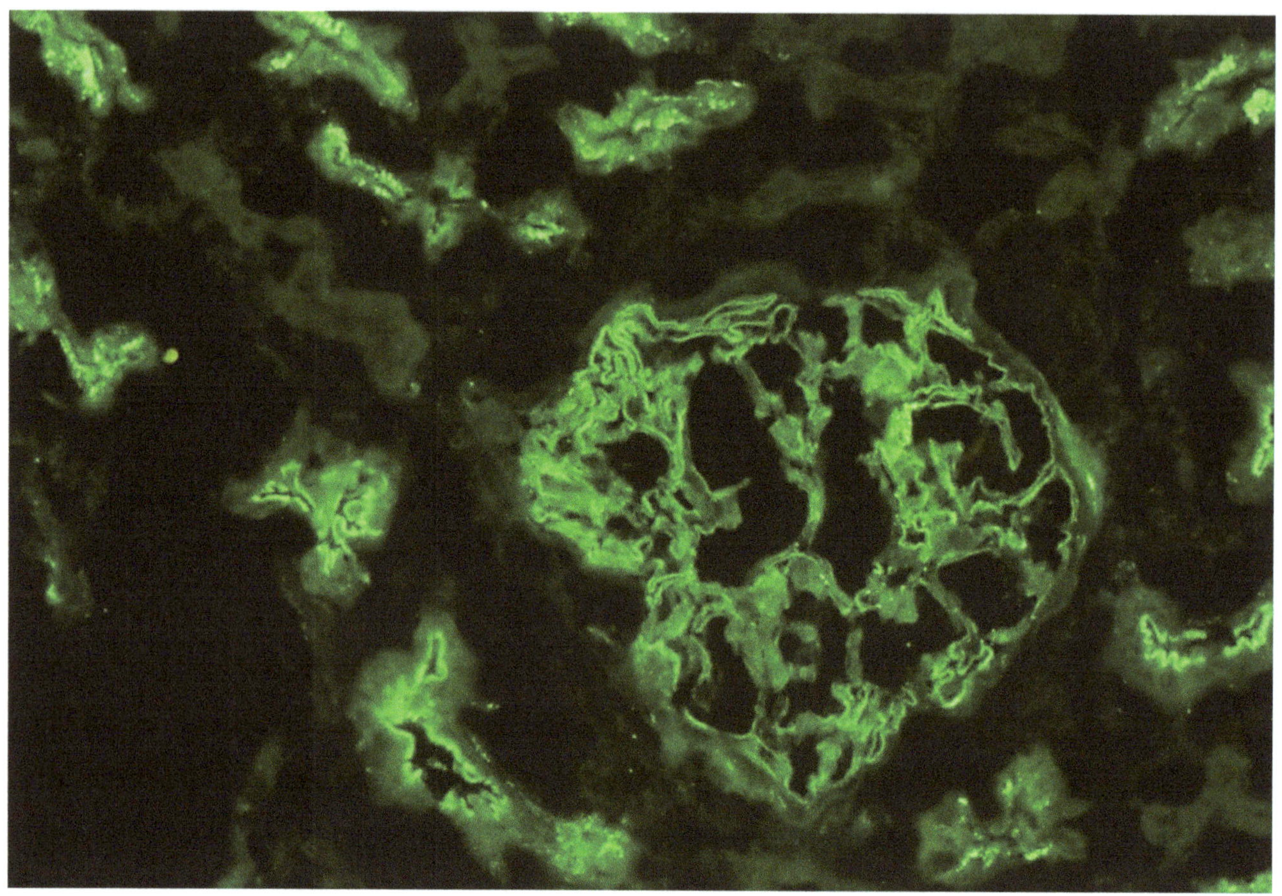

Figure 2:1.3: Immunofluorescence IgG 20x: Negative.

Interpretation:
   Minimal Change Disease (MCD).

Additional Reading:

MCD Variants:
1. IgM Nephropathy: significant IgM immune deposits on the Immunofluorescence study.
2. C1q Nephropathy: significant C1q immune deposits on the Immunofluorescence study.
3. Mesangial hypercellularity
4. MCD with tubular injury: NSAIDs induced.
5. MCD with IgA immune deposits on the Immunofluorescence study:
    a. **Minimal Change Disease (MCD) with Incidental IgA Deposits:** Diffuse foot process effacement and absent mesangial/Paramesangial electron-dense deposits.
    b. **IgA Nephropathy** (Oxford Classification: M0 E0 S0 T0-C0)**:** Diffuse foot process effacement with mesangial/Paramesangial electron dense deposits.

Electron Microscopy:

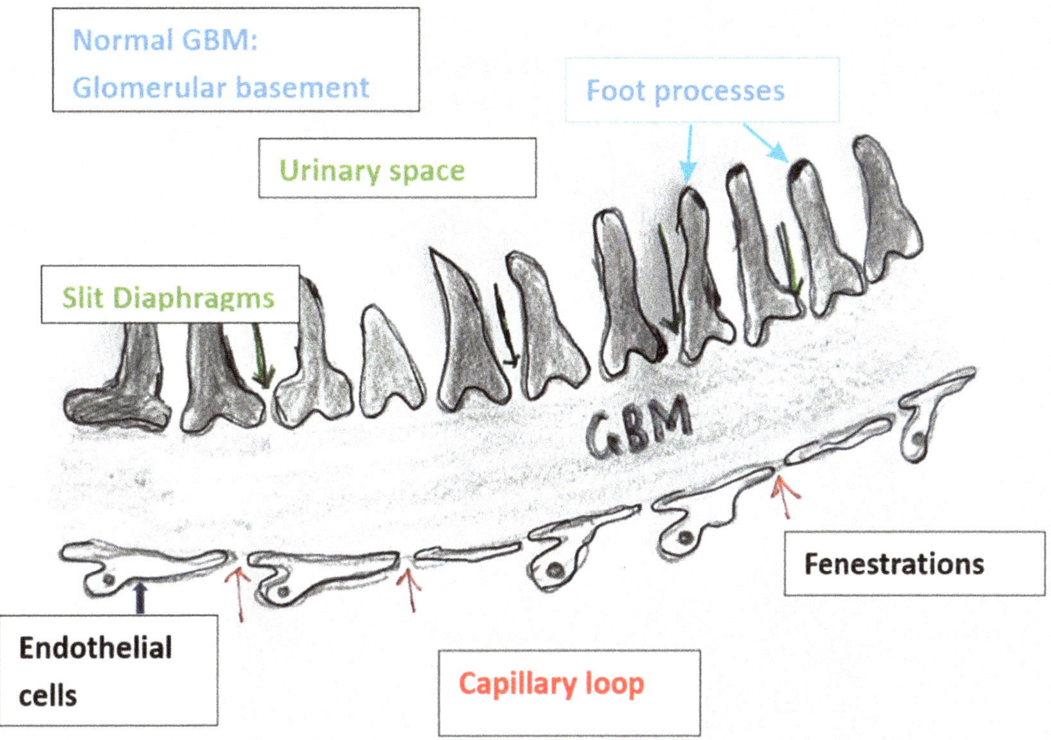

Figure 2:1.4: Diagrammatic representation of Electron microscopy: normal glomerulus.

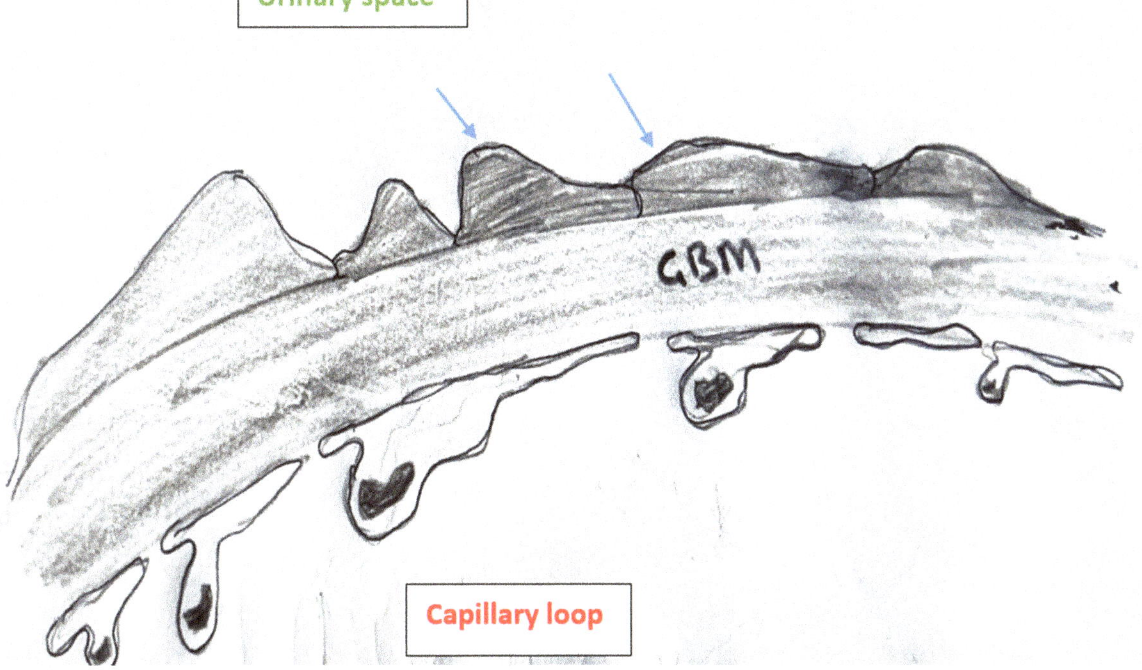

Figure 2:1.5: Diagrammatic representation of Electron microscopy: MCD: Minimal Change Disease: Diffuse foot process effacement (blue arrows) and absence of electron-dense deposits.

Pathology Pearls

*% of glomeruli expected to be sclerosed at a particular age = (Age÷2) -10

** A sample with at least 20 glomeruli is required to confidently exclude the presence of FSGS affecting 10% of glomeruli.

***In the following scenario, MCD can be considered, provided electron microscopy suggested diffuse foot process effacement:

1. If focal global glomerulosclerosis (<10%) is present without the presence of tubulointerstitial changes of chronicity,

2. Mild Focal tubular changes, including atrophy, thickening of the tubular basement membranes,

3. Mild mesangial widening, and

4. Mild mesangial hypercellularity.

****Involuted glomeruli (Figure 2:1.6): This is a pattern of glomerulosclerosis in which there is a strong staining matrix with few viable cells that can stain with podocyte or parietal cell markers. These are commonly seen in frequently relapsing nephrotic syndrome with MCD.

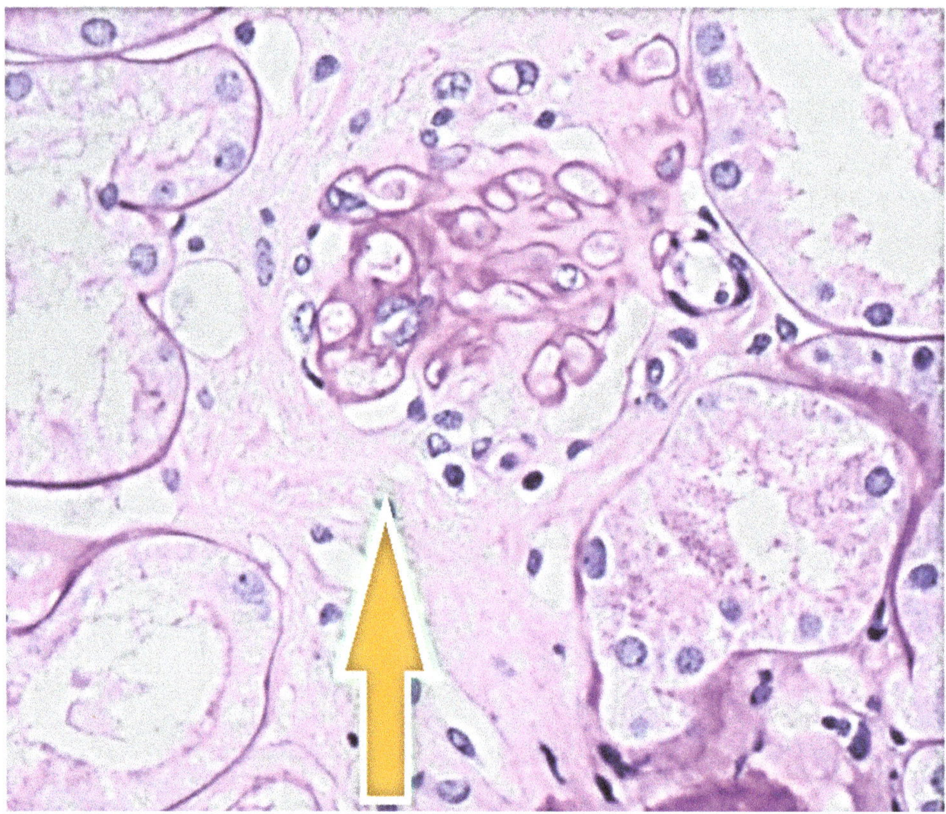

Figure 2:1.6: H&E Stain 20x: Involuted glomerulus and normal adjacent tubules with no tubular atrophy/interstitial fibrosis

References

*Smith SM, et al., Low incidence of glomerulosclerosis in normal kidneys, Arch Pathol Lab med 1989;113:1253.

**Corwin HL, et al., The importance of sample size in the interpretation of the renal biopsy. Am J. Nephrol 1988;8(2):85-89.

***International Study of Kidney Disease in Children: Primary Nephrotic Syndrome in Children: A Report for the International Study of Kidney Disease in Children. Kidney Int 1981; 20:765.

****Dijkman et al.: Glomerular involution in children with frequently relapsing minimal change nephrotic syndrome: An unrecognized form of glomerulosclerosis?- February 2007: Kidney International 71(1):44-52

CASE 2

History: A 16-year-old male was referred to the nephrology clinic due to renal dysfunction; he has been having episodes of hematuria since early childhood, especially after episodes of upper respiratory tract infection and fever. The hematuria would resolve in a day or two and was not further evaluated. He has no h/o joint pains, skin rash, or any systemic features of connective tissue disease. There is no history of any indigenous medication use. Family history of kidney disease: maternal grandfather expired due to kidney disease. He has an elder sister with no kidney disease.

BP: 150/90 mm of Hg. Pedal edema +.

Investigations: Serum creatinine 3 mg/dl. Urine analysis: Protein: 3+, RBCs: 15 to 20/HPF, Pus cells: 2 to 3/HPF, RBC casts: present. 24-hour Urine Protein: 4300 mg/day. Haemoglobin: 8 g/dl. Serum calcium: 6.8 mg /dl, serum albumin: 2.5 g/dl. C3 and C4: both normal, ANA: negative, ANCA: negative. Viral screen: negative. USG: both kidneys have raised parenchymal echotexture with normal size and decreased corticomedullary differentiation.

Clinical Diagnosis: Nephrotic syndrome with active urinary sediment with hypertension and renal dysfunction, likely chronic kidney disease.

Table 2:2.1: Differential Diagnoses.

Sr. No.	Features	IgA N	TBMD	Epstein syndrome	Fechtner syndrome	Alport syndrome
1.	Microscopic Hematuria	+	+	+	+	+
2.	Proteinuria	+	–	+	+	+
3.	Kidney Failure	+	–	+	+	+
4.	Deafness	–	–	+	+	+
5.	Anterior lenticonus	–	–	–	–	+
6.	Thrombocytopenia with Large Platelets	–	–	–	+	–
7.	Leucocyte Cytoplasmic Inclusions	–	–	–	+	–
8.	Autosomal Dominant Inheritance	–	+	+	+	–/+
9.	X-linked Inheritance	–	–	–	–	+

TBMD: Thin basement membrane disease; IgA N: IgA Nephropathy.

Light Microscopy:

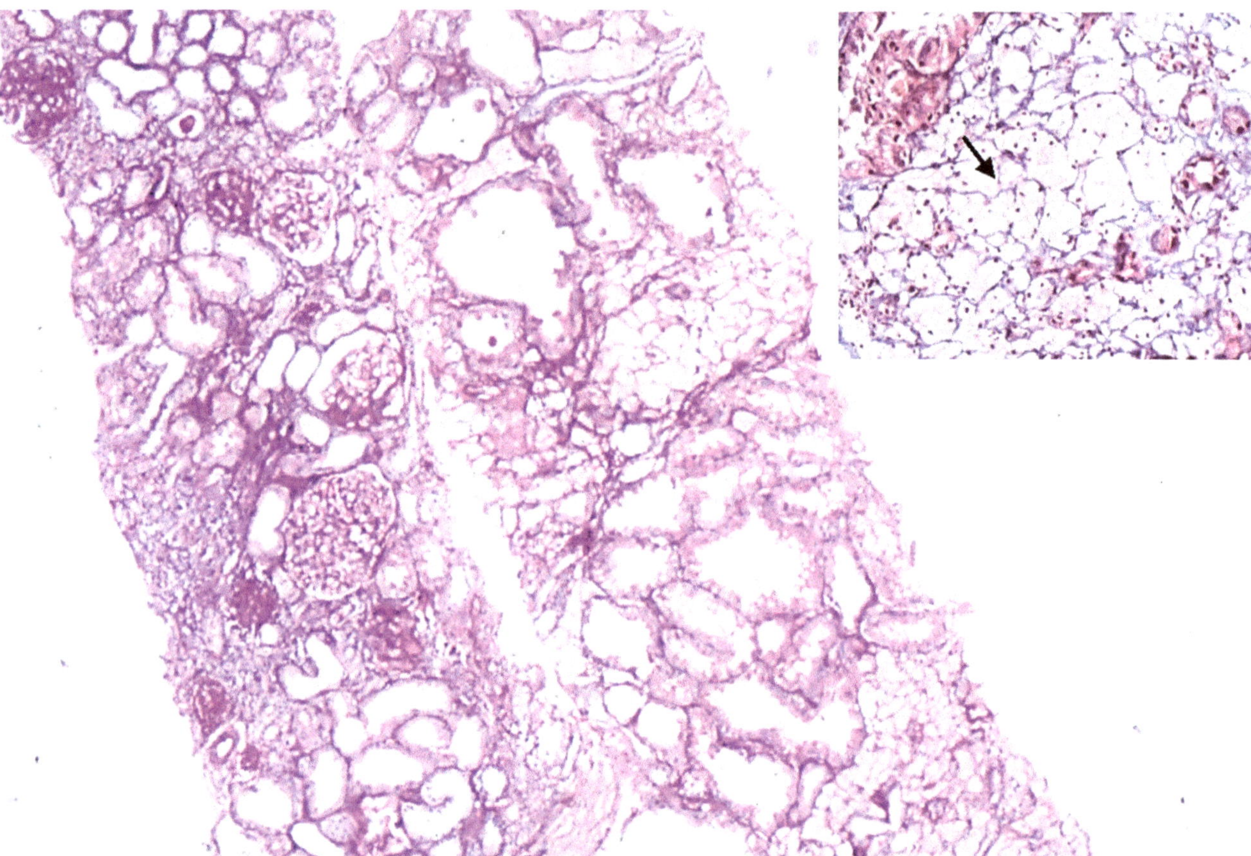

Figure 2:2.1: PAS Stain 4x: moderate tubulointerstitial changes of chronicity. (**Inset image**) MT Stain 10x: sheets of interstitial foam cells.

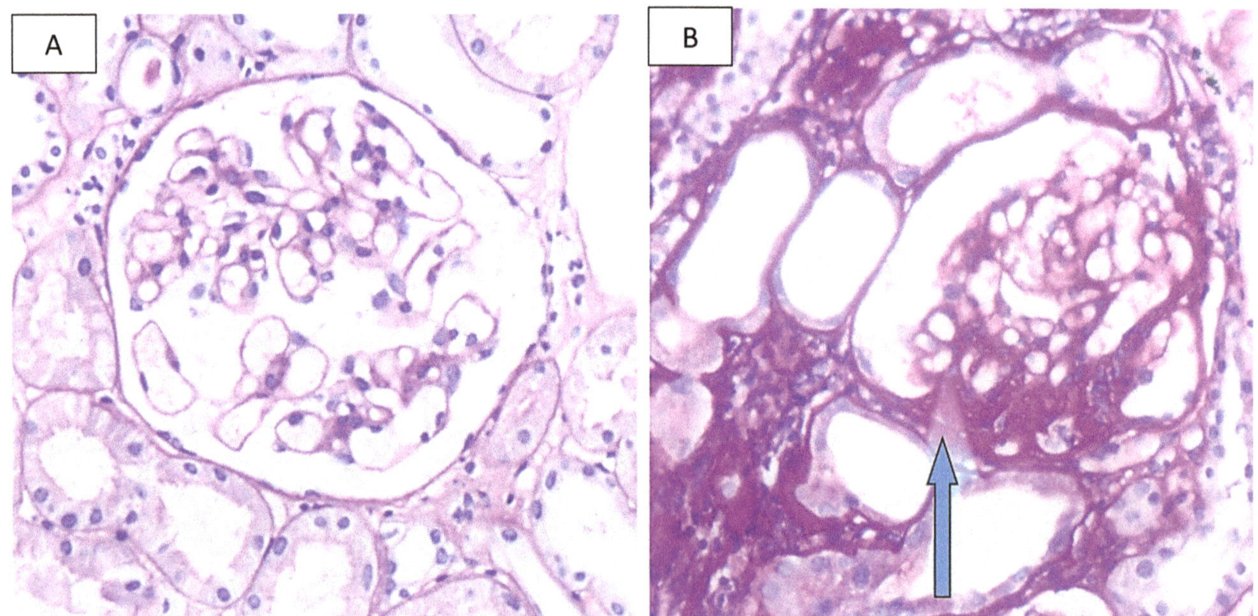

Figure 2:2.2: (a) PAS Stain 20x: mildly rigid glomerular basement membranes **(b)** PAS Stain:20x: segment of sclerosis (**blue** arrow) attached to Bowman capsule.

Immunofluorescence:

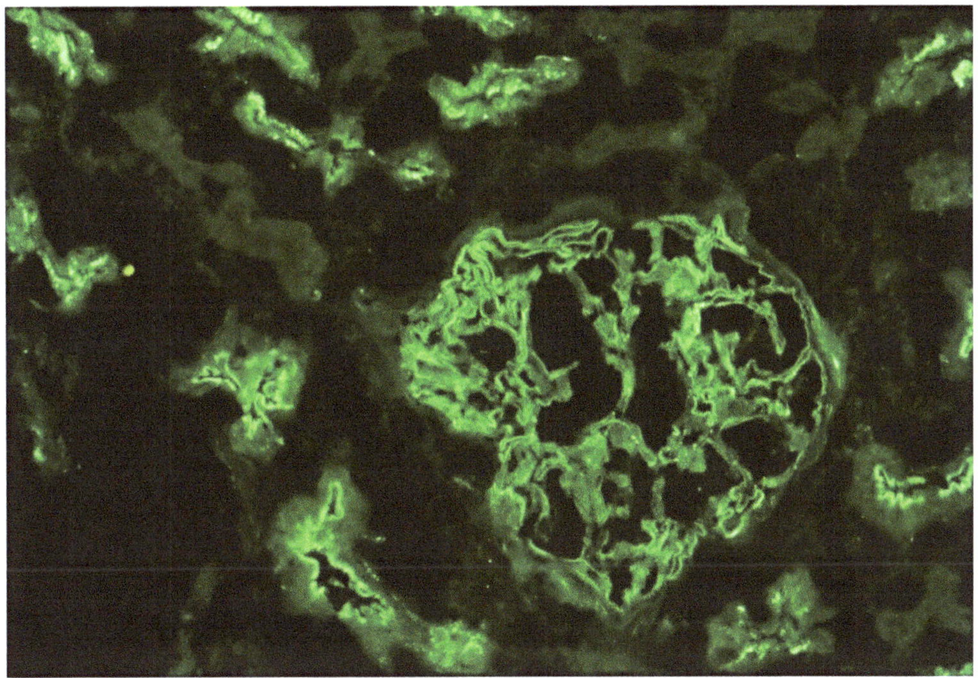

Figure 2:2.3: Immunofluorescenc IgG:20x: Glomerulus: no immune deposits.

Interpretation: Focal segmental glomerulosclerosis with moderate IF/TA and prominent interstitial foam cells.

Electron Microscopy Findings:

It shows irregularly thickened and thinned areas of glomerular basement membrane with splitting and fragmenting of the lamina densa forming a basket-weave pattern (Figure 2:2.4.c)

Normal thickness of GBM: Glomerular Basement Membrane in adults is 300 to 350 nm, slightly thicker in males than in females, and thinner in children who achieve adult thickness by age 10 to 12 years.

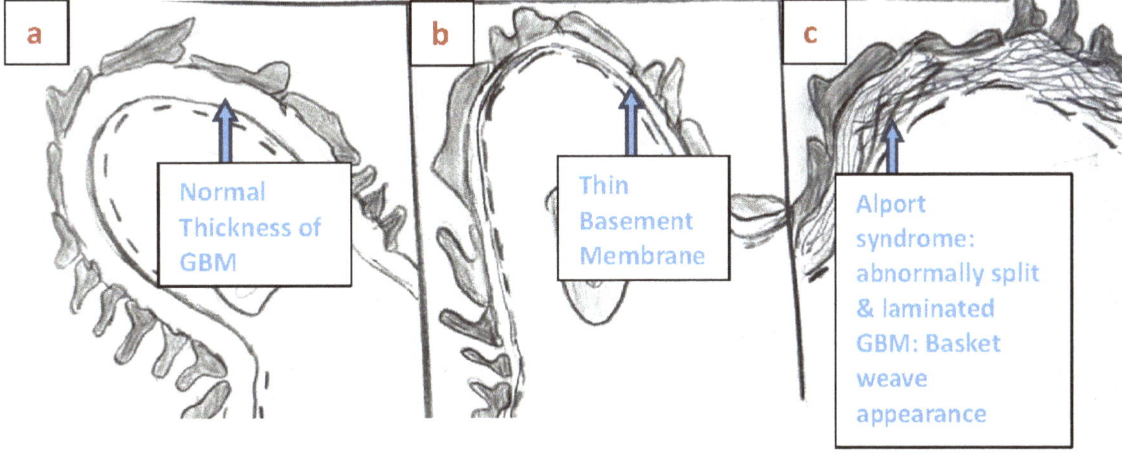

Figure 2:2.4: (a), (b), and (c) Diagrammatic Representation of Electron Microscopy of a Capillary Glomerular Basement Membrane.

Reference:

Jorgensen F, et.al: The ultrastructure of the normal human glomerulus. Thickness of glomerular basement membrane, Lab Invest 1968;18:42.

Final Diagnosis: Alport Syndrome.

On Further Evaluation: He has audiometric detection of bilateral early sensorineural hearing loss. On the slit lamp, he has anterior lenticonus. On screening family members, the Mother is found to have microscopic hematuria and subnephrotic proteinuria with normal renal function, suggesting X-linked recessive inherited Alport syndrome, with the mother having subclinical renal disease and male family members having a 50% risk of inheriting Alport disease with no transmission from father to son. Maternal grandfather transmitted the affected X chromosome to the mother of the patient. Lyonization explains variable milder phenotypic manifestation in females.

Additional Information: Alport syndrome is X-linked recessive (COL4A5 gene mutation) in 80%, autosomal recessive (COLA4A3/A4 gene mutation) in 15%, and autosomal dominant (COLA4A3/A4 gene mutation) in 5%. However, next-generation sequencing of Alport family members identifies autosomal dominant inheritance more often than believed earlier. Females and males are equally affected by autosomal recessive and dominant inherited Alport syndrome. Extra renal manifestations are less common in Autosomal dominant inherited disease. Thin basement membrane disease, a benign entity with microscopic hematuria detected usually incidentally or on screening, could be a variant of Alport syndrome.

History: An 18-year-old male presented with gross anasarca of one-month duration without a history of any preceding infection, with no history of any Indigenous medication use, no history of NSAIDs use, no history of diabetes, non-hypertensive, and without a family history of kidney disease. No systemic features to suggest any secondary glomerulonephritis (like arthritis, oral ulcers, skin rash, uveitis, poly serositis). BP: 130/80 mm of Hg.

Investigations: Urine analysis: protein: 4+, RBCs: 4 to 6/HPF, pus cells: 1 to 2/HPF, serum creatinine: 0.7 mg/dl, serum albumin: 1.4 g/dl, serum total cholesterol: 280 mg/dl, TG: 300 mg/dl, HDL: 48 mg/dl, LDL: 170 mg/dl.

Clinical Diagnosis: Adult-onset Nephrotic syndrome

Differential Diagnoses: MCD / FSGS / Membranous Nephropathy.

Light microscopy:

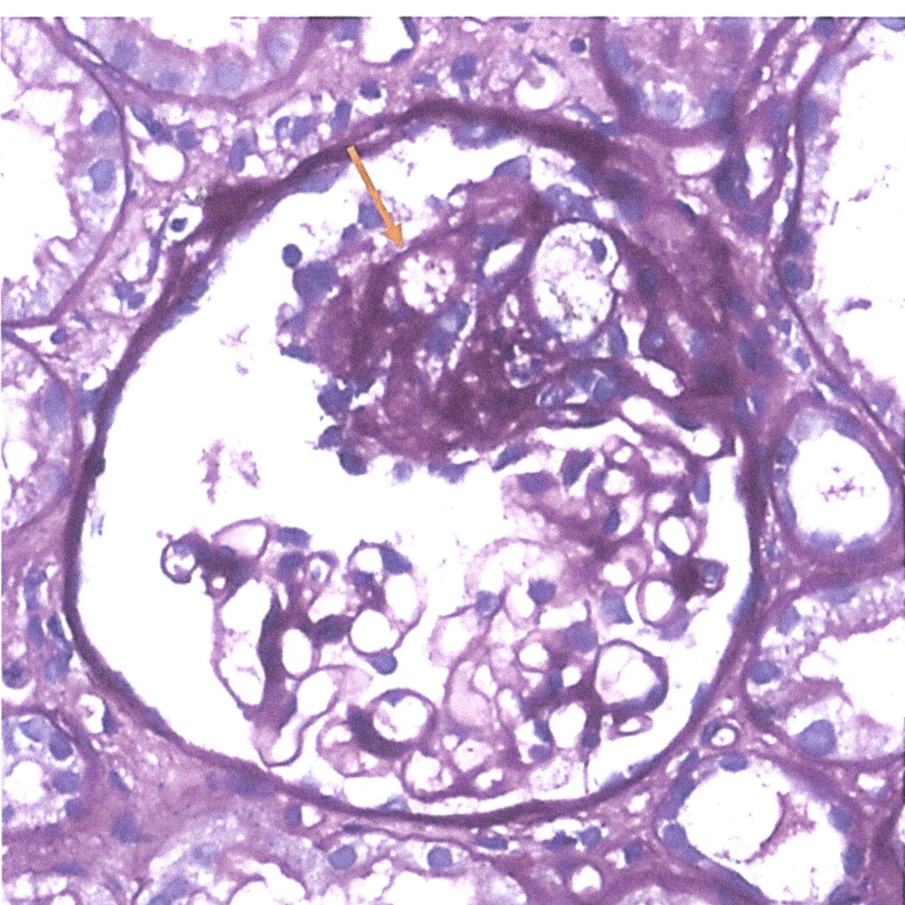

Figure 2:3.1: PAS Stain 20x: orange arrow shows segment of sclerosis with segmental endocapillary foam cells attached to Bowman capsule with capping of overlying podocytes.

Immunofluorescence:

Nonspecific IgM, C3c, C1q entrapped in the sclerosed portions of the glomeruli.

Interpretation: FSGS, NOS (Not Otherwise Specified) Variant

Electron Microscopy findings:

Diffuse foot process effacement and absence of electron-dense deposits.

Final Diagnosis: Primary FSGS, Not Otherwise Specified (NOS) Variant with mild IF/TA.

Immunofluorescence:

Nonspecific IgM, C3c, C1q entrapped in the sclerosed portions of the glomeruli.

Interpretation: FSGS, NOS (Not Otherwise Specified) Variant

CASE 4

History: 58 years old female, post-menopausal, non-diabetic & non hypertensive, nonsmoker, no other addictions, presented with progressive swelling over feet and facial puffiness for 3 weeks. No history of NSAIDS. History of using Residronate weekly once for the last 9 months for osteoporosis. No history of using any indigenous medication. BP 170/90 mm of Hg.

Investigation: urine analysis: protein: 4+, RBCs:10 to 12/HPF, Pus cells: 3 to 5/HPF, 24 urine protein: 8000 mg, serum creatinine:1.6 mg/dl, serum albumin: 2gm/dl, total cholesterol: 290mg/dl, LDL:180mg/dl.

Clinical Diagnosis: Adult-onset Nephrotic syndrome with HTN with renal dysfunction and active urinary sediment

Differential Diagnoses: FSGS/Membranous Nephropathy/IgA Nephropathy.

Light Microscopy:

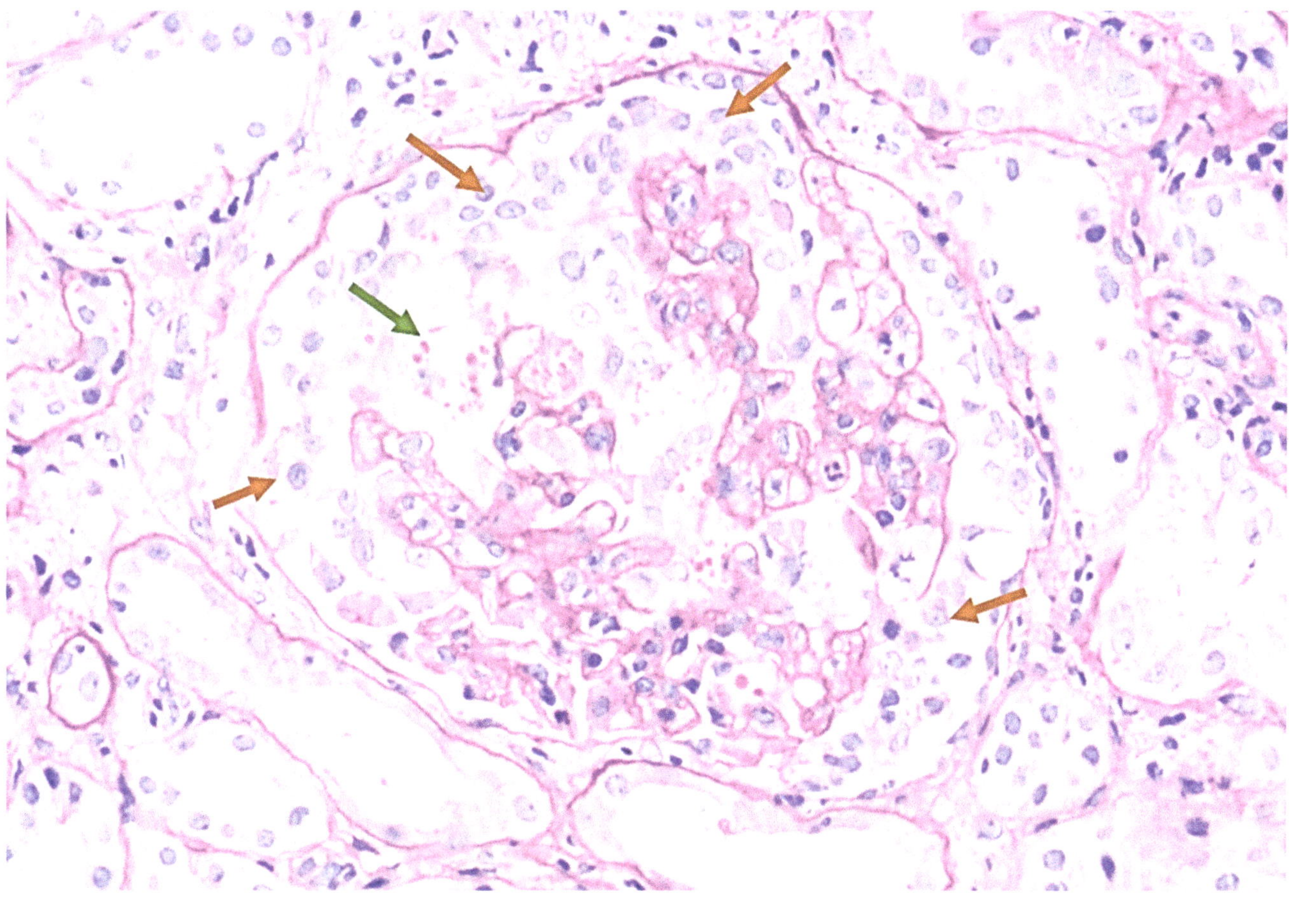

Figure 2:4.1: PAS Stain 20x: Global collapse of the tuft with hypertrophy and hyperplasia of overlying podocytes (orange arrows) with protein resorption droplets (green arrow).

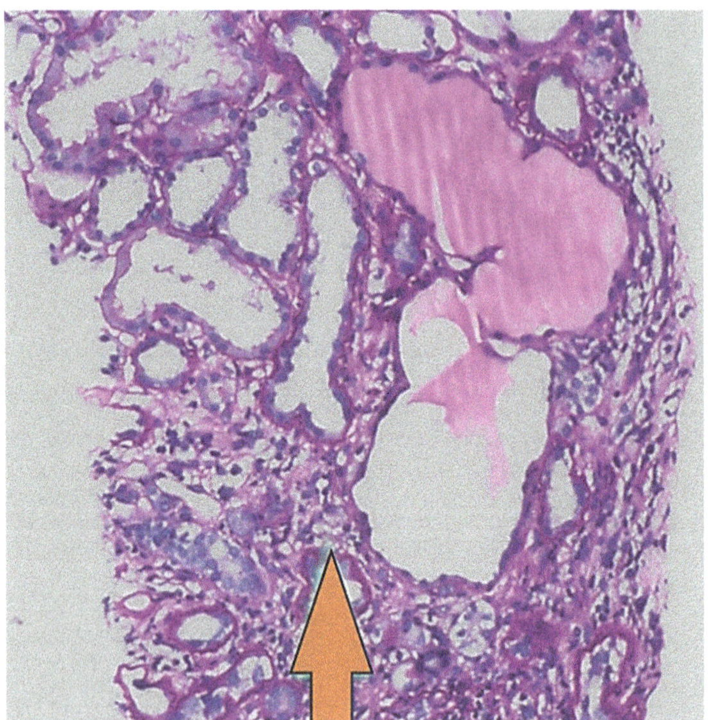

Figure 2:4.2 PAS Stain-20x: Microcystic dilatation of tubules with proteinaceous casts and moderate IFTA.

Collapsing Glomerulopathy with crumpled paper appearance

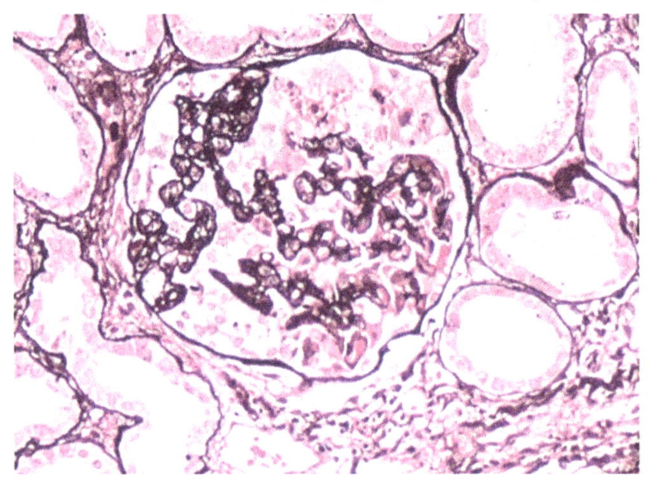

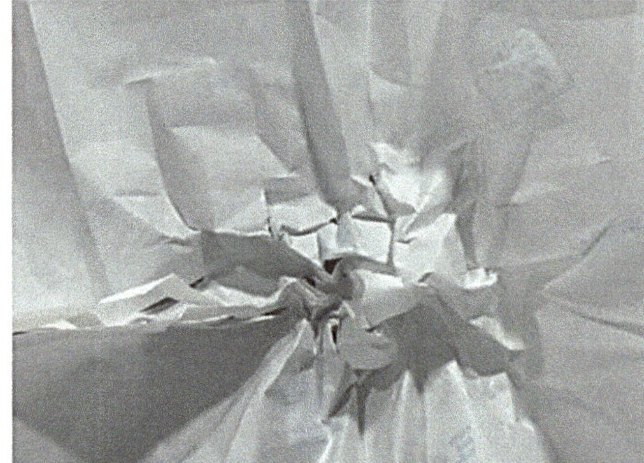

Figure 2:4.3: Crumpled paper appearance of the tuft.

Immunofluorescence: IF study shows no significant deposits.

Interpretation: FSGS, Collapsing Variant.

Electron Microscopy findings:

Diffuse foot process effacement and wrinkling of glomerular basement membrane.
Absence of electron dense deposits.

Final Diagnosis: Anti resorptive drug induced Collapsing Glomerulopathy.

Pathology Pearls

How to differentiate collapsing Glomerulopathy from a cellular crescent on the slide:

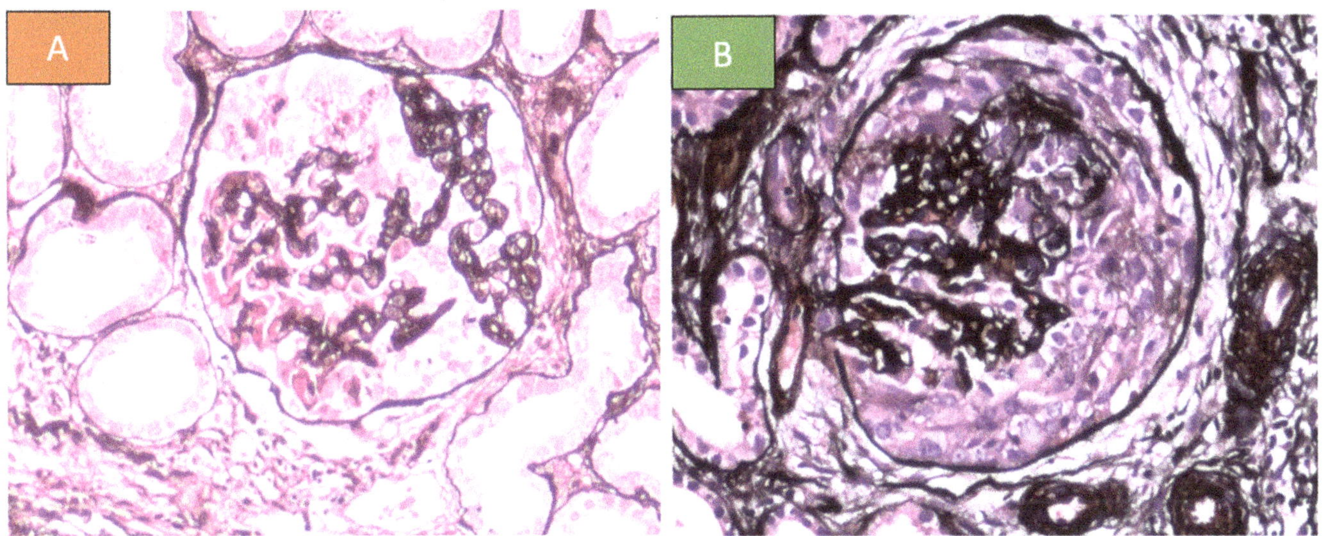

How to differentiate collapsing Glomerulopathy (a) from a cellular crescent (b) under the light microscopy:

Sr. No.	Features	Collapsing GP	Cellular crescent
1.	Intercellular Matrix	–	+
2.	Shape of cells	Polygonal	Spindle
3.	Breach of Bowman capsule	No	Often
4.	Tubular microcysts	+	–
5.	Periglomerular inflammation	–	+
6.	IHC-WT-1	Often +	–
7.	Glomerular tuft necrosis	–	+/–

IHC: immunohistochemistry, WT1: Wilms tumour 1.

Other Conditions in which Collapsing GP is seen:

1. HIVAN
2. IgA Nephropathy (Seen in 10% cases) *
3. Lupus Nephritis**
4. Diabetic Nephropathy***
5. Thrombotic Microangiopathy (TMA)****

References

* Diagnostic Pathology, Kidney Diseases, Second Edition, Colvin/Chang: IgA nephropathy page no.130.)
** Collapsing glomerulopathy in 19 patients with systemic lupus erythematosus or Lupus like disease. Salvatore SP et al. Clin J Am Soc Nephrol 2012;7(6):914-925.
*** Salvatore SP et al. Collapsing glomerulopathy superimposed on diabetic nephropathy: insights into etiology of an under-recognized, severe pattern of glomerular injury. Nephrol Dial Transplant. 2014 Feb;29(2):392-399.
**** Collapsing glomerulopathy is common in the setting of thrombotic microangiopathy of the native kidney: David Buob et al., Kidney International (2016)90,1321-1331.

CASE 5

History: 25-year-old male, nondiabetic & non hypertensive, presented with progressive puffiness of face and pedal edema for the last month with frothyuria. No history of preceding infection/ NSAIDs/ indigenous medicine use. BP: 120/80 mm of Hg.

Investigations: Urine analysis: Protein:4+ No active urinary sediment. Serum Albumin 1.8 g/dl, serum Creatinine 0.6 mg/dl.

Clinical diagnosis: Adult-onset nephrotic syndrome without hypertension/renal dysfunction

Differential diagnoses: MCD/FSGS/Membranous nephropathy.

Light Microscopy:

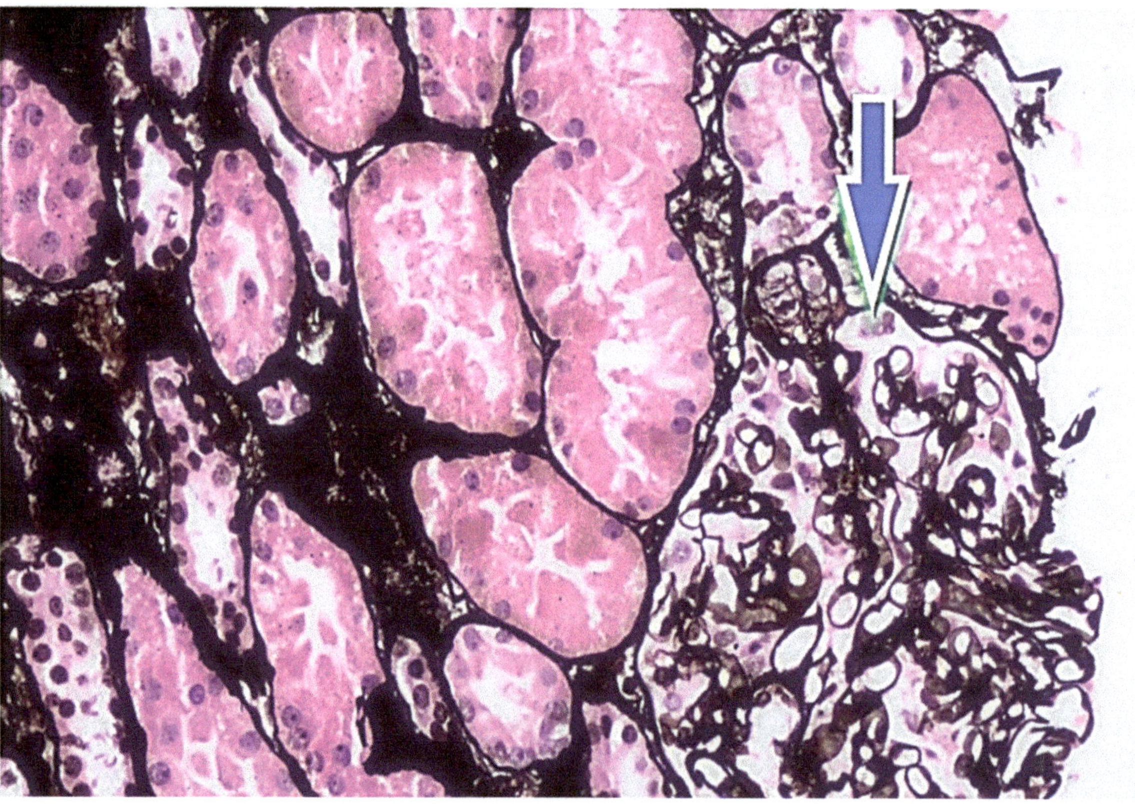

Figure 2:5.1: PASM Stain 20x: Segmental endocapillary foam cells prolapsed at the origin of proximal tubule.

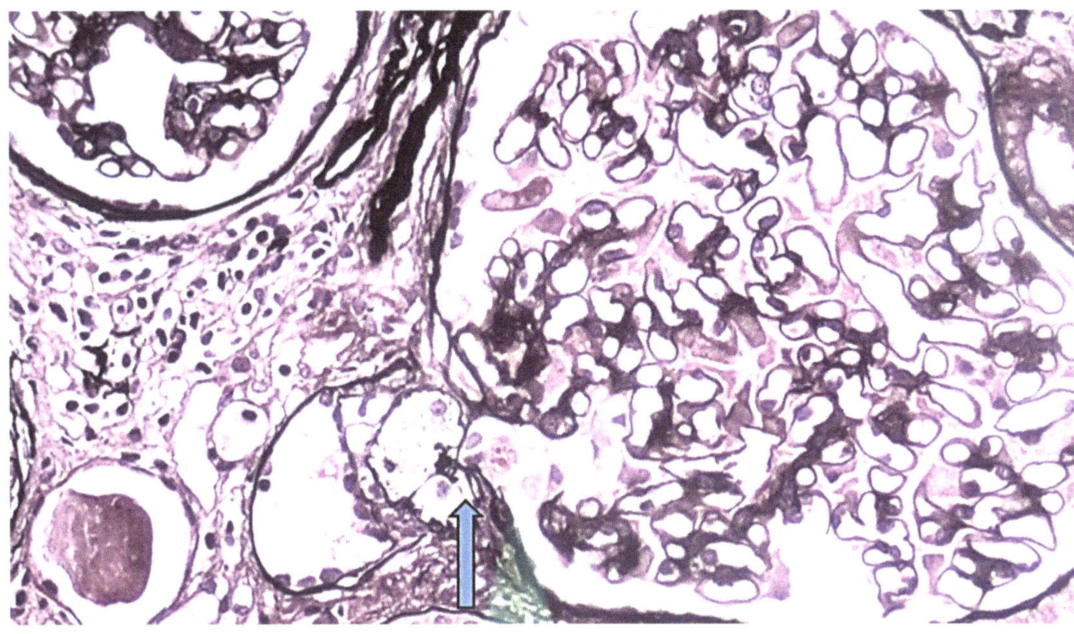

Figure 2:5.2: PASM Stain 20x: Tip lesion: Segmental endocapillary foam cells prolapsed into the tubular orifice with confluence of overlying podocytes with proximal tubular epithelial cells (Tip lesion).

Immunofluorescence: IF/TA: <05%

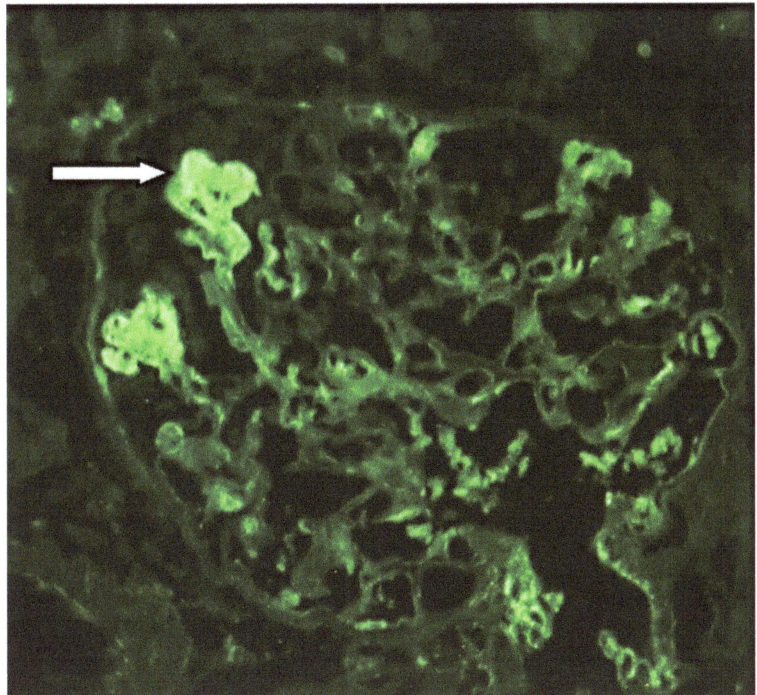

Figure 2:5.3: Immunofluorescence: IF study shows a glomerulus with minimal entrapped (arrow) deposits of IgM, C3c and C1q in the sclerosed portion of the tuft.

Interpretation: Tip Variant, FSGS

Electron Microscopy:
Significant foot process effacement without electron dense deposits.

Final Diagnosis: Focal segmental glomerulosclerosis (FSGS), Tip variant with minimal IF/TA (<05%)

Pathology Pearls

Tip lesions may also be seen in other diseases with heavy proteinuria:

1. Membranous glomerulonephritis
2. Diabetic nephropathy
3. Preeclampsia

Reference

*Heptinstall's Pathology of the kidney: seventh edition: chapter 06: Focal Segmental Glomerulosclerosis page no.218: Table 6.2: Histologic variant of FSGS: Clinical features.

Case 6

History: 45-year-old female, hypertensive for 5 years, non-diabetic, nonsmoker, no history of PIH, progressive renal dysfunction with pedal edema and frothyuria for last 2 months. No hematuria. No systemic features to suggest of any collagen vascular disease. BP: 150/90 mm of Hg.

Investigations: Serum creatinine 1.4 mg/dl a month back & now 2.4 mg/dl. Urine analysis: Protein:4+, RBC s:8 to 10/HPF, Pus cells :1 to 2/HPF, RBC Casts: 1 to 2/HPF, 24-hour Urine protein: 5600 mg/day, serum albumin 2.1 gm/dl, HBA1c:5.5%.

Clinical Diagnosis: Ault onset Nephrotic syndrome with hypertension and renal dysfunction.

Differential Diagnoses: Membranous nephropathy / FSGS/ IgA Nephropathy/ Infection related glomerulonephritis.

Light Microscopy:

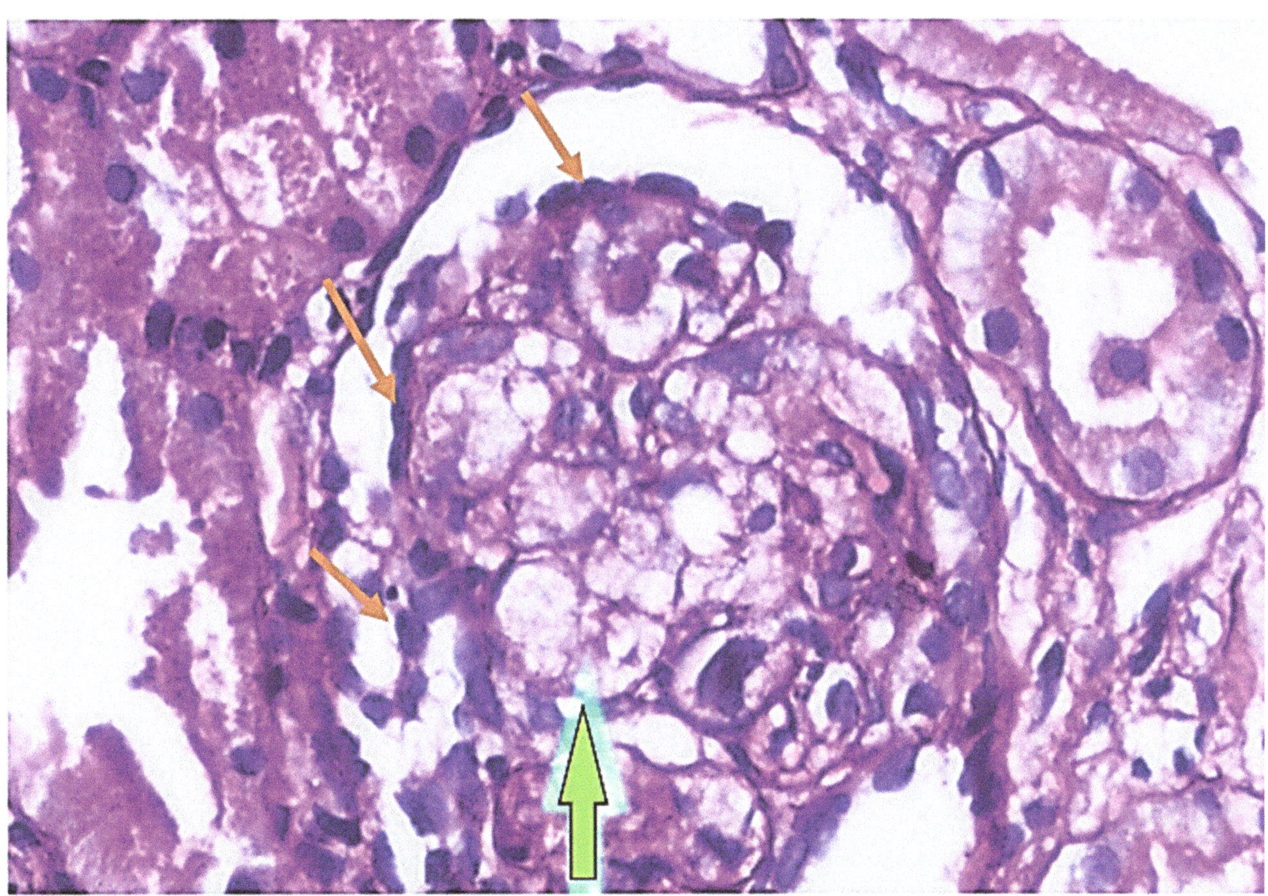

Figure 2:6.1: PAS Stain-40x: Cellular FSGS Expansile lesion with endocapillary foam cells (**green** arrow) and prominence of overlying podocytes (**orange** arrows).

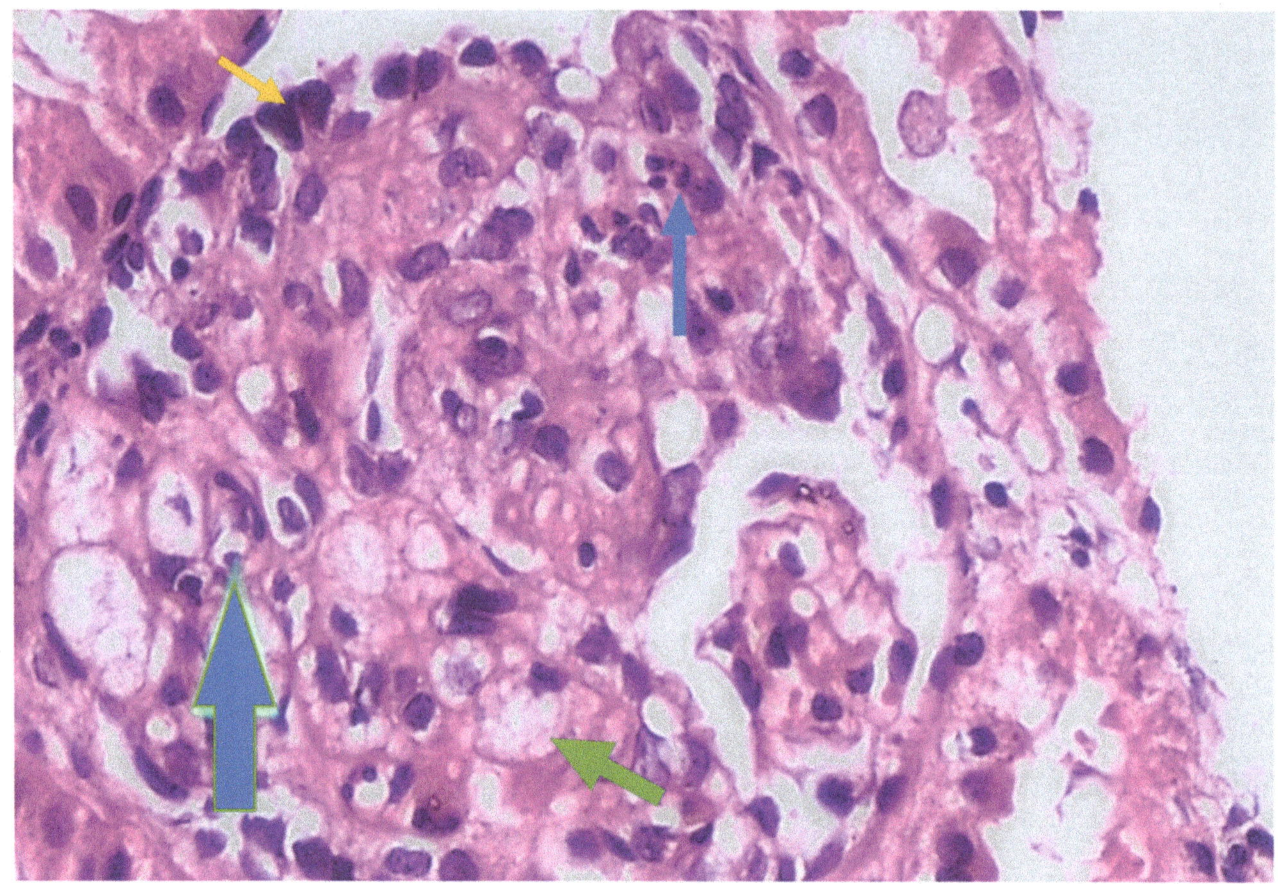

Figure 2:6.2: H&E Stain-40x: segmental endocapillary hypercellularity obliterating the capillary lumina with occasional leukocytes (blue arrows), endocapillary foam cells (green arrow) and capping of podocytes (orange arrow).

IF/TA: mild (10%).

Immunofluorescence: IF study shows no significant immune deposits.

Interpretation: Cellular Variant, FSGS

Electron microscopy:

Diffuse foot process effacement and absence of electron-dense deposits.

Final Diagnosis: Focal segmental glomerulosclerosis, Cellular variant with mild IF/TA (10%).

CASE 7

History: 50-year-old obese lady, non-smoker, with h/o hypertension for last 10 years, non-diabetic, without any history of NSAIDs or indigenous medication use. Presented with pedal edema on & off for 6 months, weight gain of 4 kgs in last 6 months. No hematuria. No other urinary complaints. Shortness of breath on exertion. No systemic features of secondary GN. BP: 160/90 mm of Hg.

Investigations: Urine analysis: Protein:2+, RBC: 5-6/HPF, RBC Casts: nil, UPCR: 2 g/g. Serum creatinine: 1.5 mg/dl. Serum albumin: 3.5 g/dl. Serum Cholesterol 190 mg/dl, Serum HDL: 36 mg/dl, Serum LDL: 140 mg/dl, Serum Triglycerides: 200 mg/dl. HBA1C: 6.4 %.

Clinical presentation: sub-nephrotic range proteinuria with hypertension and renal dysfunction with obesity.

Differential diagnoses: FSGS/Hypertensive nephropathy/IgA Nephropathy.

Light Microscopy:

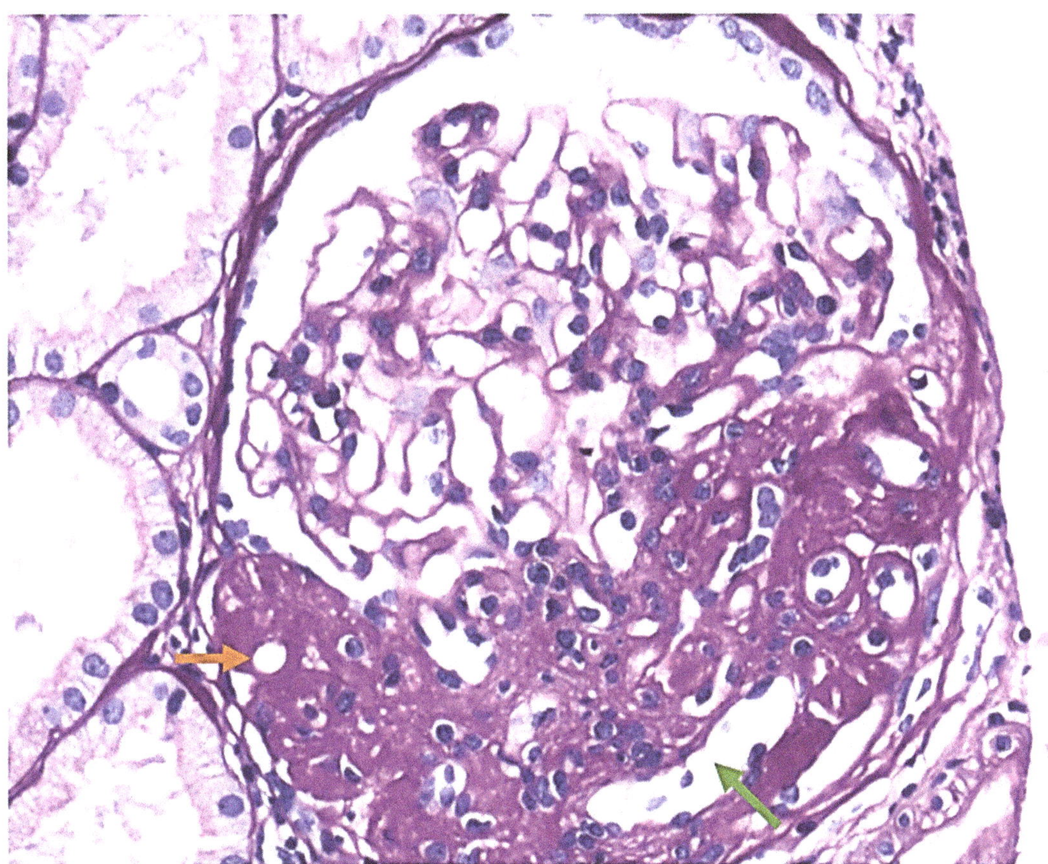

Figure 2:7.1: PAS Stain 20 x: Perihilar variant, FSGS: Segment of sclerosis attached to Bowman capsule with segmental hyalinosis (orange arrow) near the hilum (green arrow).

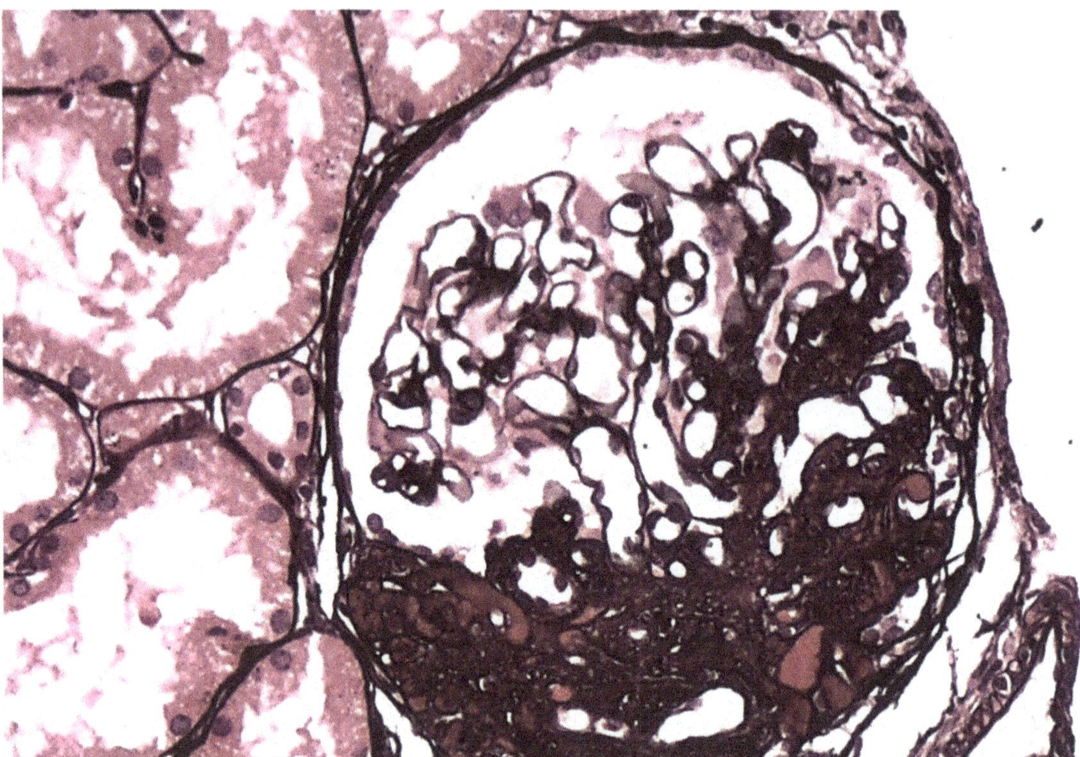

Figure 2:7.2: PASM Stain 20 x: Perihilar variant, FSGS: Segment of sclerosis near the hilum attached to Bowman capsule with segmental hyalinosis. (Note: there is no prominence of overlying podocytes)

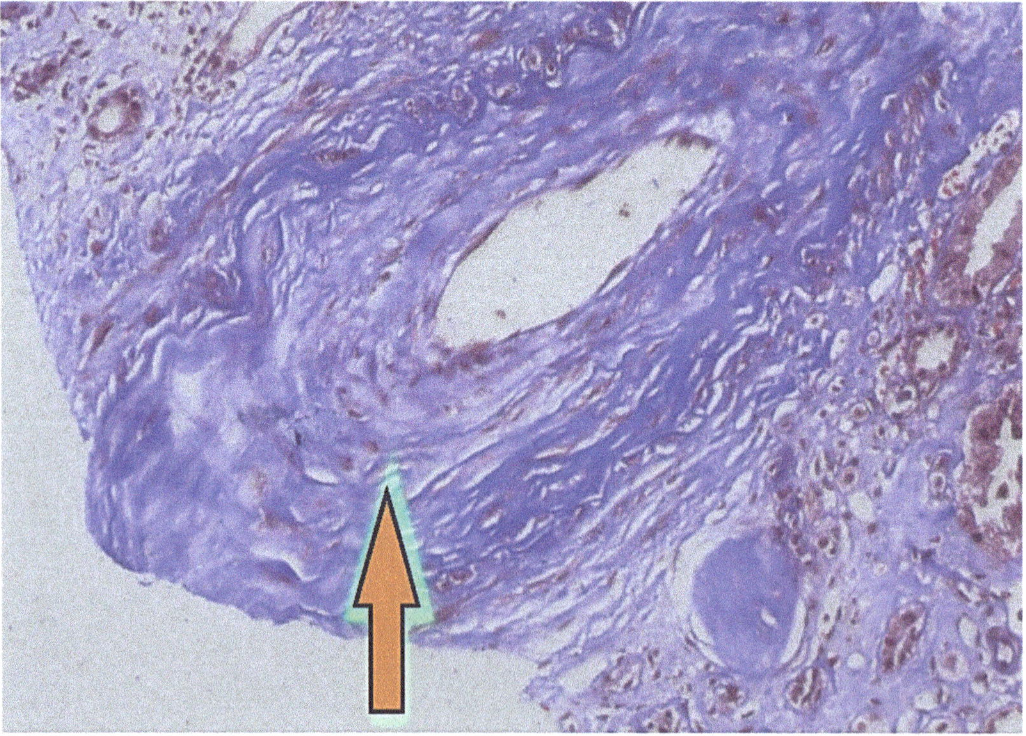

Figure 2:7.3: MT Stain 20x: Large artery, Arteriosclerosis: Intimal fibrosis with focal reduplication of internal elastic lamina focally exceeding the thickness of the media.

Immunofluorescence: IF studies shows no significant deposits.

Interpretation: Focal segmental glomerulosclerosis, perihilar variant.

Electron Microscopy:

Focal foot process effacement is seen.

Final Diagnosis: FSGS Perihilar variant secondary to chronic hypertension.

Pathology Pearls

Perihilar variant FSGS: seen in following conditions:

1. Hypertensive Nephropathy
2. Obesity Related Glomerulopathy
3. Adaptive nephropathy due to low nephron mass (Single kidney / Low birth weight/ Preterm birth / Vesico ureteric reflux etc)

CASE 8

History: 36-year-old unmarried male, non-smoker, non-alcoholic, with promiscuous behavior and history of significant weight loss in the last 6 months with progressive edema all over the body for the last month, with new onset hypertension. No systemic features of secondary GN. No h/o using any indigenous medicines / NSAIDs / recreational drugs. No h/o fever/night sweats.

Investigations: Urine analysis: protein:4+, RBCs: 10 to 12/HPF, Pus cells:4 to 5/HPF, UPCR 7.2 g/g, serum creatinine 2.0 mg/dl. Serum albumin: 2 gm/dl. HIV: Positive, HBsAg: negative, HCV: negative. TSH = 2.4 mUI/ml.

Clinical Diagnosis: Nephrotic syndrome with HTN with active urinary sediment and renal dysfunction.

Differential Diagnoses: HIVAN / Membranous Nephropathy/ IgA Nephropathy

Light Microscopy:

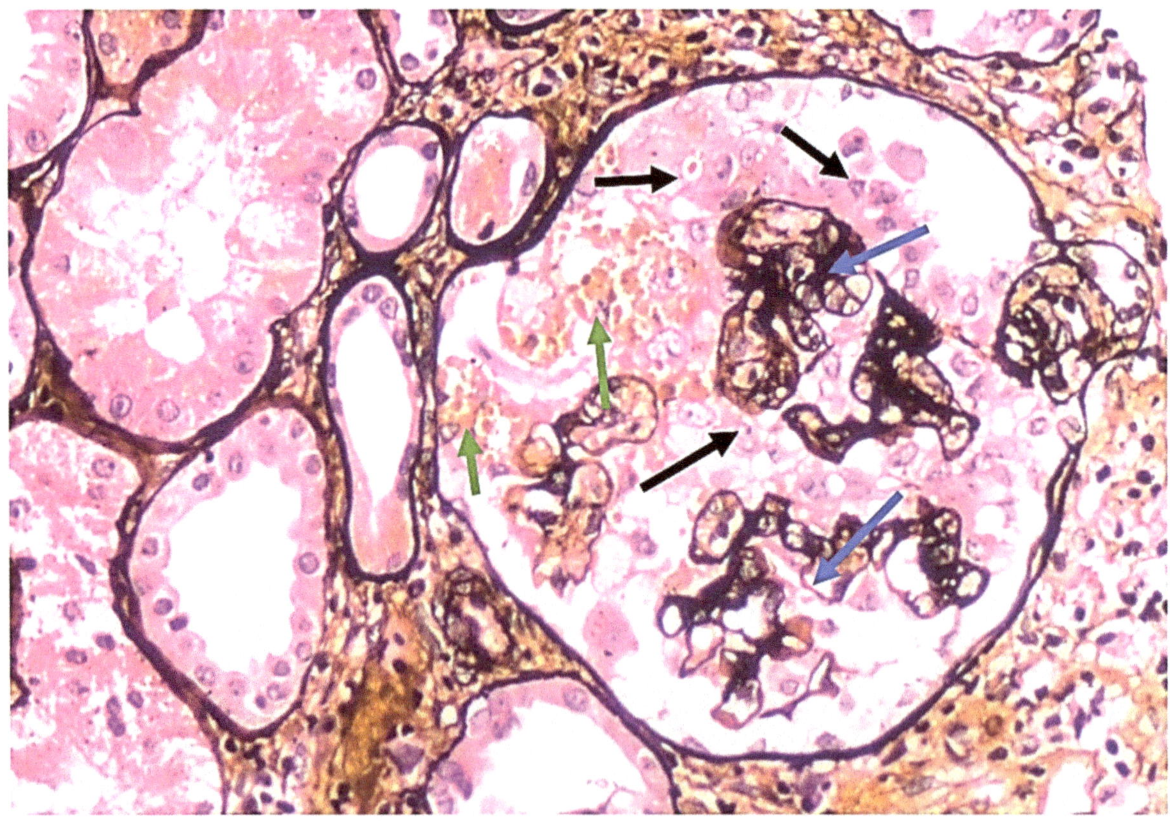

Figure 2:8.1: PASM Stain 20x: **(**blue arrows) Global collapse of the tuft with hypertrophy and hyperplasia of overlying podocytes (**black** arrows) and presence of protein resorption droplets (**green** arrows)

Immunofluorescence: IF studies shows no significant deposits.

Interpretation: FSGS-Collapsing glomerulopathy

Final Diagnosis: Human Immunodeficiency Virus Associated Nephropathy (HIVAN).

Suggested Reading:

Table 2:8.1: Columbia morphological classification of FSGS

Sr. No.	Variant	Inclusion Criteria	Exclusion Criteria
1.	**FSGS (NOS)**	At least 1 glomerulus with the segmental increase in matrix obliterating the capillary lumina.	Exclude perihilar, cellular, tip, and collapsing variants
2.	**Perihilar variant**	≥50% of glomeruli with segmental lesions must have perihilar sclerosis and/or hyalinosis	Exclude cellular, tip, and collapsing variants
3.	**Cellular variant**	At least 1 glomerulus with segmental endocapillary hypercellularity occluding lumina, with or without foam cells and karyorrhexis	Exclude tip and collapsing variant
4.	**Tip variant**	At least 1 segmental lesion involving the tip domain (outer 25% of tuft next to the origin of proximal tubule)	Exclude collapsing variant Exclude any perihilar sclerosis
5.	**Collapsing variant**	At least 1 glomerulus with segmental or global collapse and overlying podocyte hypertrophy and hyperplasia	None

***Reference**

Pathologic Classification of Focal Segmental Glomerulosclerosis: A Working Proposal: Vivette D D'Agatti et.al, Editorial, volume43, issue 2, page no.368-382, February 2004.

CASE 9

History: 35 years old male, software professional, non-obese, non-diabetic, normotensive with h/o chronic backache with history of using medicines on & off for backache, took massage therapy at a siddha medicine centre for last 2 months. He now presented with neurological symptoms of progressive weakness in lower limbs with areflexia and normal sensory assessment with pedal edema and frothyuria without any other urinary complaints for the last 4 weeks. BP: 110/70 mm of Hg.

Investigations: Urine analysis: Protein: 4+, RBCs: 8-10/HPF, RBC Casts: nil/HPF. 24-hour urine protein: 14 gm, serum creatinine: 0.9mg/dl, Serum albumin: 1.6 gm/dl.

Clinical Diagnosis: Adult-onset Nephrotic syndrome with microscopic hematuria without renal dysfunction or hypertension and with Guillain Barre Syndrome.

Differential Diagnoses: Membranous Nephropathy/ MCD/ FSGS.

Light Microscopy:

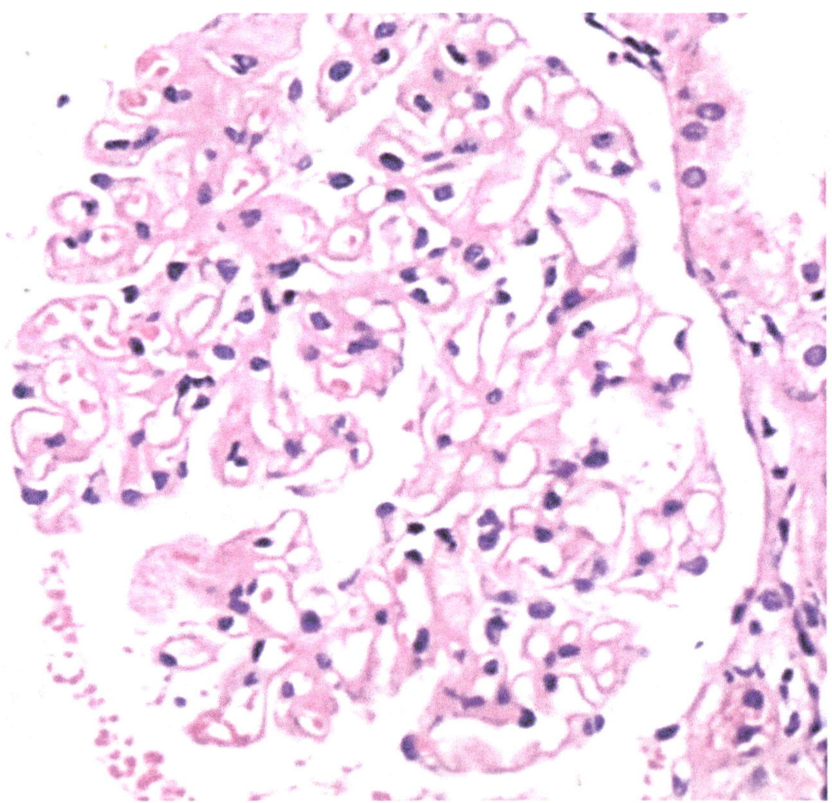

Figure 2:9.1: H&E Stain 20x: exaggerated normalcy appearance, mild diffuse thickening, and rigidity of the basement membranes.

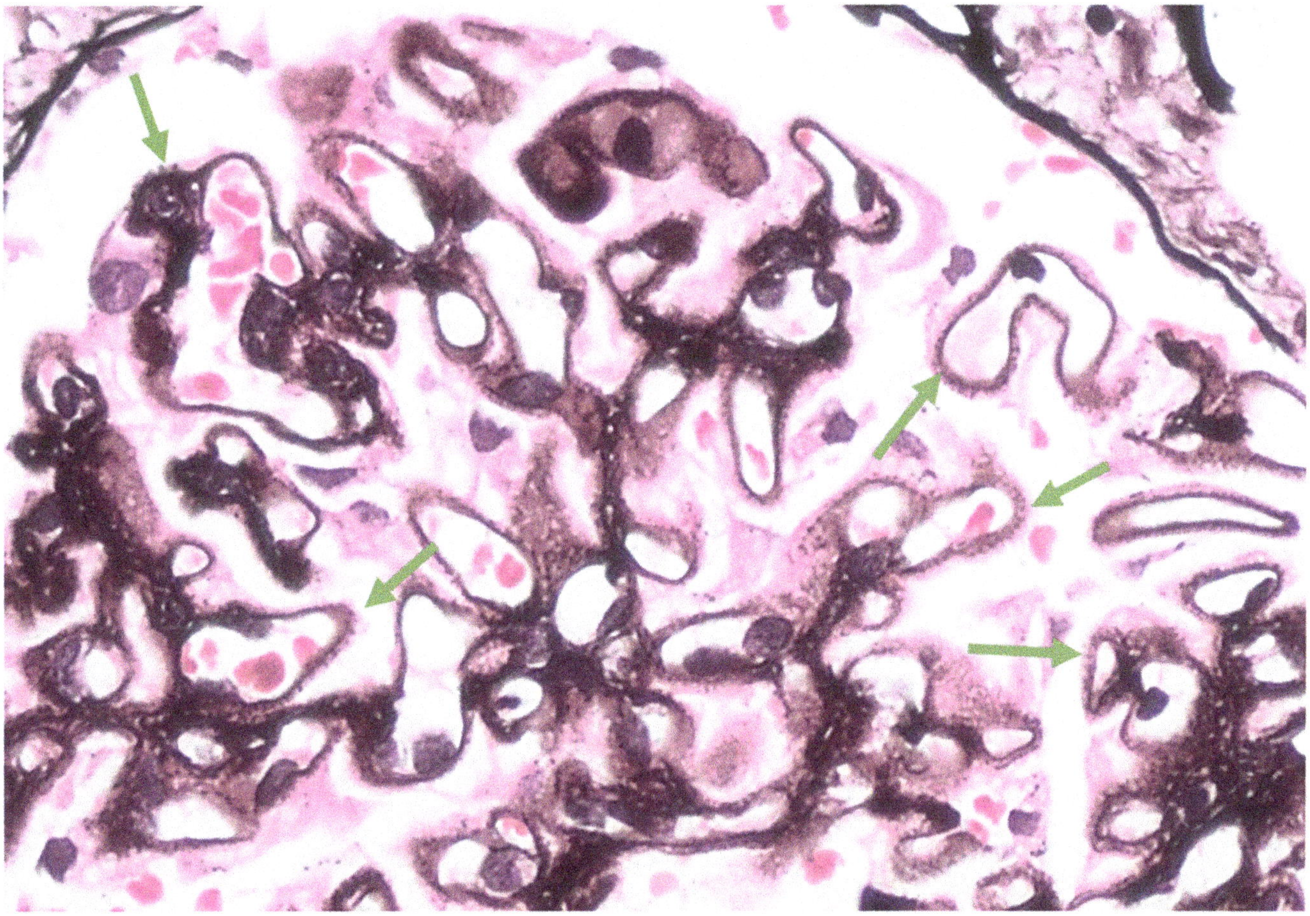

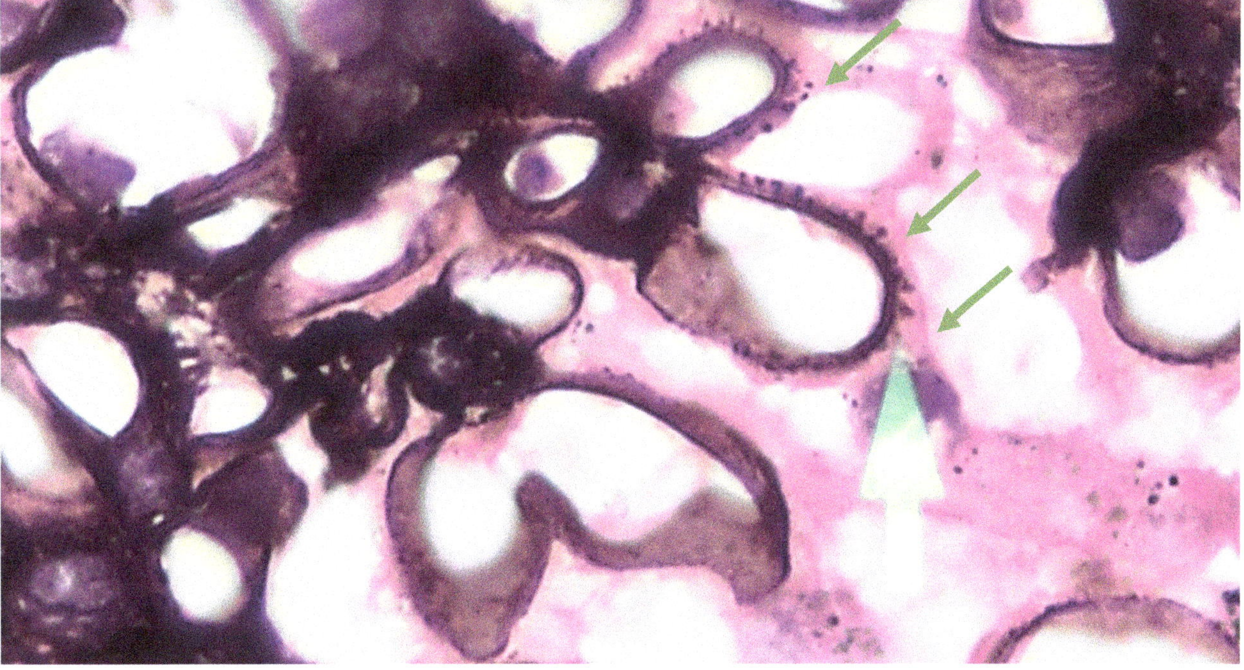

Figure 2:9.2: PASM Stain: 40x-subepithelial spikes (green arrows)

Figure 2:9.3: PASM Stain: 100x(oil immersion): subepithelial spikes (green arrows)

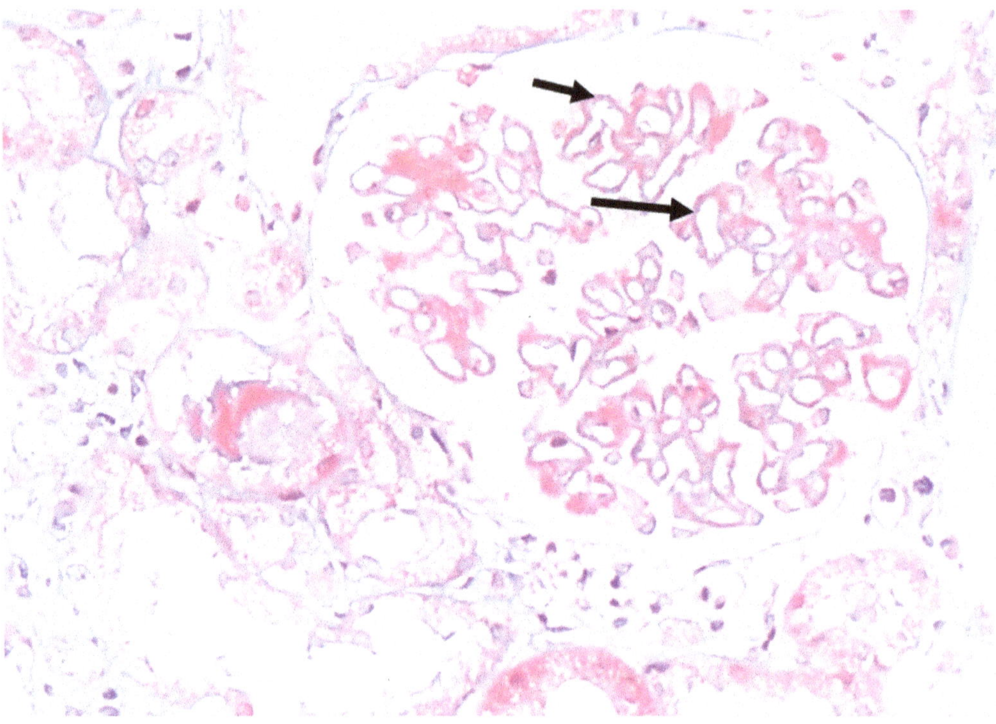

Figure 2:9.4: Masson Trichrome Stain:20x: fuchsinophilic (reddish) subepithelial deposits

Immunofluorescence:

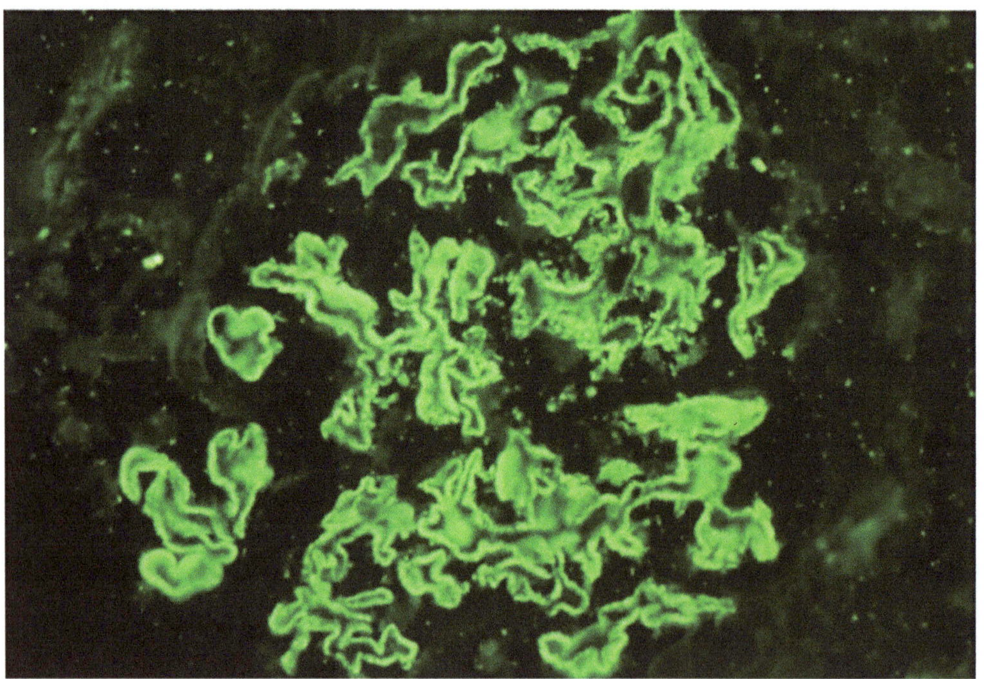

Figure 2:9.5: Immunofluorescence: IgG:20x: Glomerulus: Capillary wall fine granular immune deposits

Interpretation: - Membranous nephropathy

Supportive investigations: ANA Negative, C3 and C4 Normal, Viral markers: negative. 24 hour Urine Mercury level – 200 mcg/L .

Final Diagnosis: Mercury exposure induced Membranous Nephropathy.

Electron microscopy findings:

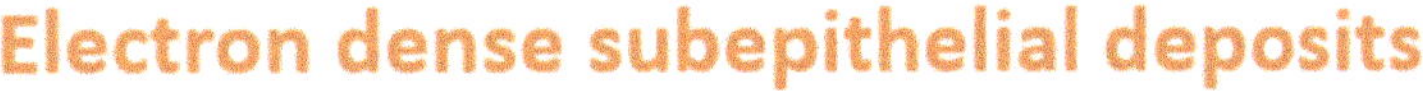

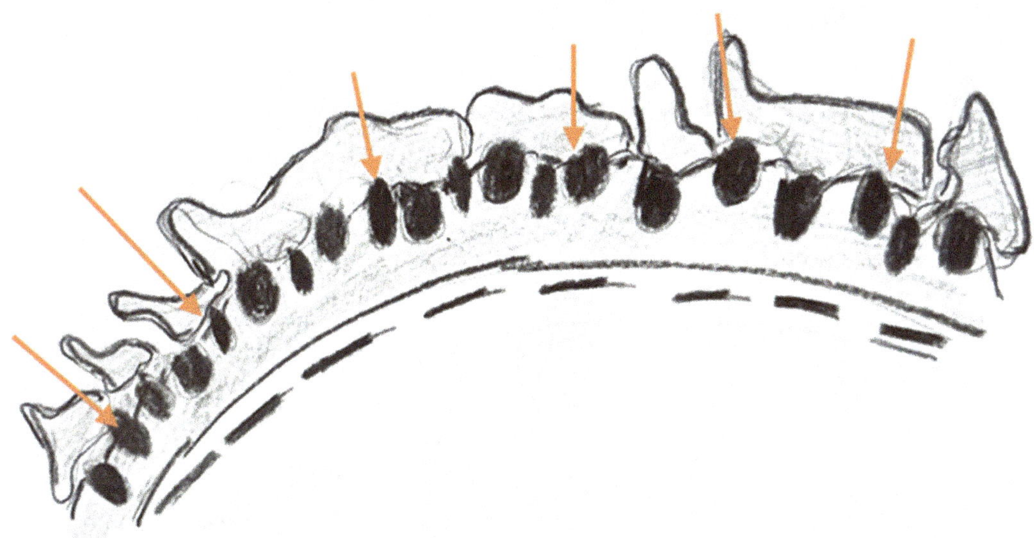

Figure 2:9.6: Diagrammatic representation of Electron microscopy: subepithelial electron dense deposits (orange arrows)

Suggested Reading:

Table 2:9.1: Scoring of the chronic lesions in individual renal tissue compartments

Tissue compartment	SCORE			
	0	1	2	3
Glomerulosclerosis (GS score)	<10%	10–25%	26%–50%	>50%
Interstitial fibrosis (IF score)	<10%	10–25%	26%–50%	>50%
Tubular atrophy (TA score)	<10%	10–25%	26%–50%	>50%
Arteriosclerosis (CV score)	Intimal thickening < thickness of media	Intimal thickening ≥ thickness of media		

1. A GS score includes the percentage of glomeruli with global and segmental sclerosis and ischemia.

2. The IF and TA scores include the percentage of the renal cortex involved by interstitial fibrosis and tubular atrophy, respectively.

3. CV score includes the severity of arteriosclerosis determined by the extent of thickening of the intima.

Table 2:9.2: Grades of chronic changes based on total renal chronicity score (0–10)

Grade	Total renal chronicity score
Minimal chronic changes	0 - 1
Mild chronic changes	2 - 4
Moderate chronic changes	5 - 7
Severe chronic changes	≥ 8

The total chronicity score is the sum of individual chronicity scores for each renal tissue compartment, as shown in Table 2:9.1:.

***Reference**

A proposal for standardized grading of chronic changes in native kidney biopsy specimens Sanjeev Sethi, et.al: Kidney International (2017) 91, 787–789.

History: 30 years old married female, non-diabetic & normotensive, non-obese, nonsmoker, non-alcoholic. She has 2 children. There is no history of pregnancy induced hypertension or abortions. She came with h/o progressive anasarca for a month and came to the emergency room with an episode of gross hematuria and acute abdomen. No other urinary complaints, no fever. There is no history of skin rash, oral ulcers, and arthralgia. BP 160/90 mm of Hg.

Investigations: Urine analysis: protein:4+, blood: 3+, Pus cells:5 to 6/ HPF, UPCR:13g/g. Serum Albumin: 1.2 gm/dl. Serum creatinine is 1.5 mg/dl.

Clinical Diagnosis: Adult onset Nephrotic syndrome with hematuria and AKI

Differential diagnoses: Membranous Nephropathy/ IgA Nephropathy/FSGS with Renal vein thrombosis.

Light microscopy:

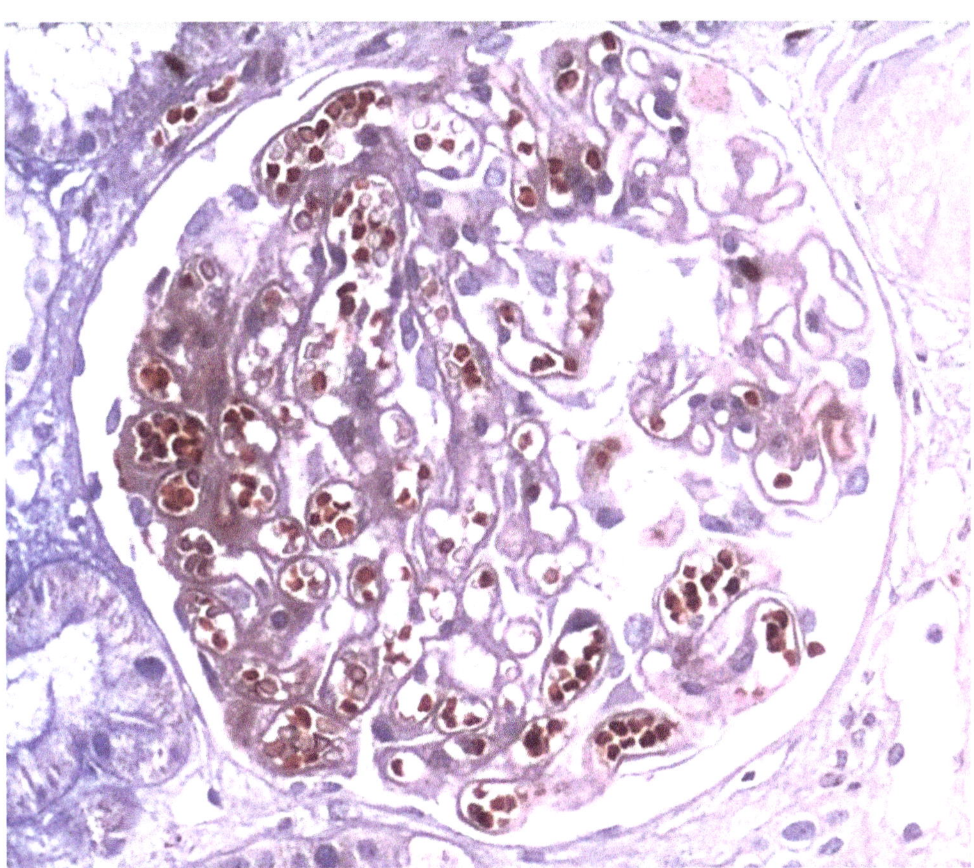

Figure 2:10.1: MT Stain: 20x: congested capillary lumina (RBCs in capillary lumina). Left Renal vein thrombosis was noted on Renal Doppler.

Immunofluorescence: Significant diffuse capillary wall fine granular immune deposits of IgG.

Immunohistochemistry (IHC): Anti-PLA2 R Ab:

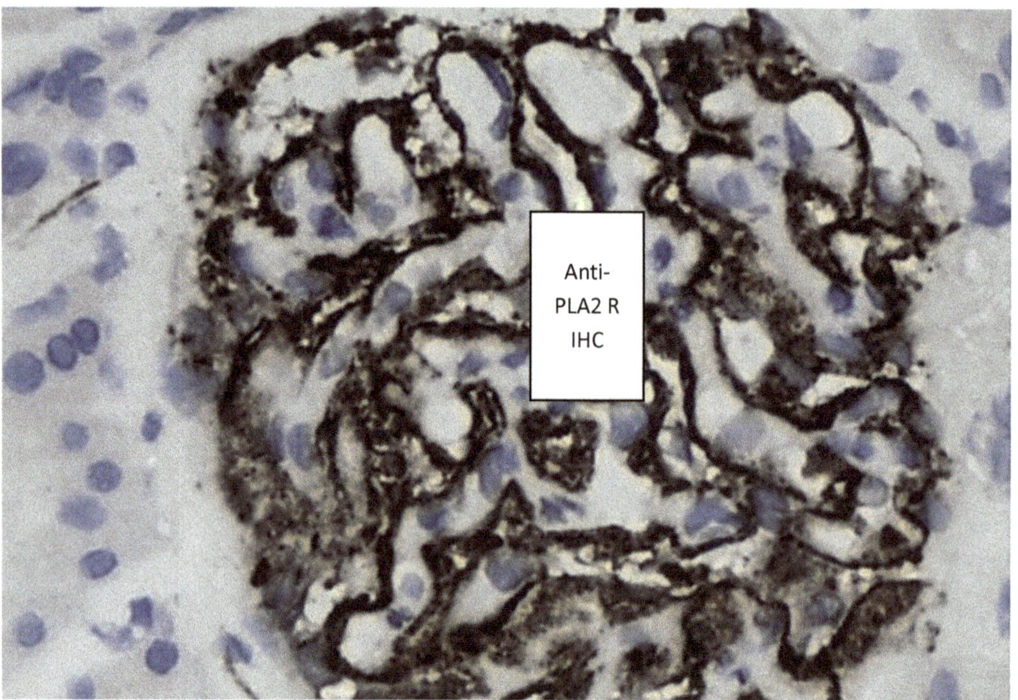

Figure 2:10.2: IHC:20x: anti-PLA2R Antibody: diffuse capillary wall granular positivity

Interpretation:

Membranous Glomerulonephritis

Additional investigations: ANA: negative, C3 & C4: normal, serum anti-PLA2R antibody: elevated, chest X-ray: normal, Renal vein doppler: suggestive of Left Renal vein thrombosis, Papanicolaou smear: negative for intraepithelial lesion or malignancy.

Final Diagnosis: Anti PLA2R Mediated Membranous Nephropathy with Renal Vein thrombosis.

***Few Antigens in Membranous Nephropathy:**

Sr. No.	Antigen	Common subclass of IgG	Commonly seen in
1.	PLA2R	IgG4	Primary membranous nephropathy
2.	NELL-1	IgG1	Malignancy/mercury induced membranous nephropathy
3.	Thrombospondin 7A	IgG 4	Malignancy in few
4.	Exostosin 1	IgG1	Lupus nephritis
5.	Semaphorin 3B	IgG1	Paediatric membranous nephropathy

***Reference**

Pierre Ronco et al., Membranous nephropathy, Nature Reviews, Disease Primers (2021)7:69.

CASE 11

History: 59 years old male, Chronic smoker, non-diabetic, hypertensive for the last 8 years, presented with a history of progressive loss of appetite for the last 6 months and 5 kg weight loss in the last 3 months. He has had a chronic cough with occasional streaks of blood in his sputum with progressive edema feet for the last 1 month. BP: 150/90.

Investigations: Urine protein 4+, RBCs:8 to 10/HPF, Pus cells :1 to 2/HPF, RBC casts: nil/HPF, UPCR 8 gm/gm with serum creatinine of 1.4 mg/dl. Serum albumin: 2.7 gm/dl. Dyslipidemia +.

Clinical Diagnosis: Adult onset Nephrotic syndrome with active sediments in urine with hypertension and renal dysfunction with significant weight loss.

Differential diagnoses: Membranous nephropathy/Amyloidosis/ANCA Vasculitis.

Light Microscopy:

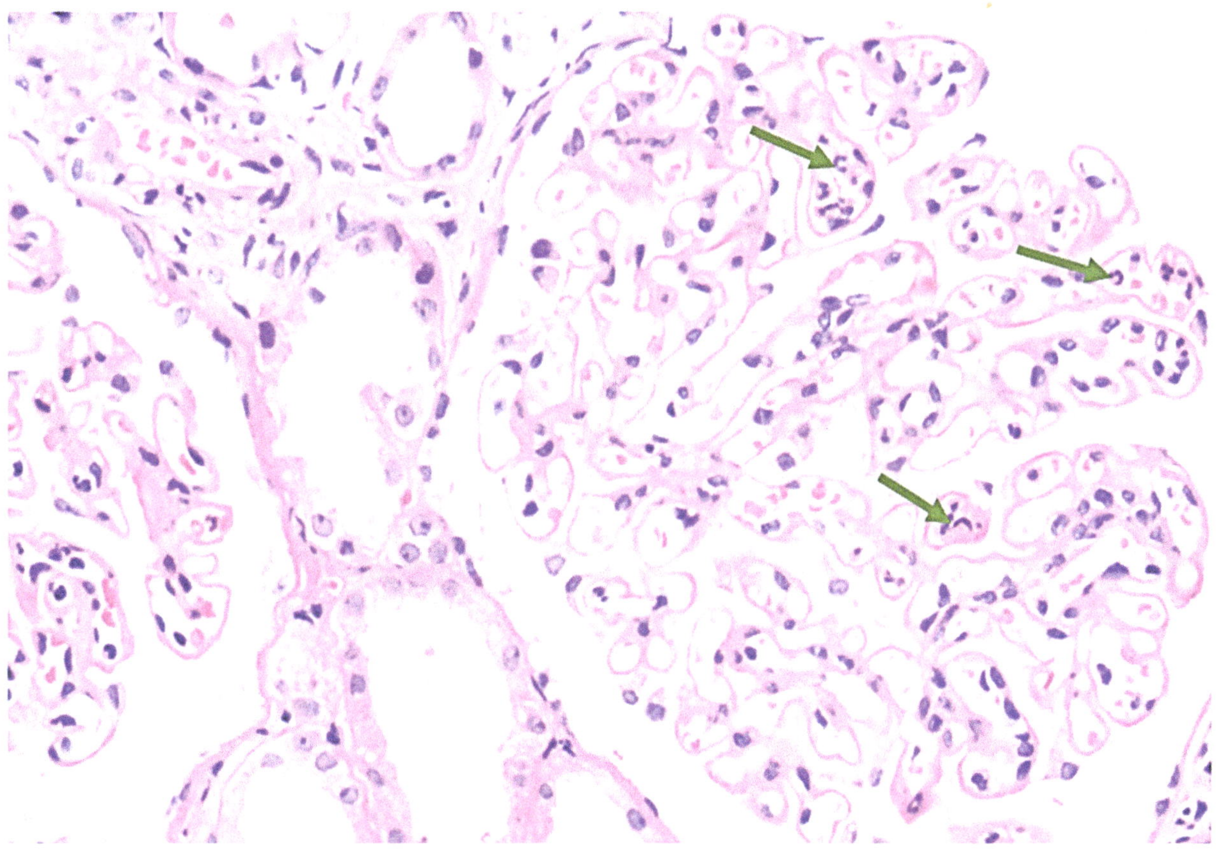

Figure 2:11.1: H&E Stain 20x: Glomerulus: Few neutrophils in the capillary lumina and mild diffuse uniform thickening and rigidity of the basement membranes (green arrows).

Immunofluorescence:

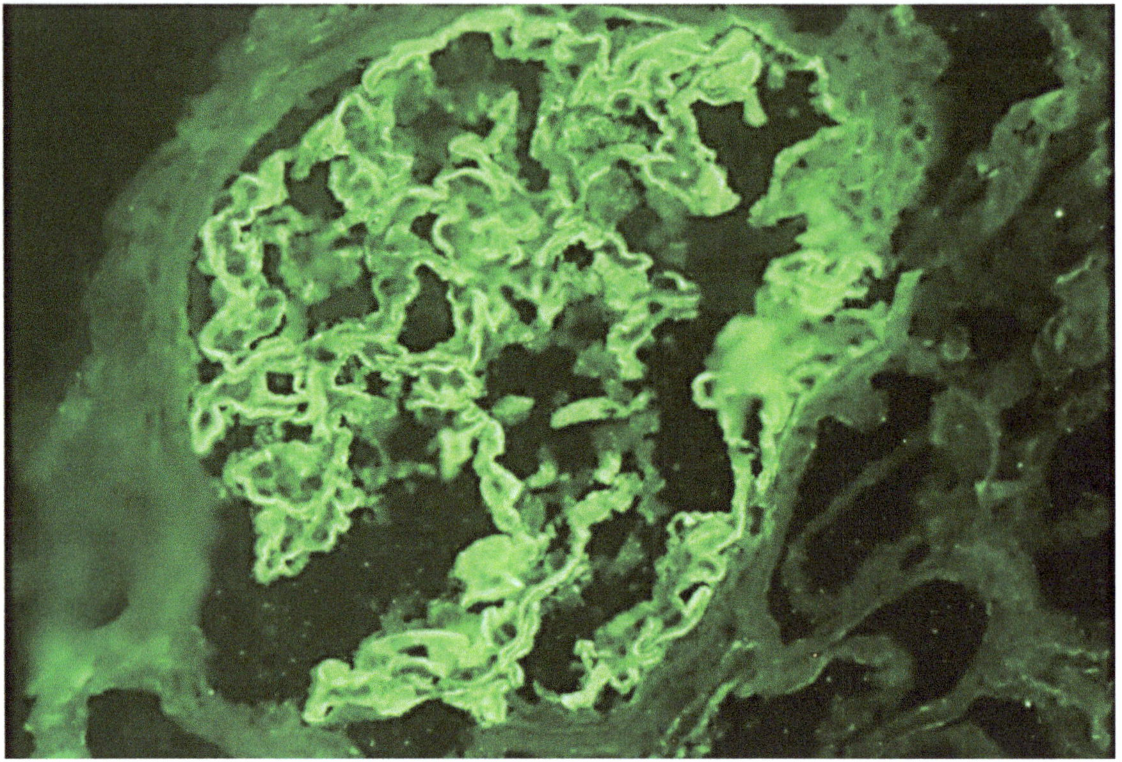

Figure 2:11.2: IgG:20x: Diffuse Capillary wall fine granular immune deposits.

Interpretation: Membranous Nephropathy.

Supportive investigations: ANA: negative, C3 and C4 Normal, ANCA: Negative, Anti GBM: negative, Viral screening: negative. CT Chest revealed: endo bronchial mass lesion suggestive of Lung malignancy.

Final Diagnosis: Malignancy associated Membranous Nephropathy.

***Suggested Reading:**

The finding of an increased number of inflammatory cells within the glomeruli, in the absence of endocapillary proliferation or membranoproliferative features, favoured a secondary form of MGN related to malignancy over primary MGN: Lefaucheur C, Stengel B, Nochy D, et al. Membranous nephropathy and cancer: epidemiologic evidence and determinants of high-risk cancer association. Kidney Int 2006; 70:1510-1517.

CASE 12

History: 45 years old female nondiabetic and normotensive with bilateral silicone breast implants placed 12 years ago. She had joined a physical training program for weight loss 3 months back, she started having joint pains in large joints with on & off pedal edema with no other complaints. No h/o NSAIDS/Indigenous medicine use. B.P.:140/90mm of Hg.

Investigations: Urine analysis: protein: 3+, RBCs: 6-7 /HPF & no RBC casts. Serum creatinine: 1.5 mg/dl. Serum albumin: 3.6 gm/dl.

Clinical Diagnosis: Nephrotic range proteinuria with hypertension, microscopic hematuria and renal dysfunction

Differential diagnoses: Lupus nephritis/Membranous nephropathy/FSGS/IgA Nephropathy

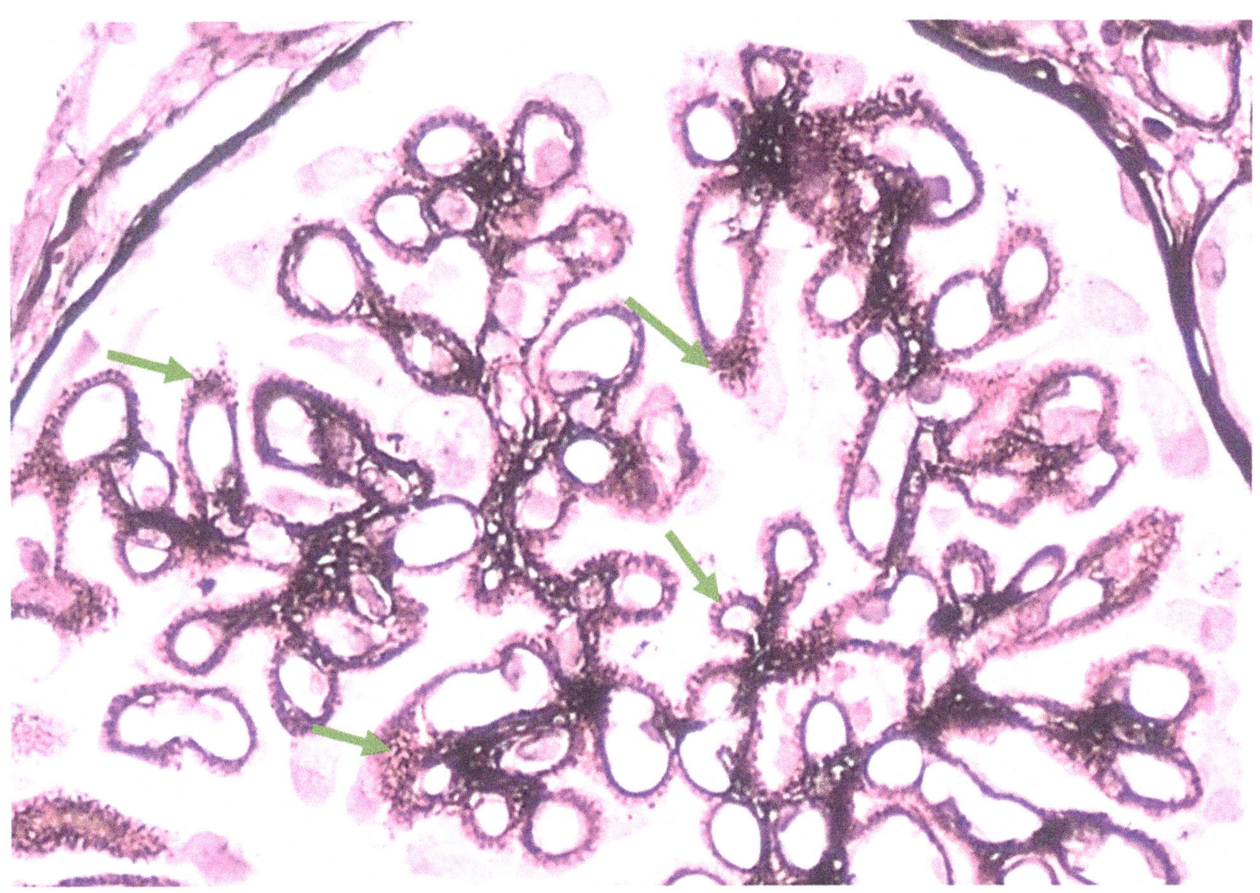

Figure 2:12.1: PASM Stain: 40x: Silver positive subepithelial spikes

Immunofluorescence: Significant diffuse capillary wall fine granular immune deposits of IgG.

Interpretation: Membranous nephropathy

Supportive investigations: Viral markers: negative. C3 & C4 normal, ANA profile Negative. Rheumatoid factor: Negative. Papanicolaou smear: negative for intraepithelial lesion or malignancy.

Stool for occult blood negative. Chest x-ray and Mammogram: Negative for any malignancy. ESR: 70 mm at the end of one hour.

MRI B/L Breasts: Intracapsular Implant rupture noted.

Final Diagnosis: Secondary Membranous nephropathy – part of ASIA Syndrome/ Shoenfeld's syndrome due to breast implant rupture with chronic silicone exposure.

Suggested reading:

ASIA Syndrome Following Breast Implant Placement Roberta Fenoglio MD, Irene Cecchi MD and Dario Roccatello MD, IMAJ 2018; 20: 714–716.

Case 13

History: 55-year-old male with a history of pedal edema on & off for the last 2 months without any urinary complaints and complaining of numbness in his right leg below the ankle with weakness and neuropathic pain in right foot for the last 1 month. He recently developed numbness in his left hand, weak hand grip, and wrist drop. He has purpuric skin lesions on both legs. With some joint pains without any swelling or tenderness of joints. BP 170/90 mm of Hg.
- No oral ulcers / Raynaud's phenomenon/ skin ulcers
- Poor appetite and history of significant unintentional weight loss (5% body weight in last 6 months) and anemia.

Investigations: Urine analysis: protein:3+, blood: 2+, RBC casts: 3-5/HPF, UPCR: 3.4 g/g, serum creatinine = 1.6mg/dl, Serum albumin = 3.5 gm/dl. Hemoglobin: 8.9 g/dl, TLC: 4500/cu mm, Platelet count:1.3 Lakh/cu mm.

Clinical Diagnosis: Nephrotic range Proteinuria with active urinary sediments with hypertension and renal dysfunction with asymmetrical sensory motor neuropathy and skin lesions suggesting an underlying vasculitic pathology.

Differential diagnoses: ANCA vasculitis/Cryoglobulinemic GN

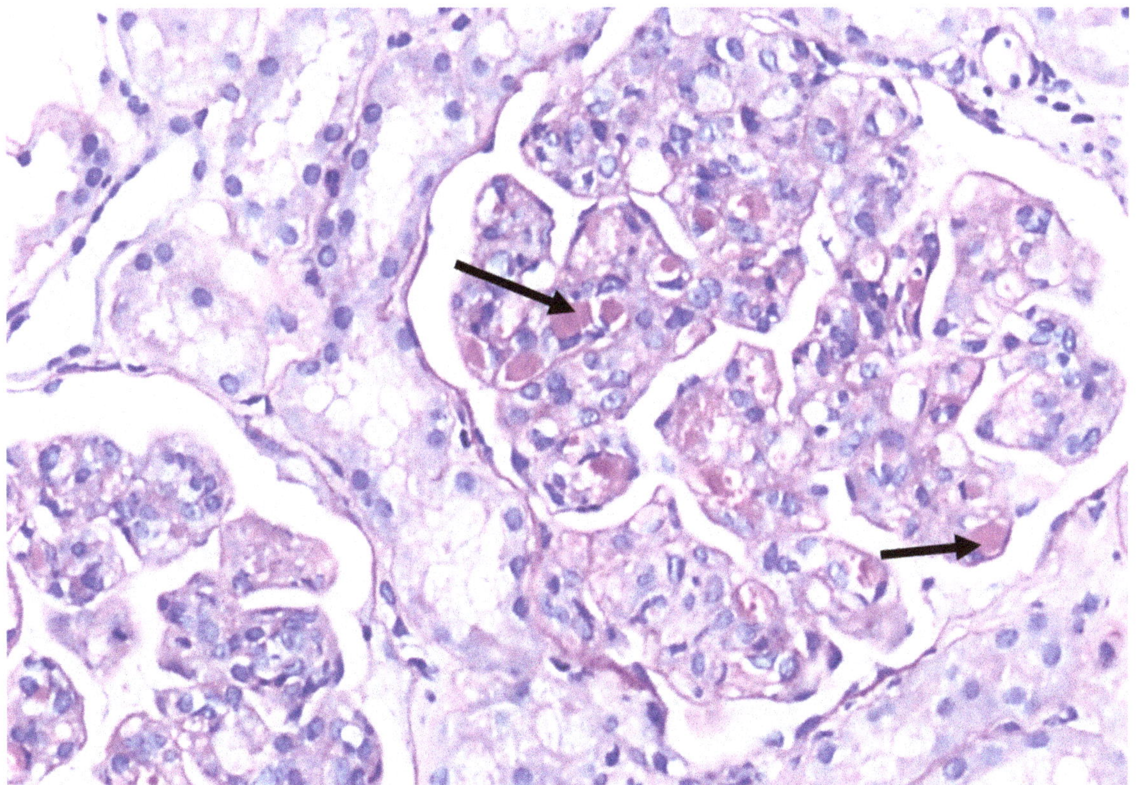

Figure: 2:13.1: PAS Stain 20x: PAS positive pseudothrombi and enlarged hypercellular glomeruli.

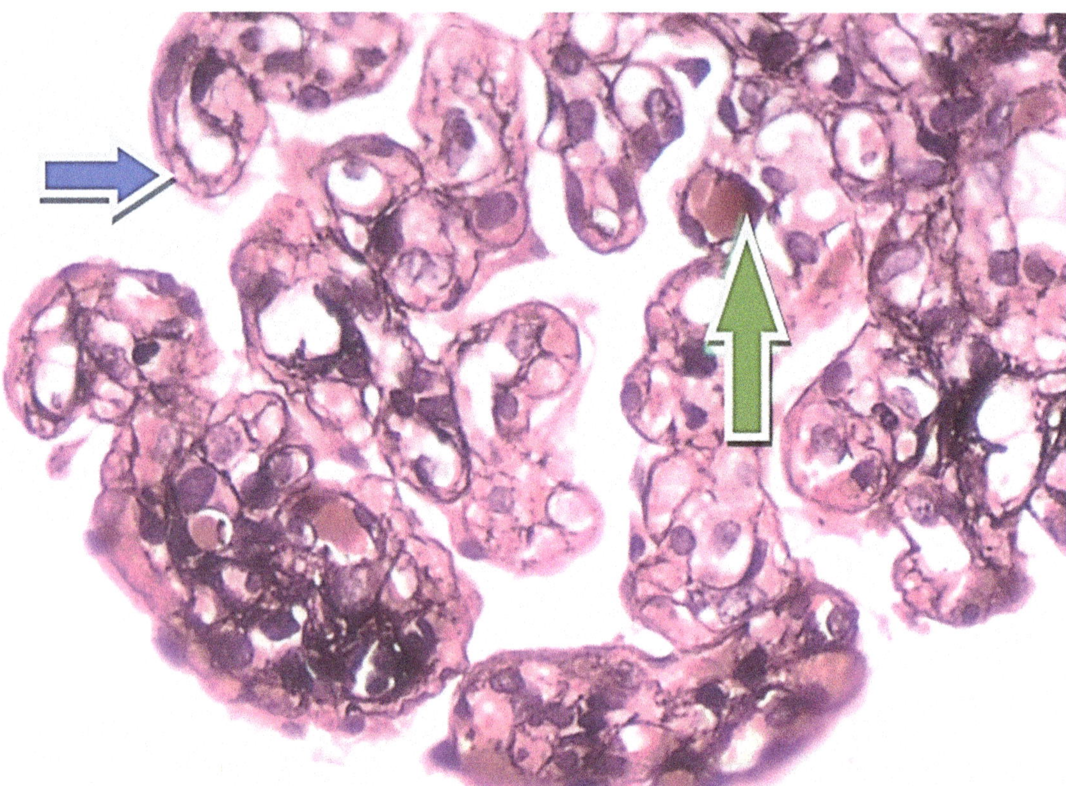

Figure: 2:13.2: Silver stain:40x: pseudo thrombi (**green arrow**) and GBM duplication (**blue arrow**) Tram -track appearance.

Immunofluorescence:

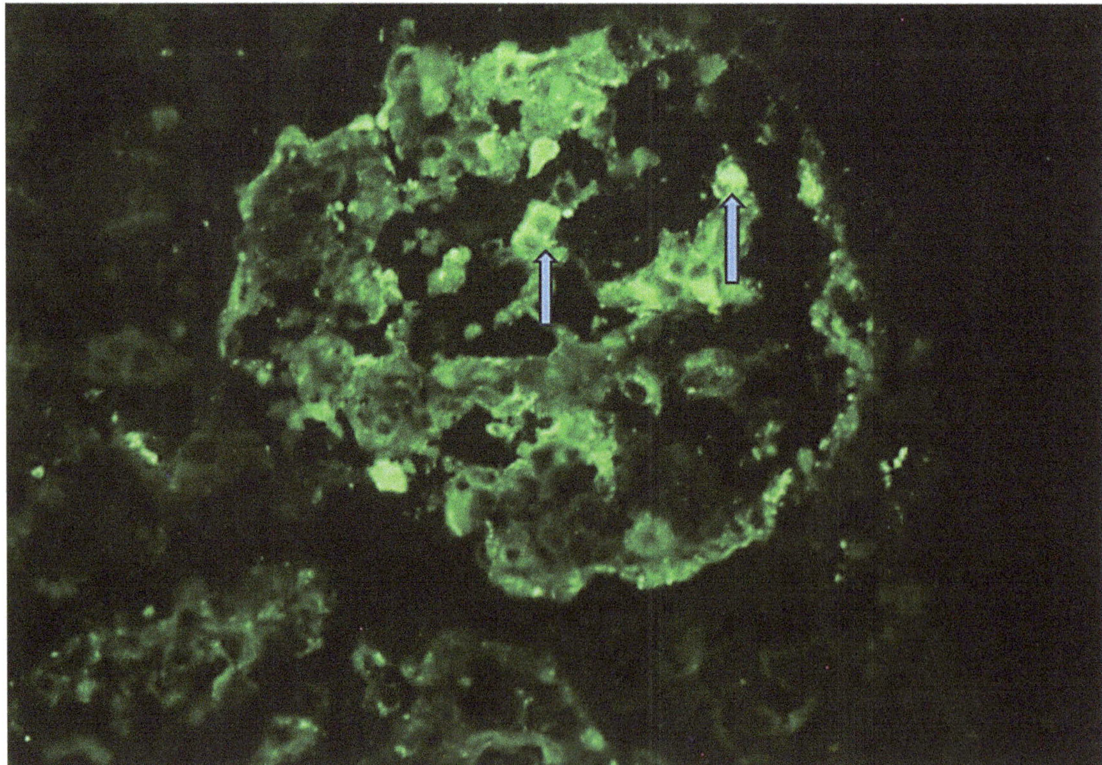

Figure 2:13.3: Immunofluorescence :20x: Pesudo-thrombi positive for IgM.

Also IgG and C3c is positive along the capillary wall and mesangium.

Electron microscopy findings:

GBM duplication with mesangial cell-interposition and mesangial and subendothelial electron-dense deposits, showing microtubules as a substructure.

Interpretation: Membranoproliferative Pattern of Glomerulonephritis with Pseudothrombi.

Supportive Investigations: Nerve conduction study: suggestive of sensory motor neuropathy in the right upper limb and lower limb.

HIV, Hbs Ag and HCV: Negative, LFT normal, Rheumatoid factor Positive, C3 level normal & C4 Low, ANA Negative. ANCA: negative. Serum Protein electrophoresis: M band seen.

Cryglobulin detection test: Positive

10 ml blood prewarmed to 37°C without anticoagulants. After clotting at 37°C for 30-60 min, the serum is separated by centrifugation at 37°C, placed in a Wintrobe tube, and refrigerated at 4°C to allow the precipitation of cryoglobulin. The precipitates are seen within 24 hours and then a diagnosis of type I Cryoglobulinemia is considered. Sometimes precipitates may be seen in 2-3 days time for mixed cryoglobulinemia and in up to 7 days in Type 2 and Type 3 Cryoglobulinemia.

Cryocrit: Measured as a percentage of the precipitate volume to the original serum volume at 4°C. cryocrit over 0.5-1% or cryoglobulin concentration >50 mcg/L is considered significant.

Final diagnosis: Cryoglobulinemic Glomerulonephritis with MPGN Pattern and Mononeuritis Multiplex due to vasculitis due to underlying Paraproteinemia.

CASE 14

History: A 16-year-old female was diagnosed 1 year back with post-infectious GN. She was managed observantly and symptomatically and had resolution of her nephritic presentation over 3-4 months. She has now again presented with facial puffiness, pedal edema, shortness of breath on exertion, no hematuria, and no systemic features of collagen vascular disease. BP is 160/90 mm of Hg.

Investigations: Urine analysis: protein:3+, blood:3+, RBC casts 3-4/HPF. UPCR: 6 g/g. Serum creatinine: 2.0mg/dl, serum albumin: 3.4 gm/dl.

Clinical Diagnosis: Nephrotic - Nephritic syndrome / Nephrotic range proteinuria with active urinary sediments with hypertension and renal dysfunction.

Differential diagnoses: Lupus Nephritis/ Infection related GN/ MPGN

Light microscopy:

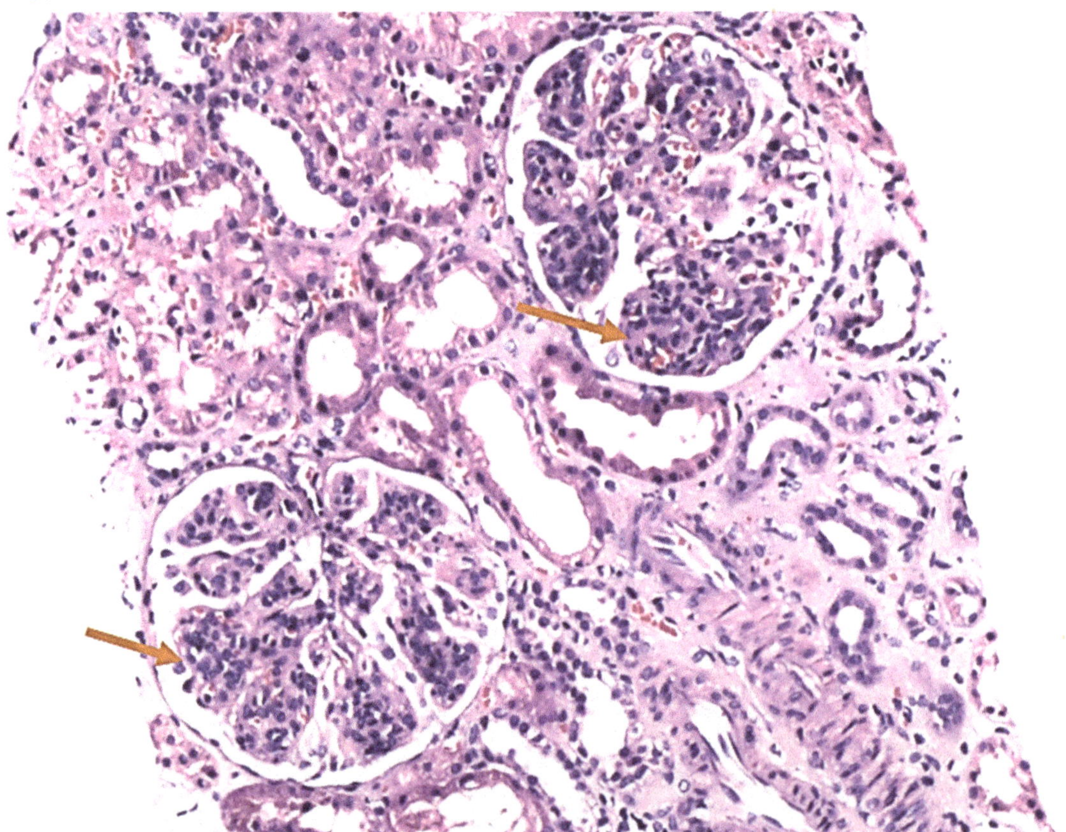

Figure 2:14.1: H&E Stain 10x: Enlarged and hypercellular glomeruli show lobular accentuation of tufts.

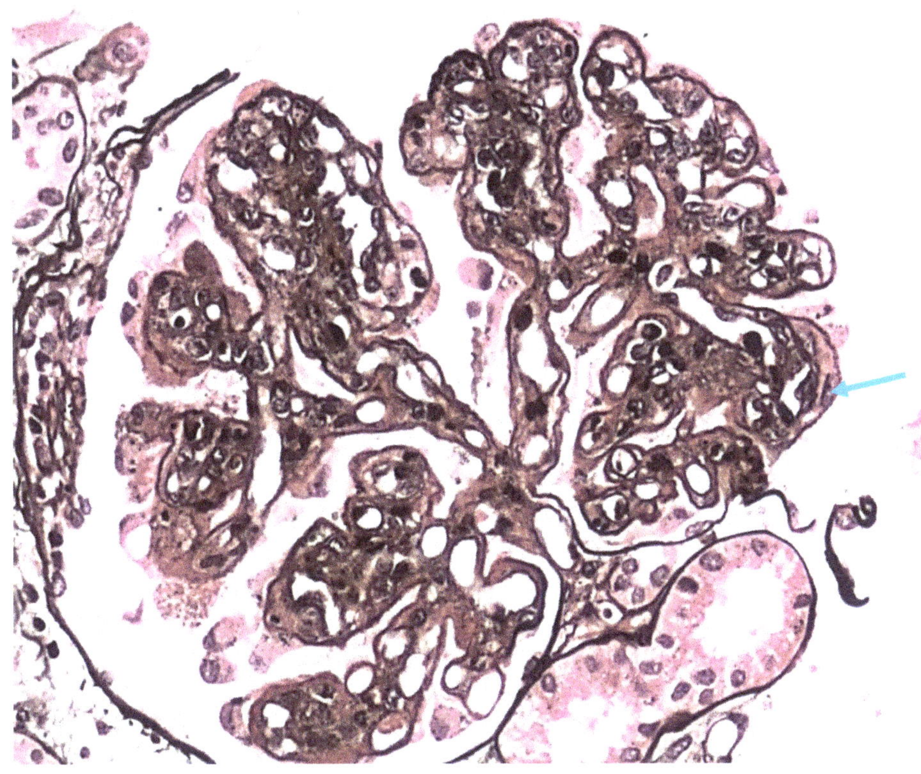

Figure 2:14.2 PASM Stain 20x: MPGN pattern of GN: GBM Tram-track appearance with mesangial cell interposition(blue arrown).

Immunofluorescence:

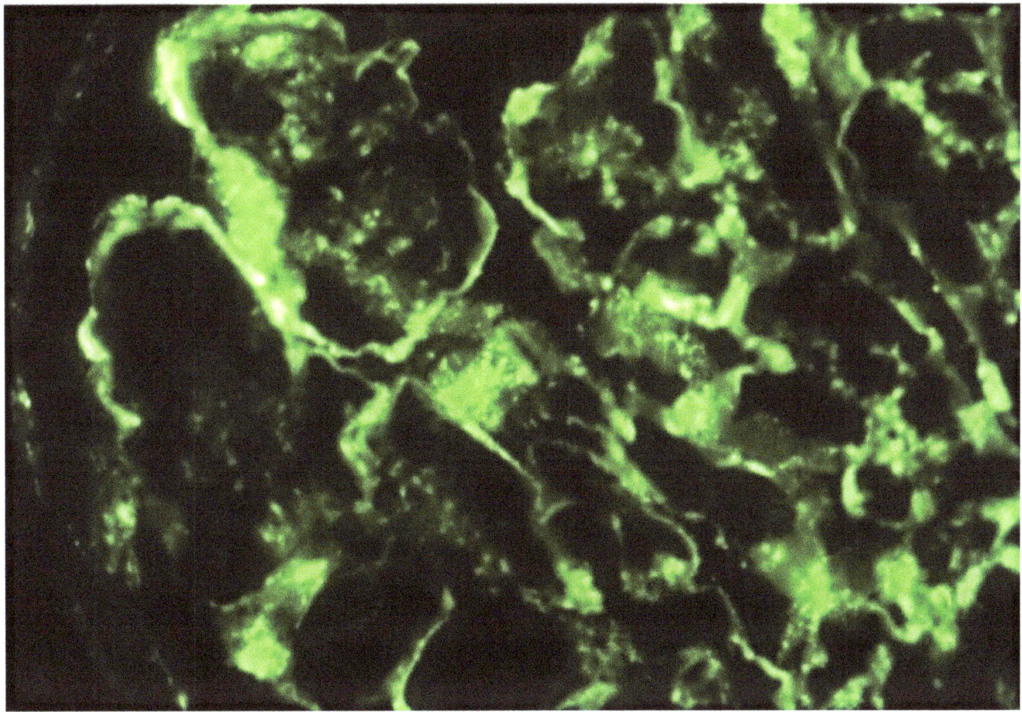

Figure 2:14.3: Immunofluorescence: IgG: 40x: capillary wall linear smooth and granular immune deposits of IgG &C3c.

Interpretation: Membranoproliferative pattern of glomerulonephritis.

Additional investigations: Viral markers: Negative. ANA Negative. C3 is low, and C4 is normal. ASO Negative. Serum Protein electrophoresis: M band is not seen.

For any MPGN pattern of GN, the following 3 etiologies need to be ruled out:

1. Neoplastic: e.g. MGRS
2. Autoimmune: e.g. SLE
3. Infection: e.g. Hepatitis B virus, Hepatitis C virus.

Electron Microscopy findings:

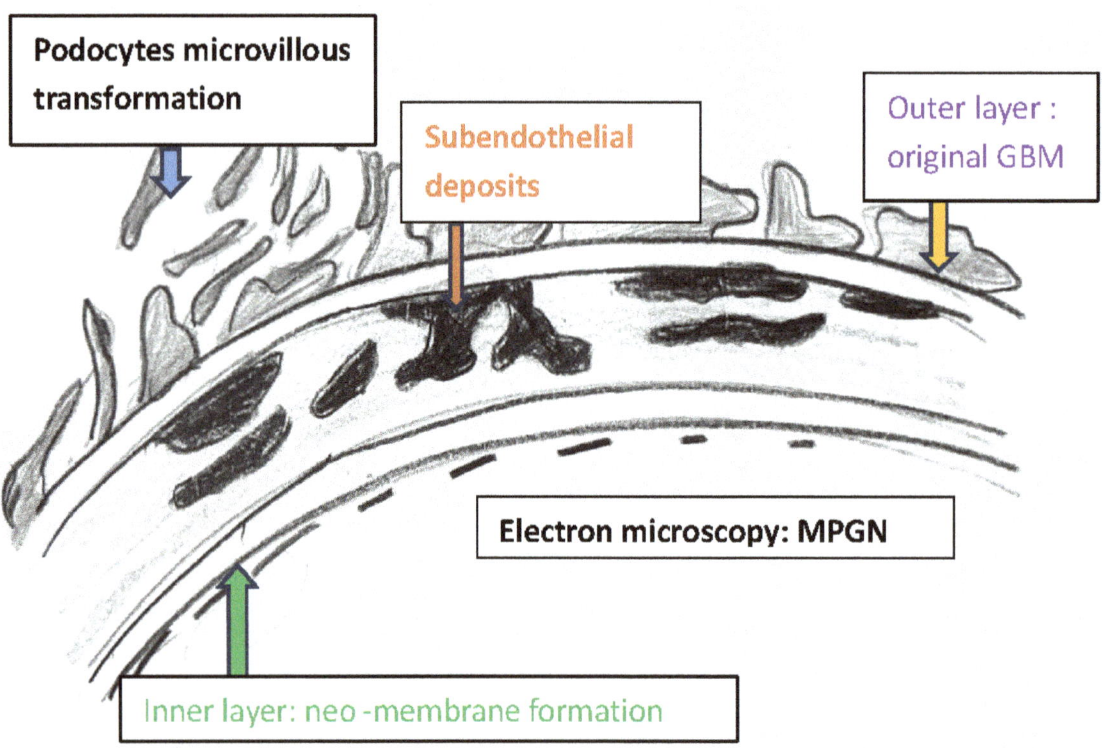

Figure 2:14.4: Diagrammatic representation of EM: MPGN: GBM duplication, mesangial and subendothelial electron dense deposits

Pathology Pearls

* Smooth outer contour of the deposits provides a useful clue indicating that the deposits are subendothelial (rather than subepithelial).

Reference

*Heptinstall's Pathology of Kidney, Seventh edition, Chapter 08: Membranoproliferative Glomerulonephritis - Immunofluorescence Microscopy: page no.310.

CASE 15

History: 36 years male, non-diabetic with recent onset hypertension. He had 1 episode of gross hematuria 6 months back, resolved without any medication, and now has a second episode of gross hematuria, preceded 3 days by URTI. He has no rash or arthralgia. No history of drug abuse. There is no history of NSAIDS abuse and no history of bleeding from any other sites. No dysuria or fever. No abdominal pain but bilateral flank pain for a week. BP 170/100 mm of Hg.

Investigations: Urine analysis: 4+ protein, plenty of RBCs and 2-3 RBC casts/ HPF, UPCR 4.8 g/g, serum creatinine: 2 mg/dl.

Clinical Diagnosis: Nephrotic range Proteinuria with hypertension and episodes of gross hematuria with renal dysfunction.

Differential diagnoses: IgA Nephropathy/ Infection related GN/ C3GN/ MPGN.

Light microscopy:

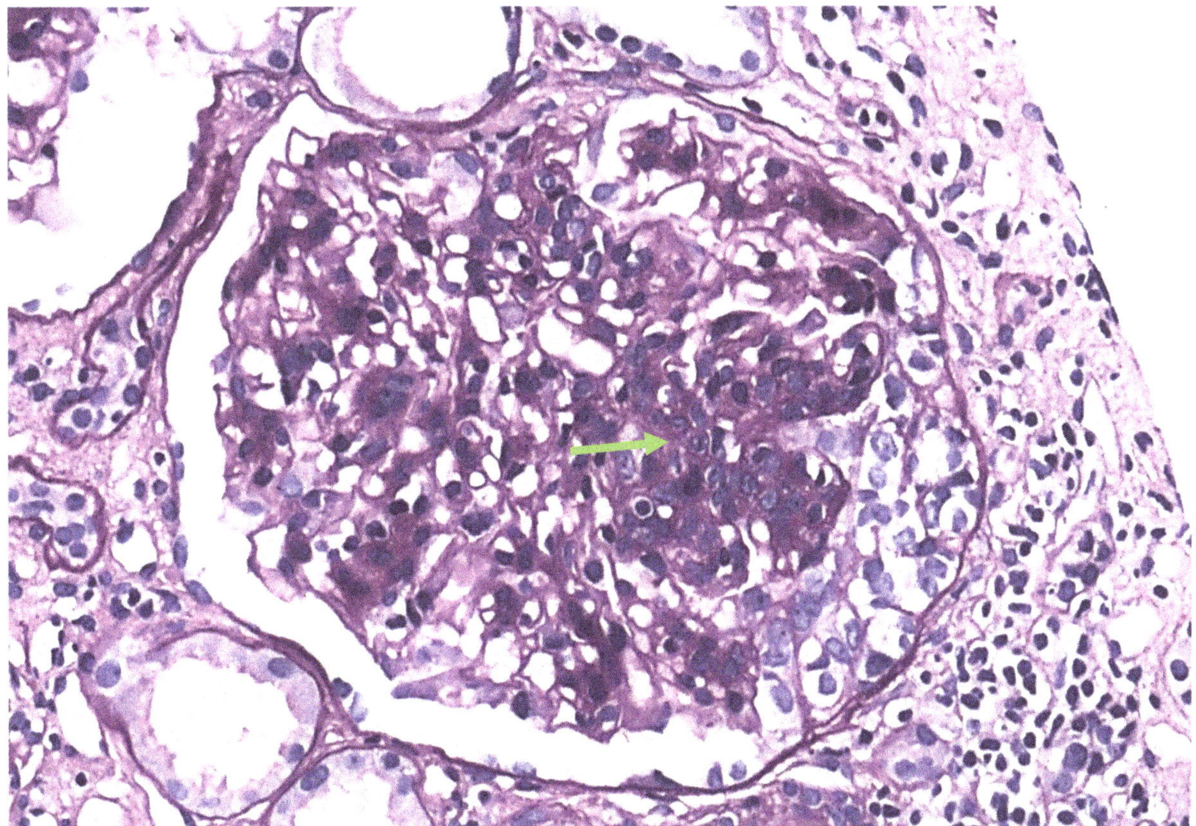

Figure 2:15.1: PAS Stain 20 x: Marked mesangial hypercellularity (green arrow) and segmental cellular crescent (red arrow).

Mesangial hypercellularity: The mesangial hypercellularity has to be scored in the PAS stain and away from the vascular pole of the glomerulus.

Grades	Number of mesangial cells
Mild	4 to 5
Moderate	5 to 7
Marked	≥8

Immunofluorescence:

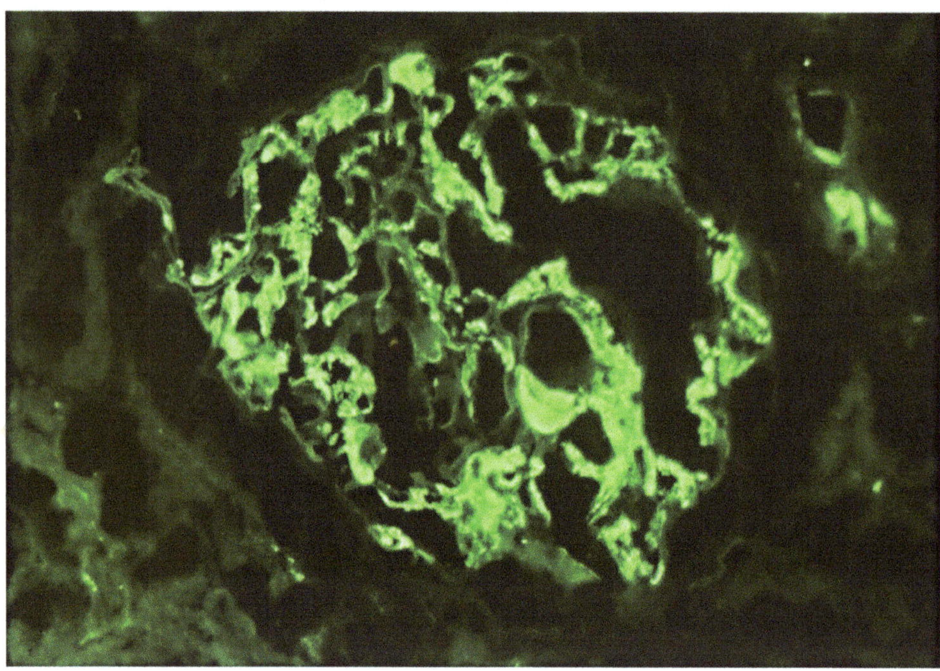

Figure 2:15.2: Immunofluorescence:20x: IgA: significant mesangial coarse granular immune deposits.

Interpretation: IgA Nephropathy.

Primary diagnosis: IgA nephropathy

Pattern of injury: Marked mesangial hypercellularity and focal cellular crescent.

Oxford classification: M1 E0 S0 T0- C1.

Additional findings: mild arteriolar hyalinosis and arteriosclerosis

Electron microscopy findings:

Paramesangial and /or mesangial electron dense deposits.

Final diagnosis: Mesangial Proliferative GN with focal crescent and IgA deposits in mesangium seen on IF Study consistent with an IgA Nephropathy.

Suggested Reading: Renal biopsy report in IgA nephropathy: IgA N: adequate biopsy: minimum 8 glomeruli are required.

Table 2:15.1: Oxford classification: MEST-C score:

Features			
Mesangial hypercellularity (M)	≤50% of glomeruli: M0	>50% of glomeruli:M1	
Endocapillay hypercellularity (E)	Absent: E0	Present: E1	
Segment of sclerosis (S)	Absent S0	Present: S1	
Interstitial fibrosis/tubular atrophy (T)	≤25% of the cortex: T0	26% to 50% of the cortex: T1	>50% of the cortex: T2
Cellular and/or fibrocellular crescents. (C)	No crescents: C0	C1 (crescent in <25% of glomeruli)	C2 (crescents in ≥25% of glomeruli)

Pathology Pearls

* The interstitial infiltrate shows few eosinophils in IgA N.

** C4d staining in IgA Nephropathy indicates poor prognostic factor.

***A low C3/C4 shows more severe clinical symptoms and chronic renal injury and could be a risk factor for patients developing to ESRD.

****Pattern of glomerular IgA deposition: If IgG is also present with IgA and is showing glomerular capillary wall deposits, it may have a worse prognosis than mesangial deposits alone.

*Diagnostic Pathology, Kidney Diseases, Second Edition, Colvin/Chang :IgA nephropathy page no.130.)

**GLOSEN: Association of C4d deposition with clinical outcomes in IgA nephropathy. Clin J Am Soc Nephrol May 9(5) :897-904,2014.

*** Relationship between serum C3/C4 ratio and prognosis of immunoglobulin A nephropathy based on propensity score matching: Yan Zhang, et.al: Chin Med J (Engl). 2020 Mar 20; 133(6): 631–637.:

****Bellur SS, et al, Working Group of International IgA Nephropathy Network and Renal Pathology Society. Immunostaining findings in IgA Nephropathy correlation with histology and clinical outcome in the Oxford classification patient cohort. Nephrol Dial Transplant.2011;26:2533-2536.

History: 15-year-old boy with a history of non-palpable, nonpruritic erythematous papular skin rash appearing on the trunk and lower limbs and resolving spontaneously over 1-2 weeks, on and off for the last 6 months. On routine evaluation was found to have microscopic hematuria which persisted in repeat evaluation even after 6 months. He is not hypertensive. There is no history of abdominal pain/arthritis/ oral ulcers. Skin biopsy of the erythematous lesion done a month back had shown leucocytoclastic vasculitis. He has no pedal edema. BP is 120/80 mm of Hg.

Investigations: Urine analysis: Protein: 2+, UPCR: 1.2, serum creatinine: 0.9 mg/dl. Serum albumin 3.6 gm/dl.

Clinical diagnosis: Subnephrotic proteinuria with persistent microscopic hematuria with cutaneous vasculitis lesions without hypertension and renal dysfunction.

Differential diagnoses: Henoch Schonlein Purpura (HSP) Nephritis/ microscopic polyangiitis/Lupus nephritis.

Light microscopy:

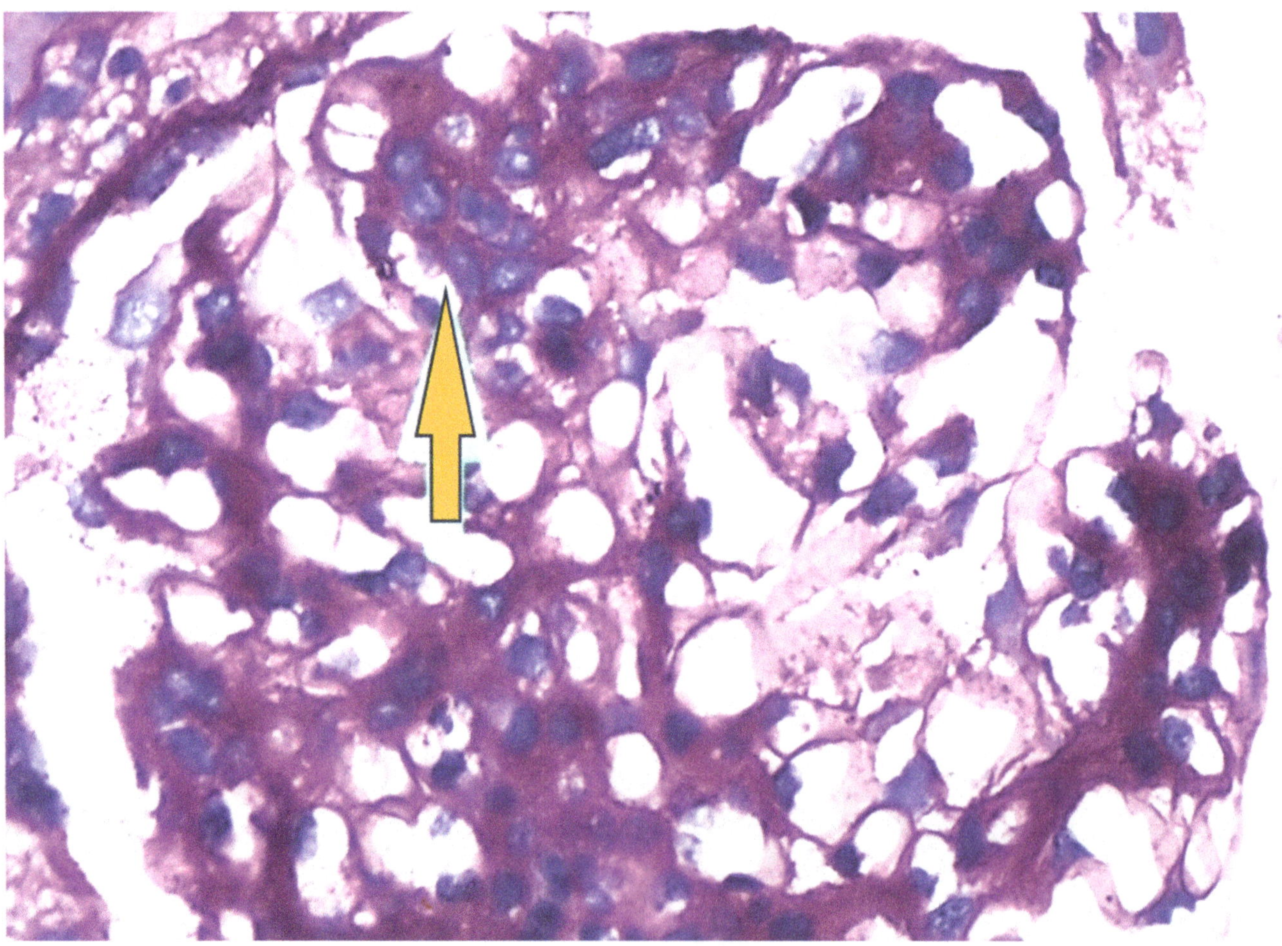

Figure 2:16.1: PAS Stain: 40x: moderate mesangial hypercellularity.

Immunofluorescence:

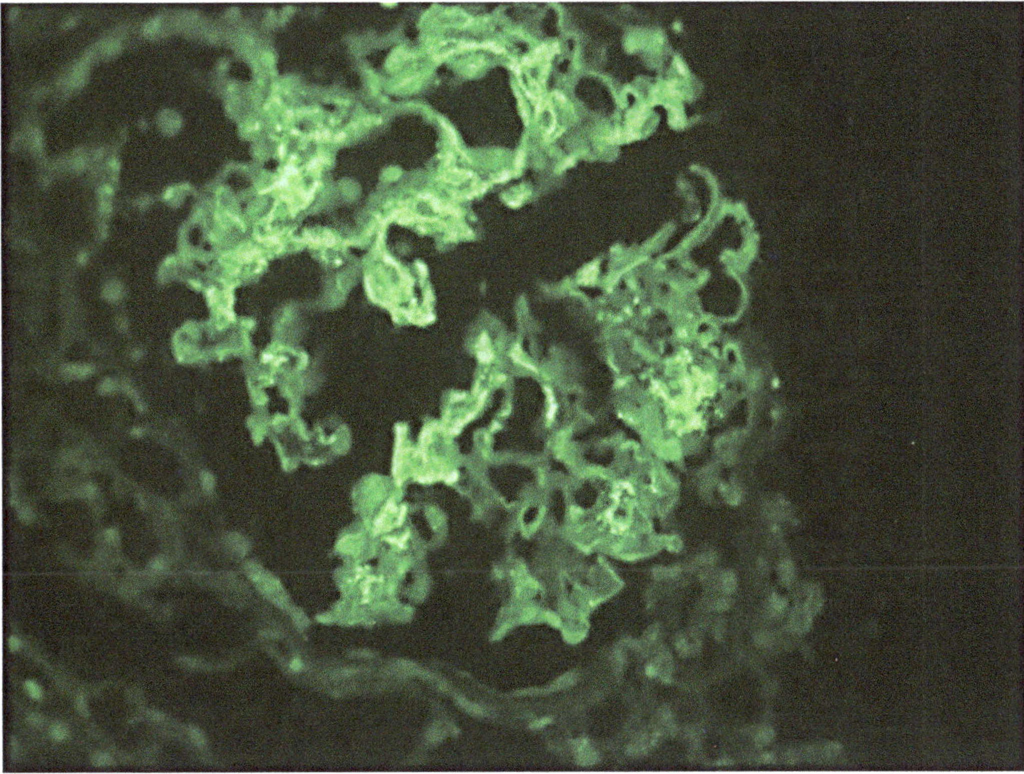

Figure 2:16.2: Immunofluorescence: IgA: significant Mesangial coarse granular deposits.

Interpretation: Mesangial proliferative GN with IgA deposits in mesangium – suggestive of IgA Nephropathy.

Final diagnosis: Henoch Shonlein Purpura—HSP nephritis ISKDC Class: II.

Suggested Reading: International Study of Kidney Disease in Childhood (ISKDC) Histologic Classification of IgA Vasculitis (Henoch-Schonlein Purpura) Nephritis:

Class	Features
I	Minimum Histologic alterations
II	Pure mesangial proliferation
III (a)	Focal mesangial proliferation with <50% crescents
III (b)	Diffuse mesangial proliferation with <50% crescents
IV (a)	Focal mesangial proliferation with 50% to 75% crescents
IV (b)	Diffuse mesangial proliferation with50% to 75% crescents
V (a)	Focal mesangial proliferation with > 75% crescents
V (b)	Diffuse mesangial proliferation with > 75% crescents
VI	Membranoproliferative-like glomerulonephritis

CASE 17

History: 50-year-old male, a chronic alcoholic with cirrhosis of the liver for the last 2 years who was managed with diuretic for ascites and underwent variceal banding 6 months back. He started to have worsening pedal edema and ascites with progressively rising serum creatinine over the last 3 weeks. Now BP is 140/90 mm of Hg; earlier, it used to be around 100/60 mm of Hg. No other systemic features to suggest a collagen vascular disease. No hepatic encephalopathy episodes. No history of using NSAIDs. No fever.

Investigation: Urine analysis: blood:3+, protein:2+, dysmorphic RBCs: 35 % on phase contrast microscopy. Serum creatinine is 3.5mg/dl.

Clinical diagnosis: Acute Glomerulonephritis with underlying Liver cirrhosis due to alcoholic liver disease.

Differential diagnoses: IgA Nephropathy/ Membranous nephropathy/MPGN.

Additional investigations: HIV, HBsAg, and HCV–negative. C3 & C4 Normal, ANA Negative.

Light microscopy: Membranoproliferative pattern of Glomerulonephritis (MPGN).

Immunofluorescence: Significant mesangial and some capillary wall and coarse granular immune deposits of IgA and C3c.

Interpretation: Membranoproliferative GN with IgA deposits.

Final diagnosis: IgA nephropathy secondary to liver cirrhosis (Oxford classification: M1 E1 S0 T0-CO).

Pathology Pearls

Table 2:17.1: Differentiation between Primary IgA N & Cirrhosis associated IgA N:

Sr. No.	Features	Primary IgA N	Cirrhosis associated IgA N
1.	Microscopic hematuria	+	-
2.	Light microscopy: most common pattern	Mesangial proliferation	Mesangial proliferation, Rare: MPGN pattern
3.	Crescents	+	+/-(rare)
4.	Immunofluorescence: C3c	+	Often absent
5.	Immunofluorescence: C1q	Often absent/weak	Often +
6.	Electron microscopy study: Electron lucent areas in deposits	-	+: of 50 to 100nm in diameter, not bound by membrane, either isolated or in clusters

Reference:

Heptinstall's Pathology of Kidney, Seventh edition, Chapter 12; IgA Nephropathy and IgA Vasculitis: page no.497.

History: An 8-year-old male presented to his pediatrician with periorbital swelling, gross facial puffiness, and pedal edema for the last 4 days. There is no history of fever or recent vaccination. There is a history of cutaneous infection 3 weeks back. He had a boil over his buttock, which resolved over 10 days. Now, the Urine is high-coloured. There is no history of kidney disease in the family or in any of his siblings. BP: 140/90 mm of Hg.

Investigations: Urine analysis: protein:3+, RBCs: 25 to 30 / HPF, RBC casts: 2-3/HPF, UPCR: 2.6, serum creatinine: 1.2 mg/dl.

Clinical diagnosis: Nephritic Syndrome

Differential diagnoses: Infection related GN/ IgA N/ MPGN.

Light microscopy:

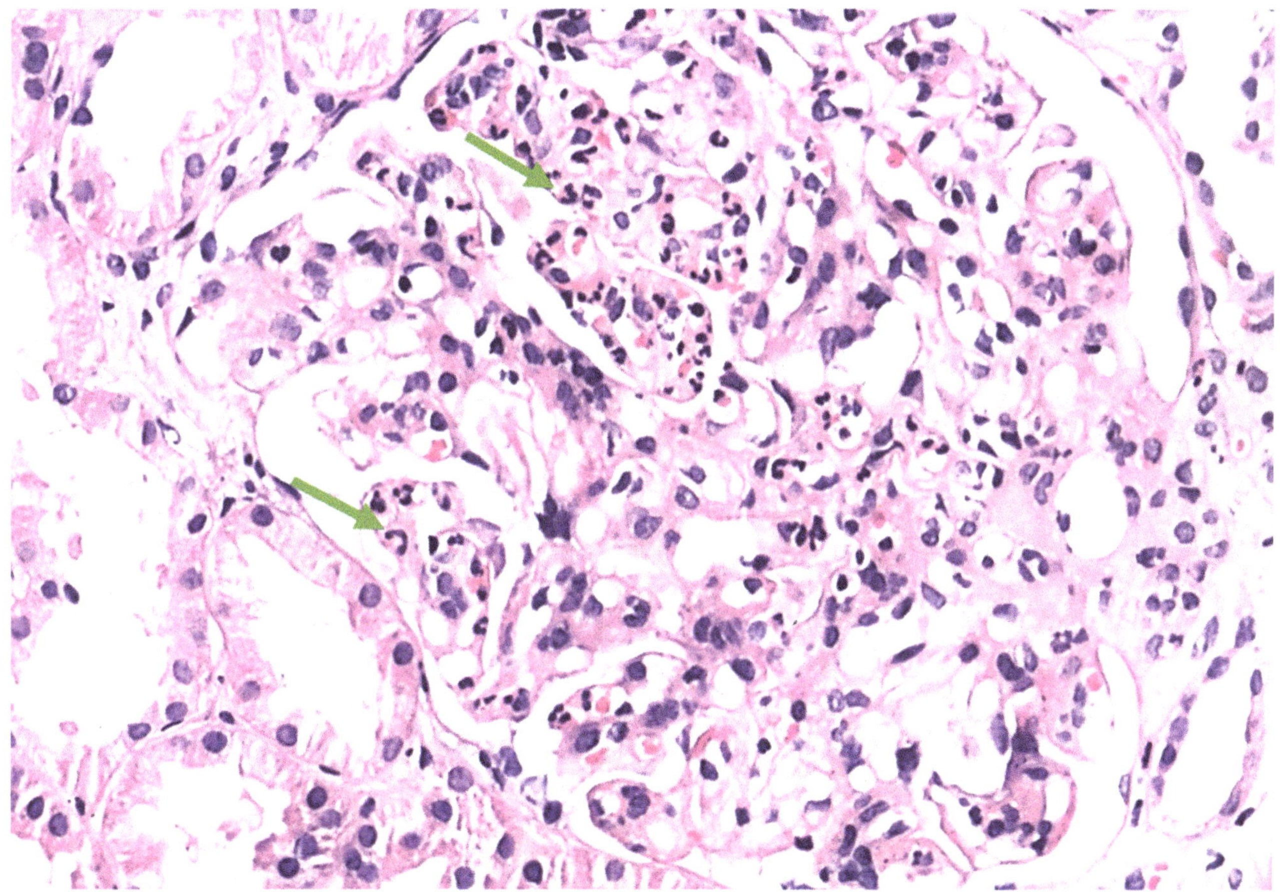

Figure 2:18.1: H&E Stain 20x: Enlarged and hypercellular glomeruli with diffuse endocapillary hypercellularity obliterating the capillary lumina with neutrophils (green arrow).

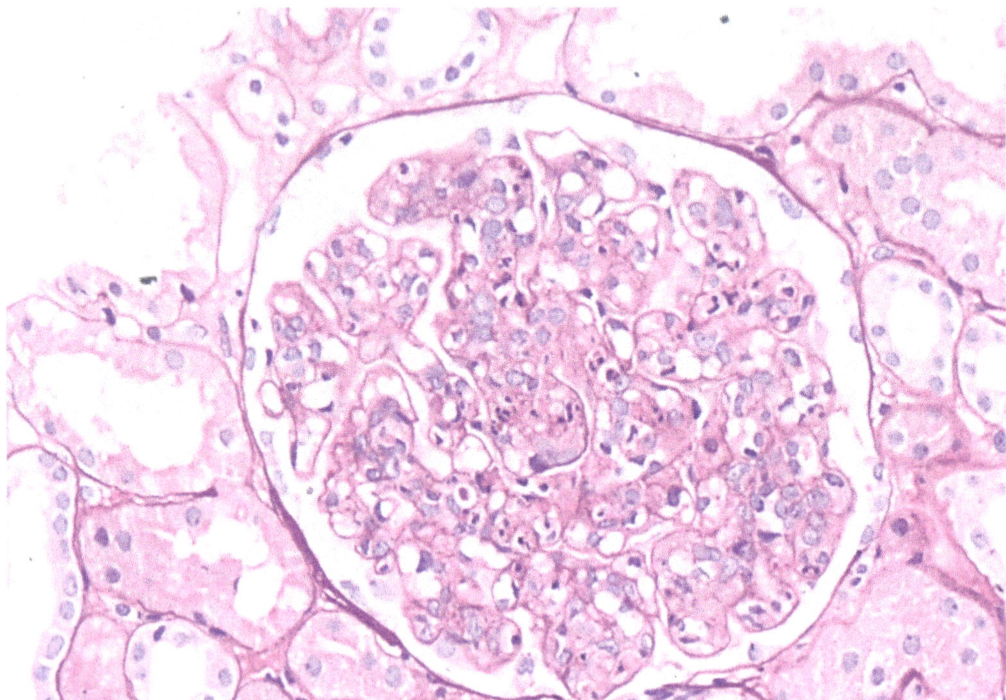

Figure 2:18.2: PAS Stain 20x: Diffuse endocapillary hypercellularity with no evidence of basement membrane thickening/duplication/segmental lesions/crescents.

Immunofluorescence:

Significant diffuse capillary wall and mesangial coarse granular immune deposits of IgG and C3c.

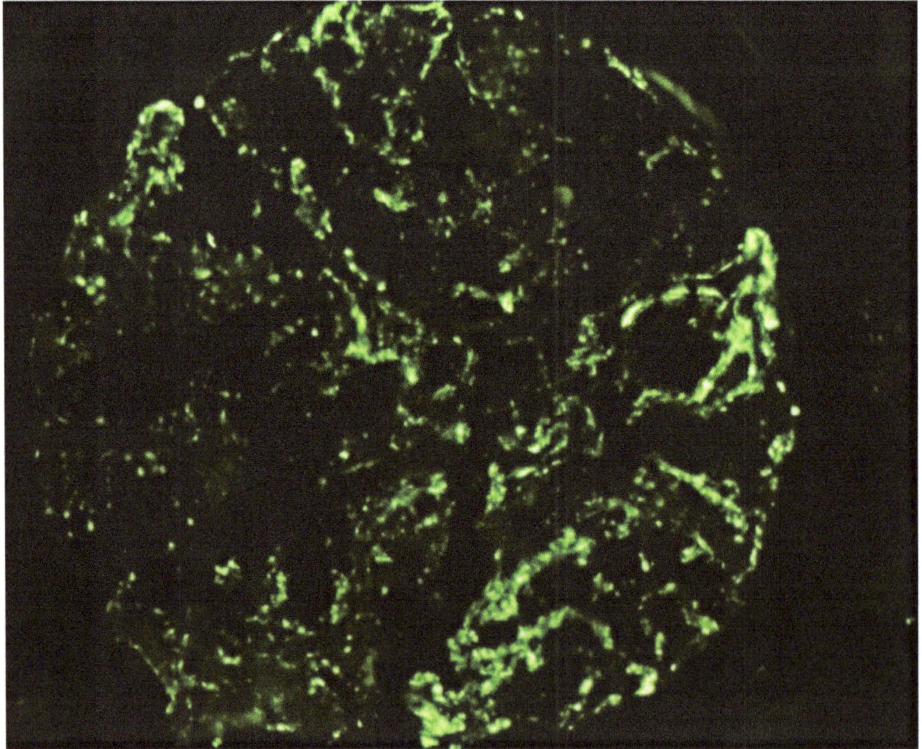

Figure 2:18.3: Immunofluorescence C3c: 20x: Glomerulus with significant capillary wall and mesangial coarse granular, lumpy-bumpy immune deposits (starry sky appearance).

Additional investigations: C3 is low, C4 is normal, ANA: negative, ASO: elevated.

Electron microscopy: Subepithelial electron dense humps

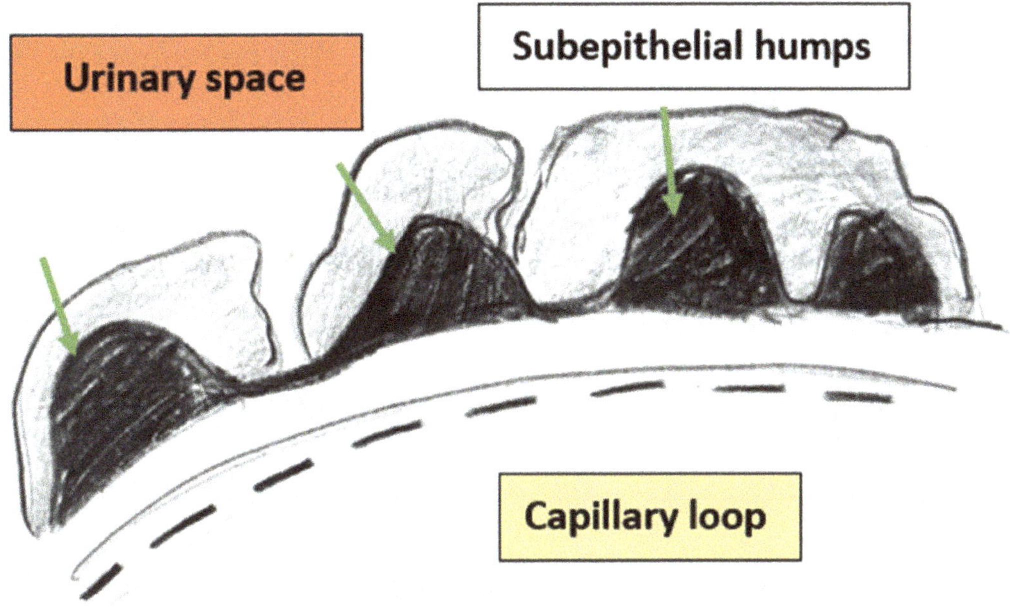

Figure 2:18.4: Diagrammatic representation of Electron microscopy: IRGN.

Final diagnosis: Infection related GN (Post infectious glomerulonephritis: PIGN)

CASE 19

History: 40-year male, non-diabetic, non-hypertensive, nonsmoker, and non-alcoholic, with no significant past medical history, presented with frothyuria, pedal edema, and hypertension for the last month. There is a history of upper respiratory tract infection 2 weeks prior to the onset of these symptoms. No systemic features of secondary glomerulonephritis. No family history of renal disease.

B.P.: 180/90 mm of Hg.

Investigations: Serum creatinine: 2.1mg/dl, Urine analysis: Protein: 3+, RBCs: 8-10/HPF, Urine PCR: 9.03 g/g, ASO titre: elevated. Serum Cholesterol 260 mg/dl, LDL: 190 mg/dl, Triglycerides: 300mg/dl, HDL: 38mg/dl. Serum Albumin: 2.9 g/dl

Clinical diagnosis: Nephrotic syndrome with active urinary sediment with hypertension and renal dysfunction.

Differential diagnoses: Infection related GN/ IgA N/MPGN.

Light microscopy:

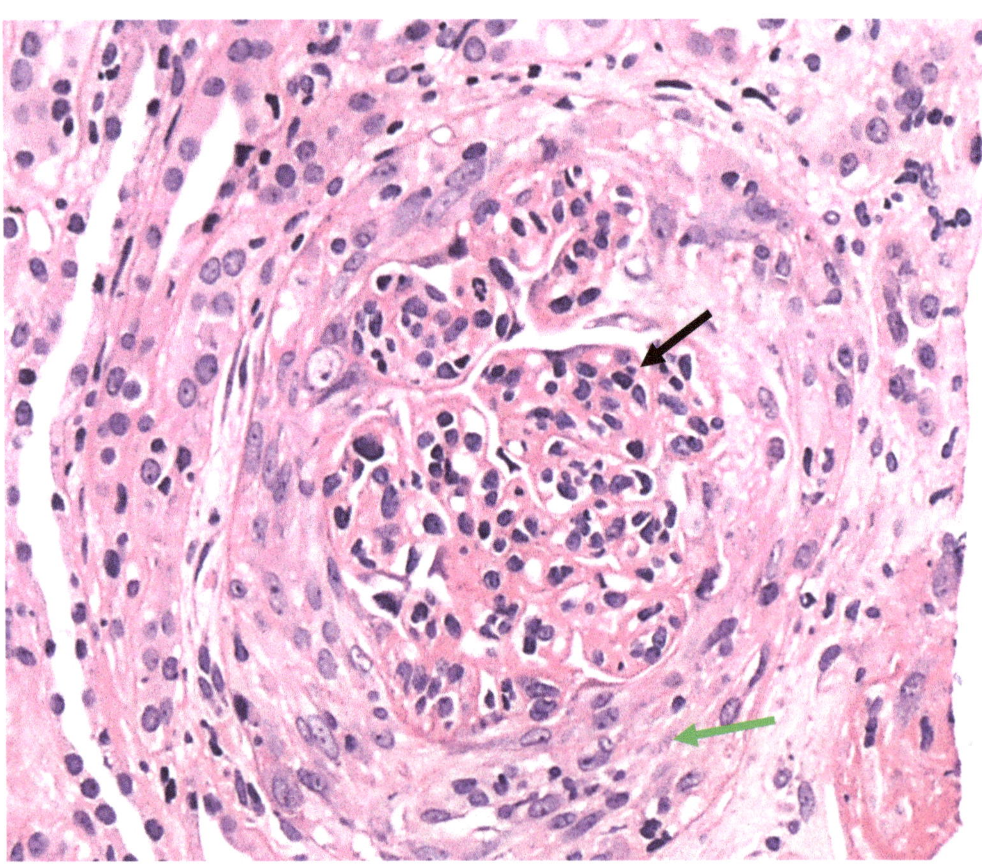

Figure 2:19.1: H&E Stain:20x: Hypercellular glomerulus with diffuse mesangial and endocapillary hypercellularity obliterating the capillary lumina with ocasniol neutrophils (**black** arrow) a circumferential cellular crescent (**green** arrow).

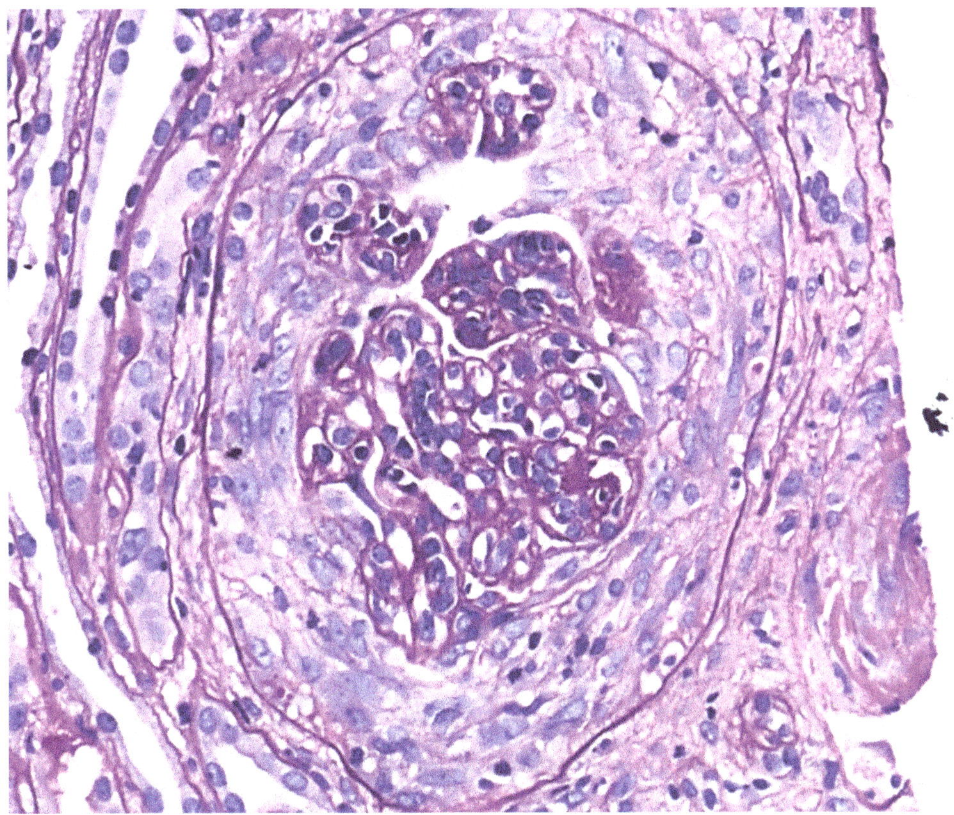

Figure 2:19.2: PAS Stain: 20x: Circumferential cellular crescent.

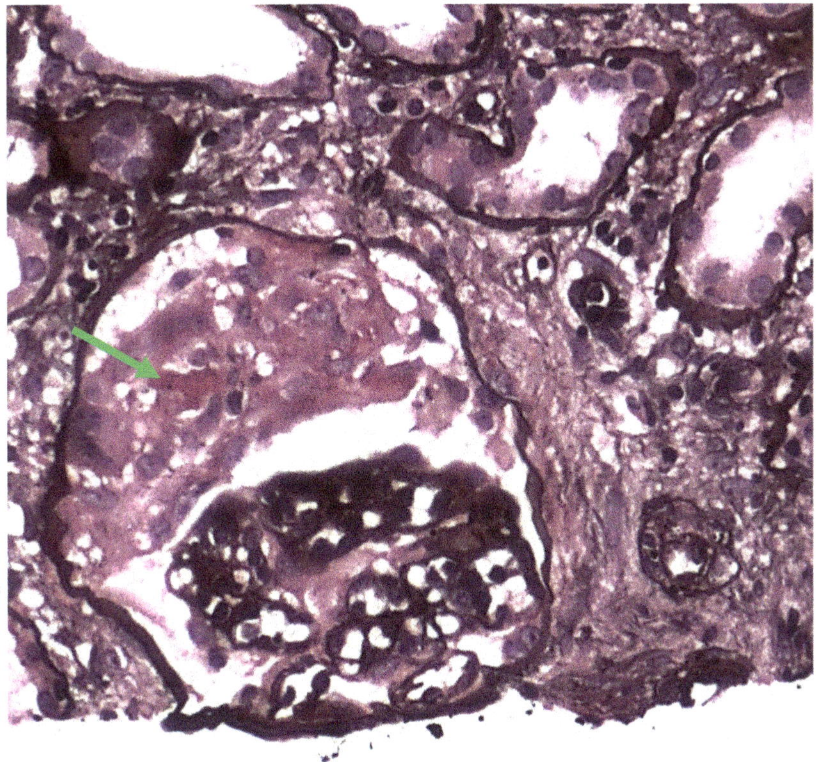

Figure 2:19.3: PASM Stain: 20x: Fibrin strands interspersed with cells of cellular crescent.

Immunofluorescence:

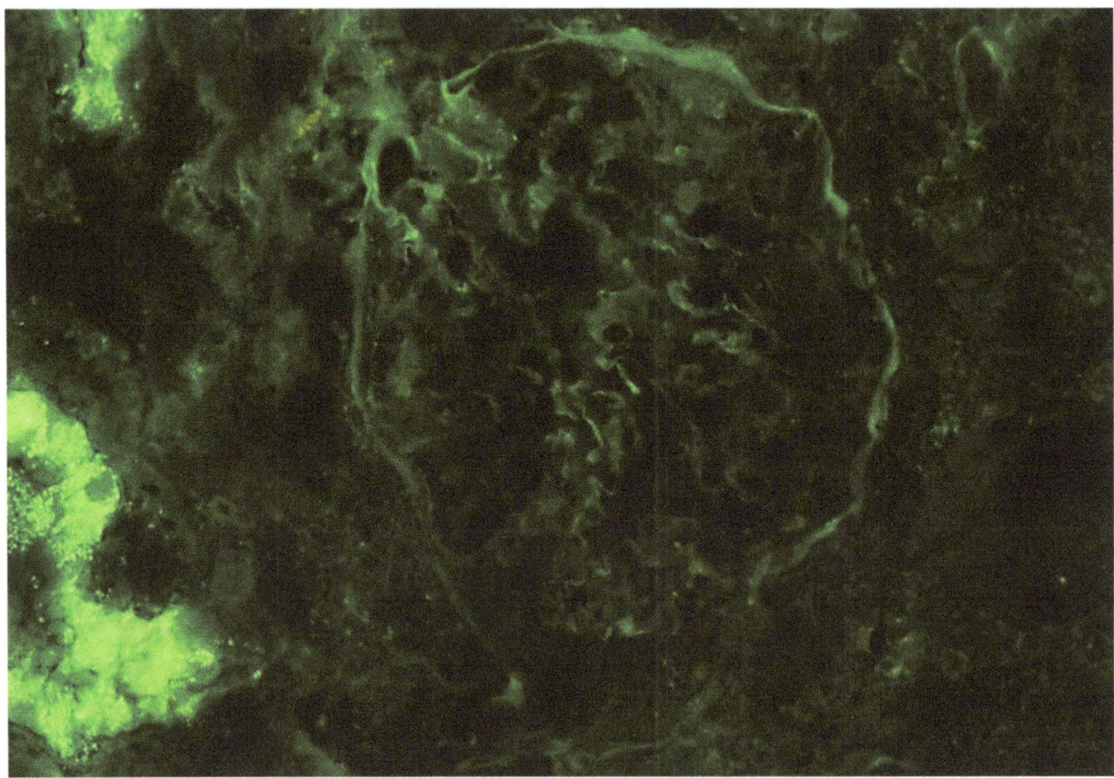

Figure 2:19.4: Immunofluorescence: 20x: IgG: negative

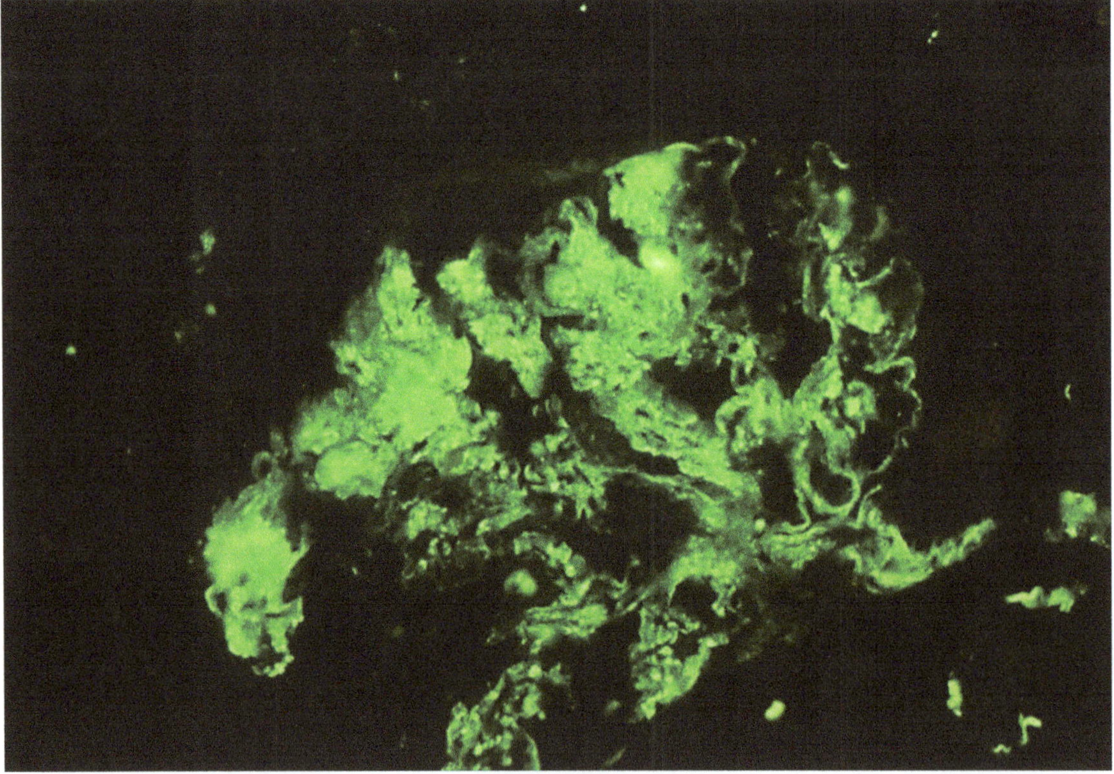

Figure 2:19.5: Immunofluorescence 20x: C3c: Significant capillary wall and mesangial coarse granular deposits

Electron Microscopic findings: Subendothelial and Mesangial electron dense deposits seen. No intramembranous sausage like osmiophilic deposits characteristic of DDD are seen. No subepithelial humps are seen.

Final diagnosis: C3 glomerulonephritis

Pattern of injury: Crescentic, diffuse proliferative.

Table 2:19.1: Additional evaluation in the above case.

Test	Result	Comment
C3	Low	Suggests: Alternate complement pathway unregulated activation
C4	Normal	
ANA	Negative	
Serum Immunofixation electrophoresis/ FLC ratio	Normal	A paraprotein/Light chain can trigger alternate complement pathway activation.
Factor H	Low	Genetic mutation or autoantibody can cause deficiency of this regulator of alternate complement pathway.
Factor B, I, MCP	Normal	Genetic mutation or autoantibody can cause deficiency of these regulators of alternate complement pathway.
C3 Nephritic factor (C3Nef)	Normal	It's an autoantibody that stabilizes the C3 convertase (C3bBb). Seen in 80% of DDD and 40% of C3GN cases
C5 Nephritic factor(C5Nef)	Normal	It's an autoantibody that stabilizes the C3 convertase ([C3b]2Bb) in the presence of properdin. It is commonly seen in C3GN.
C4NeFs	Normal	autoantibodies that stabilize the classical and lectin pathway C3 convertase. Rare seen with C3GN
Anti factor H antibody	Elevated	Suggests an auto immune aetiology,
Antibody for factor B, C3b	Normal	These also can be the cause, although less common.
Test	Result	Comment
Genetic testing for mutations: Clinical exom sequencing / Whole exom sequencing	Genes encoding factor H, factor I, C3, and complement factor H-related (CFHR) proteins (CFHR1-5) : normal	Seen in approximately20% cases with C3GN.

Final Diagnosis in this case: Crescentic C3GN – Due to Factor H auto antibody.

Pathology Pearls

Dense Deposit Disease: On Immunofluorescence: Mesangial ring pattern can be seen with capillary wall deposits of C3c.

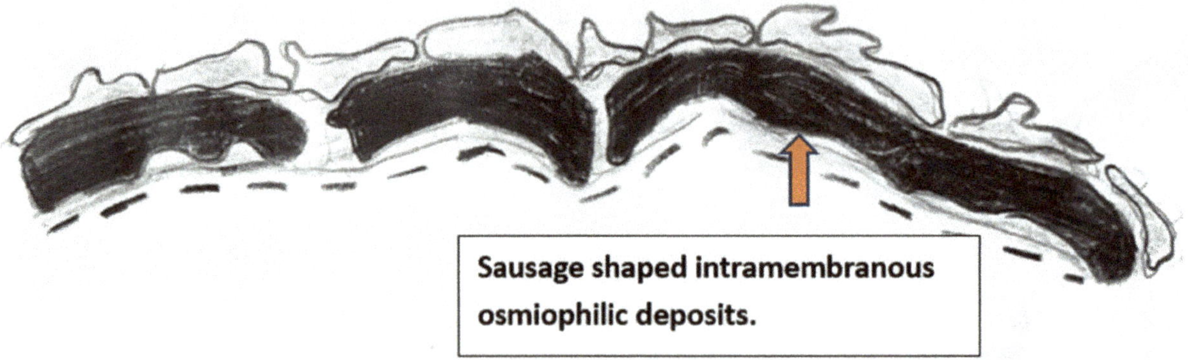

Figure 2:19.6: Diagrammatic representation of EM: DDD.

Table 2:19.2: Distinction: DDD & C3GN.

Features	Post streptococcal GN (PSGN),	Staphylococcus associated GN	DDD	C3GN
Persistent / recurring course of GN	-	-	++	++
Low C3	Transient	Transient	Persistent	Persistent
Immunofluorescence	IgG & C3c	IgG & C3c	Only C3c: mesangial ring pattern	Only C3c
Electron microscopy	Subepithelial humps	Subepithelial humps	Sausage shaped intramembranous osmiophilic deposits.	Mesangial, subendothelial & occasional subepithelial electron dense deposits.

CASE 20

History: 56-year-old male, diabetic for 15 years, hypertensive, non-smoker, presented with progressive edema feet and decreasing urine output along with shortness of breath on exertion for the last 1 week. There is a history of diabetic foot ulcer infection 1 month back, which is now better. He has no fever or active infection at present. BP is 170/100. He has diminished sensations in both feet for the last 1 year. He has diabetic retinopathy-related treatment done in both eyes. No h/o NSAIDs/indigenous medicine use. No vascular procedure in recent times. No lower tract urinary complaints. No systemic features to suggest collagen vascular disease.

Investigations: urine analysis: protein:4+, RBCs: 8-10/HPF, RBC casts: 3-4, UPCR: 6 g/g. serum creatinine is 6 mg/dl. Previous Serum creatinine 6 months back was 1.5mg/dl, USG KUB: Normal size prostate and no post void residue, no Hydroureteronephrosis.

Clinical Diagnosis: AKI with Nephrotic range proteinuria.

Differential diagnoses: Diabetic nephropathy with atherosclerotic renal artery stenosis / Post infectious GN.

Light microscopy:

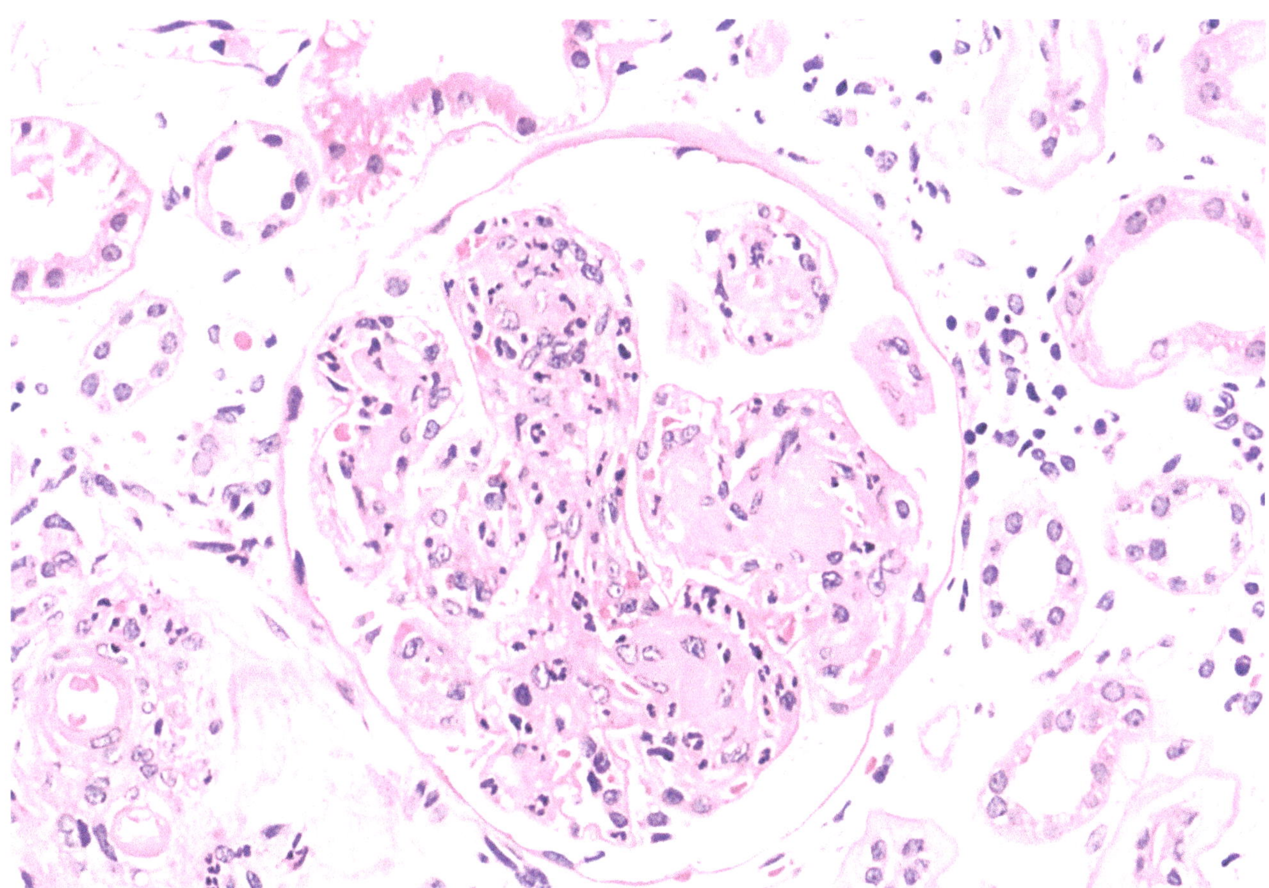

Figure 2:20.1: H&E Stain: 20x: Diffuse proliferative and exudative GN with diabetic nephropathy.

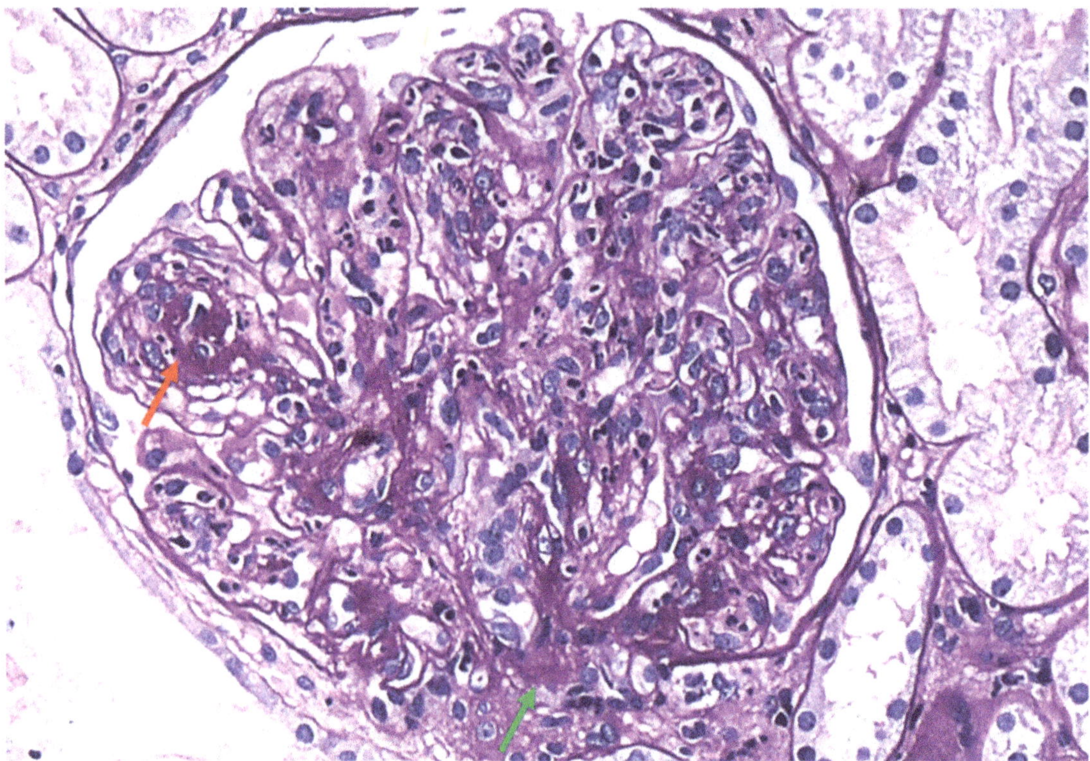

Figure 2:20.2: PAS stain:20x: The glomerulus with prominent PAS positive mesangial widening focally exceeding the diameter of adjacent capillary lumina and forming Kimmelstiel-Wilson (KW) nodule (Red arrow), Arteriolar hyalinosis (green arrow).

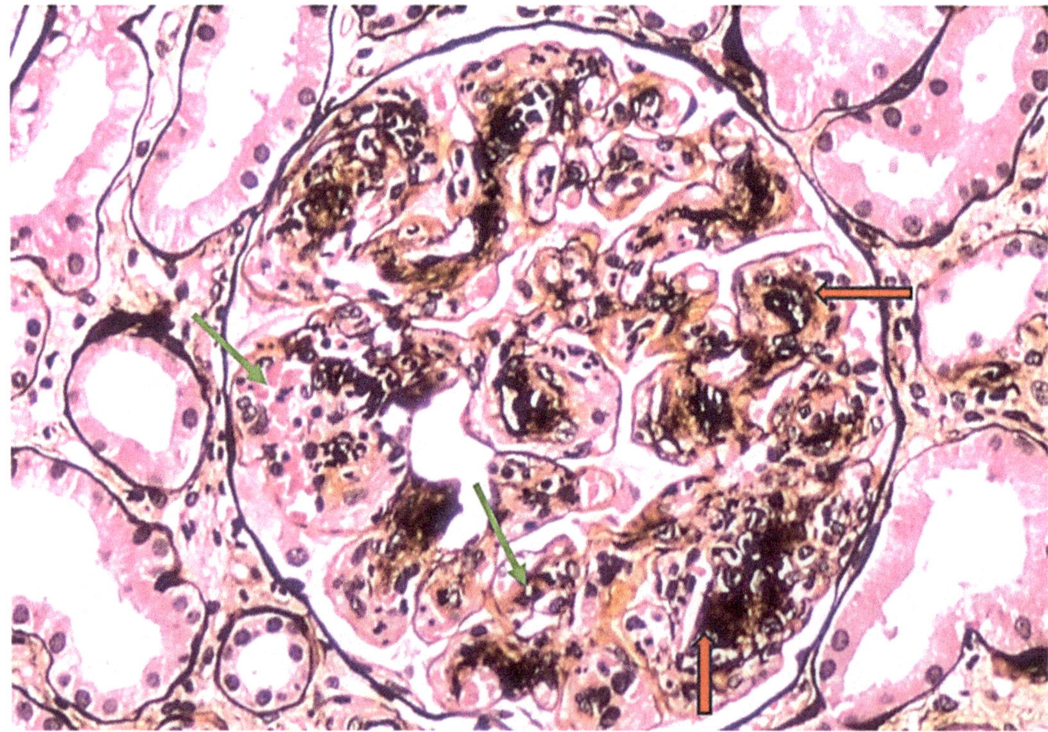

Figure 2:20.3: PASM stain: 20x: Hypercellular glomerulus: Diffuse endocapillary hypercellularity with neutrophilic infiltrate (green arrows) Silver-positive mesangial widening with (KW) nodules (red arrows). There is no evidence of basement membrane duplication/segmental lesions/crescents.

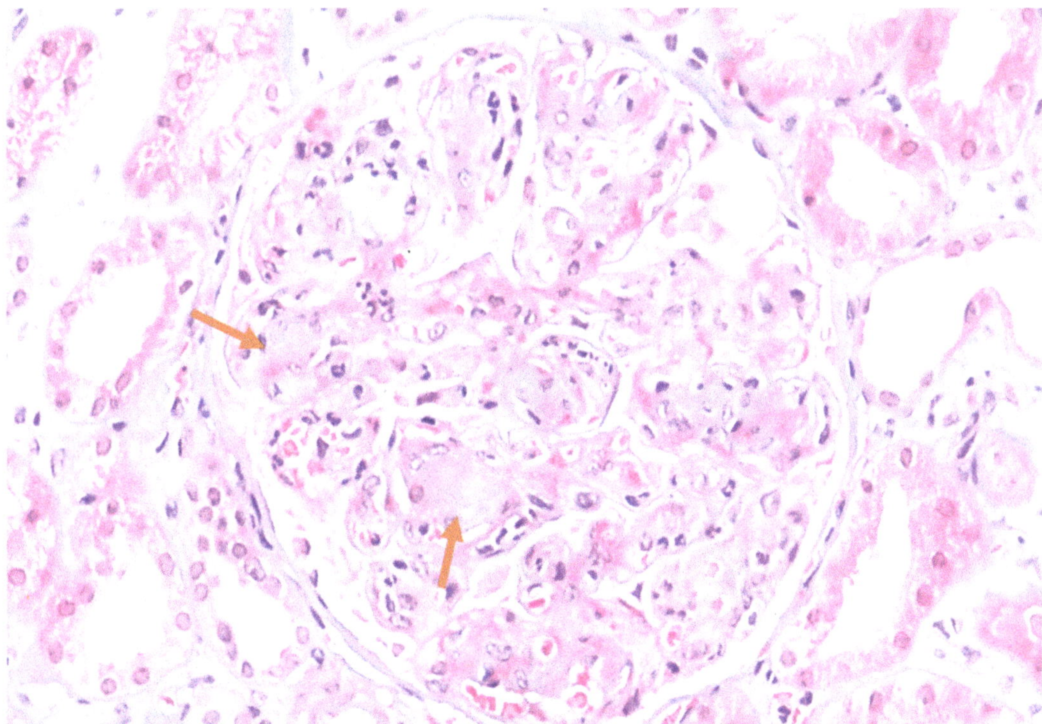

Figure 2:20.4: MT stain:20x: Hypercellular glomerulus and KW nodules (orange arrows).

Immunofluorescence:

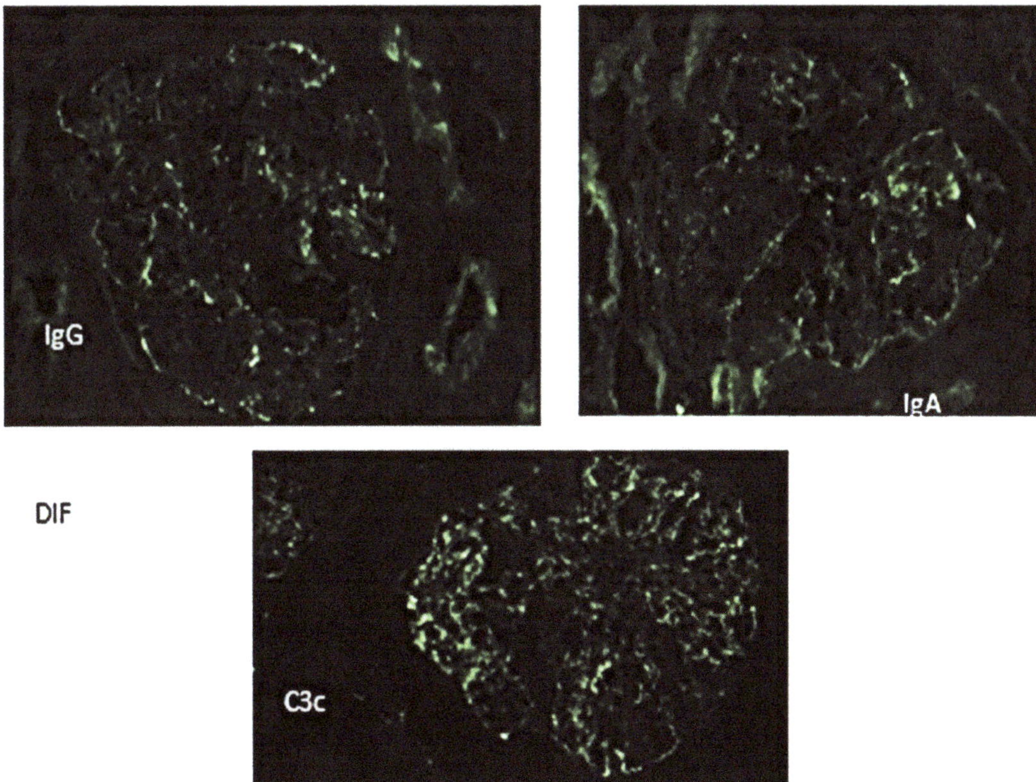

Figure 2:20.5: Immunofluorescence: Diffuse capillary wall and mesangial coarse granular immune deposits significant IgG and C3c and minimal IgA.

Interpretation: Diffuse proliferative glomerulonephritis with diabetic nephropathy and IgA co deposition in capillary loops.

Additional investigations: Viral screen is negative, C3 low, C4 normal, ANA: Negative, ANCA: Negative. SPEP: Negative.

Final diagnosis: IgA codominant PIGN, commonly associated with Staphylococcal infection-related glomerulonephritis. There are background changes of Nodular diabetic Nephropathy.

CASE 21

History: 60 years old female, presented with rapidly progressing renal failure with decreased urine output, shortness of breath & hypertension. Her BP is 176/100 mm of Hg. She has been diabetic for 5 years but well-controlled. She has no systemic features of connective tissue disorder. No history to suggest any active infection. She had chest pain a month back, for which she had undergone a coronary angiogram, which turned out to be normal. She has no skin lesions or arthritis. No redness of eyes.

Investigations: Serum Creatinine: 7 mg/dl, Urine analysis: Protein: 3+, RBCs: plenty/HPF, RBC Casts: 4-5 /HPF, Urine protein to creatinine ratio: 5 g/g. Viral markers: negative.

Clinical diagnosis: Rapidly progressive glomerulonephritis.

Differential diagnoses: Immune-complex mediated GN/pauci-immune GN/atheroembolic disease.

Light microscopy:

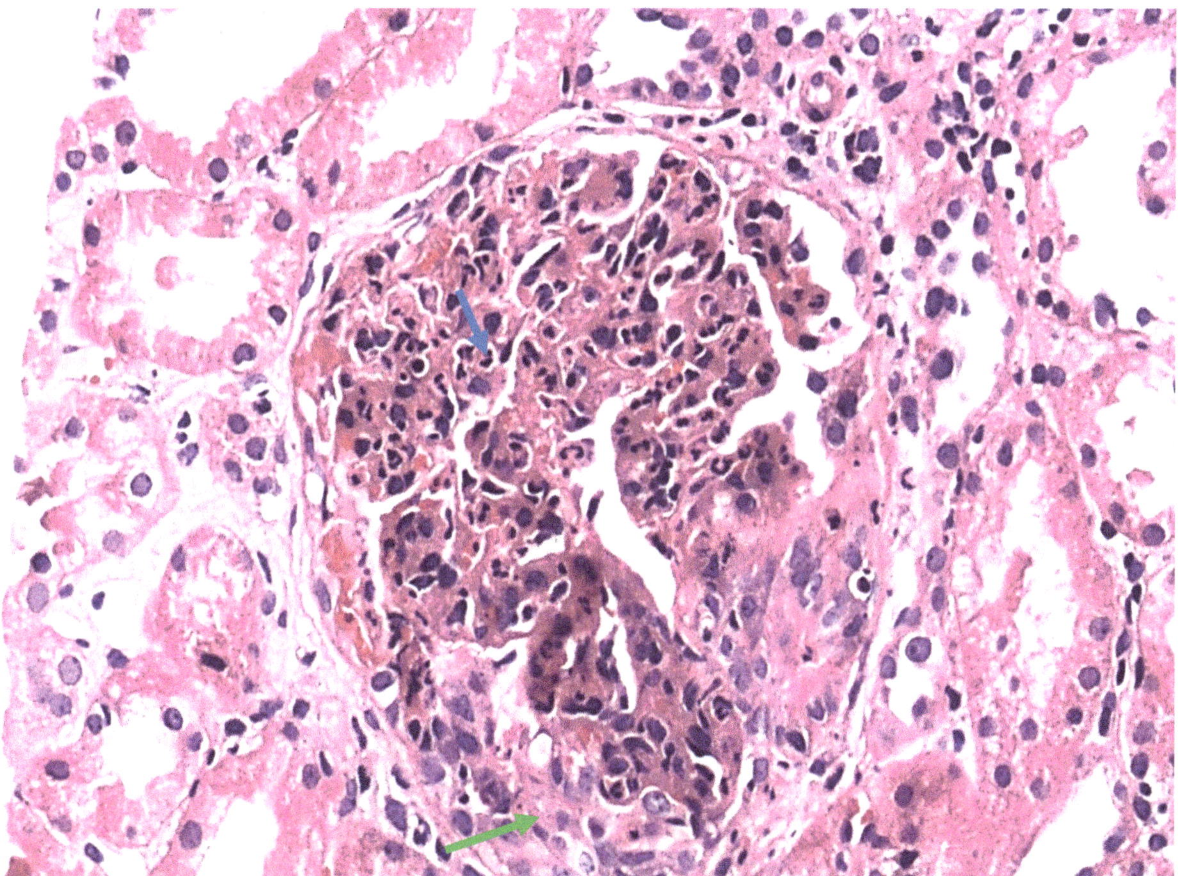

Figure 2:21.1: H&E Stain: Diffuse proliferative and exudative glomerulonephritis with neutrophilic infiltrate (blue arrow) and segmental cellular crescent (green arrow).

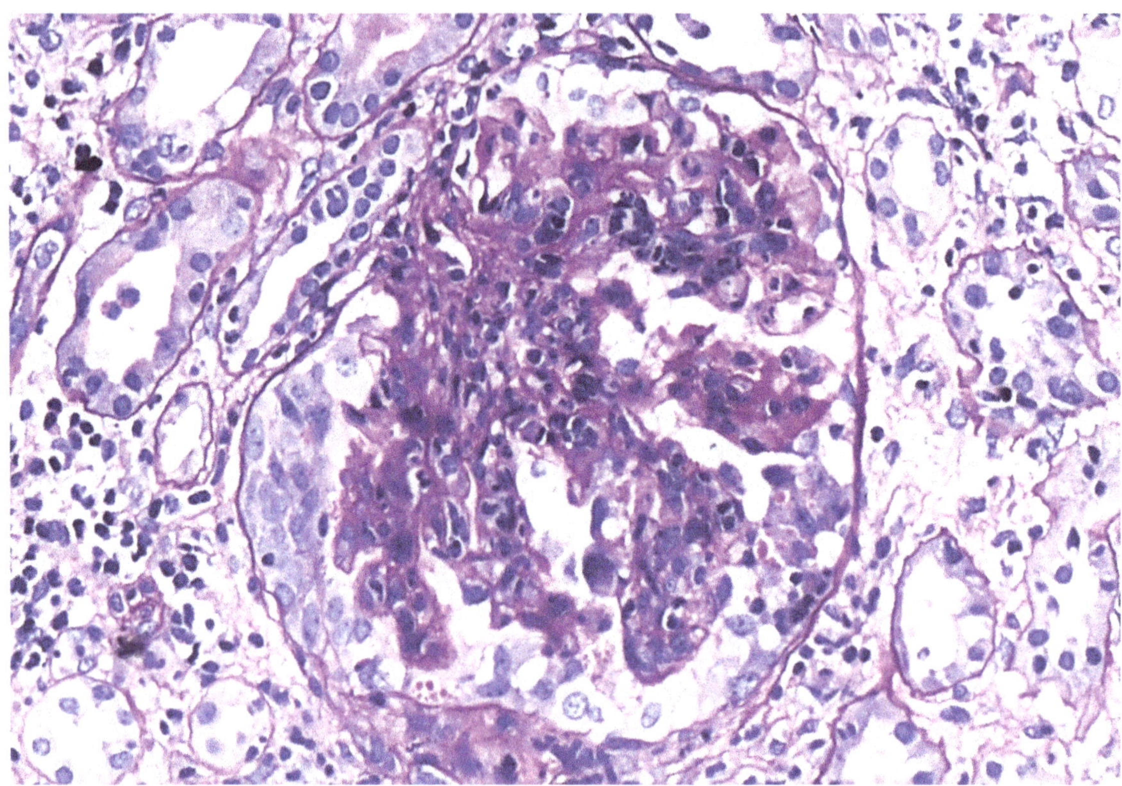

Figure 2:21.2: PAS Stain: 20x: Endocapillary hypercellularity with segmental cellular crescent.

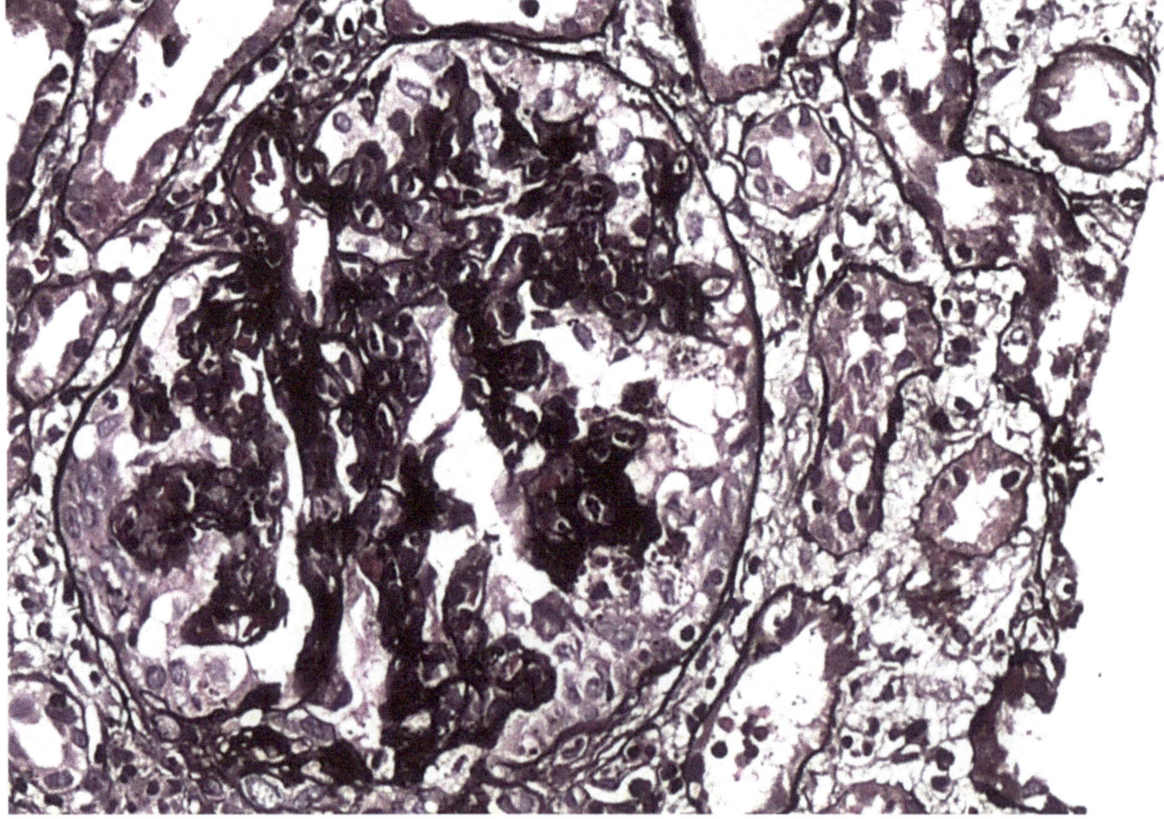

Figure 2:21.3: PASM Stain: 20x: Endocapillary hypercellularity with segmental cellular crescent.

Immunofluorescence:

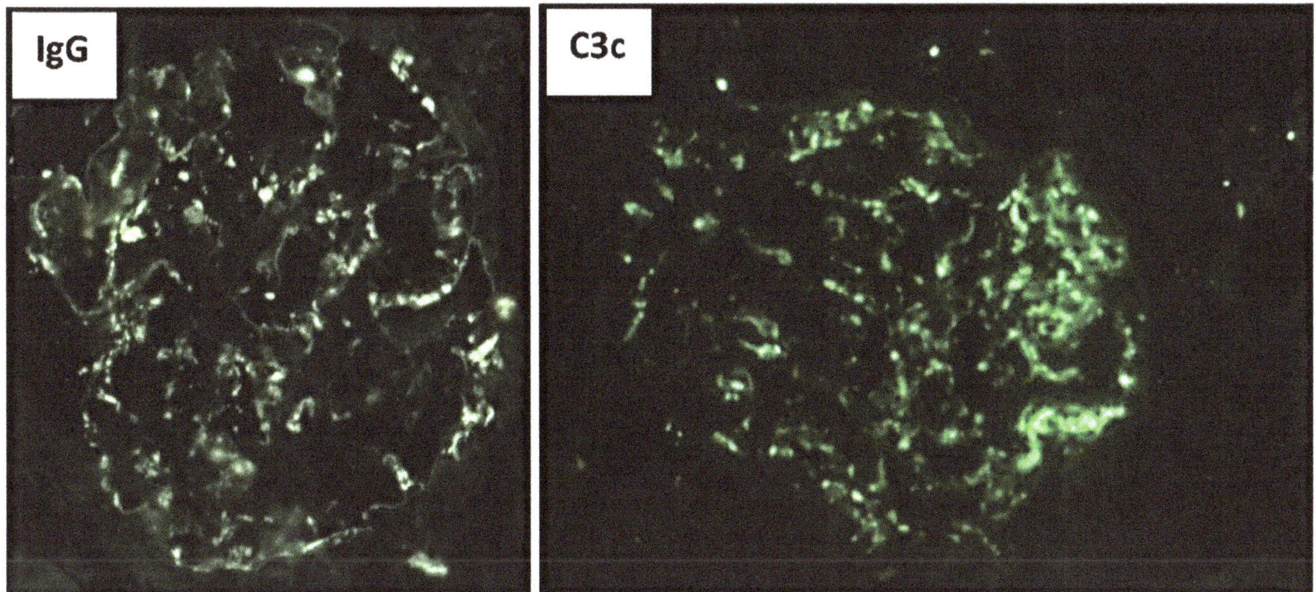

Figure 2:21.4: **(a)** Capillary wall and mesangial coarse granular immune deposits of IgG.
(b) Capillary wall and mesangial coarse granular immune deposits of C3c.

Interpretation: An Immune complex mediated diffuse proliferative and exudative GN with crescents.

Supportive investigations:

C3 is low, C4 is normal, ANA is negative, C-ANCA is positive, P-ANCA is Negative, and the anti-GBM antibody is Negative. 2D-ECHO revealed vegetations on the tricuspid valve, and a blood culture sent before pulse steroids came out positive for staphylococcus aureus.

Note: Sub acute Bacterial endocarditis can sometimes be so innocuous that it gets picked retrospectively after searching for source of infection in cases of Infection related GN.

Final Diagnosis: An Immune complex mediated diffuse proliferative and exudative GN with crescents secondary to sub-acute bacterial endocarditis due to staphylococcus aureus, possibly due to the vascular intervention a month back.

CASE 22

History: 61 years male, diabetic for 10 years and Hypertensive for 3 years. He has long-standing sub-optimal glycaemic control and chronic kidney disease diagnosed a year back. He now presented with progressive worsening anasarca. He has no lower urinary tract symptoms. No preceding infection. No history of any vascular intervention. No history of NSAIDS or any indigenous medicine use. No systemic symptoms to suggest a secondary GN other than diabetic nephropathy. BP: 170/90 mm Hg.

Previous baseline investigations: Diabetic retinopathy is present. Six months back, the serum creatinine was 1.5, and the UPCR was 1.2 g/g. The HBA1c was 8. The viral markers for HIV, HBV, and HCV were negative.

Current investigations: UPCR of 8 g/g, Serum creatinine: 4 mg/dl, Urine analysis: Protein:4+, RBCs: 3-4/HPF, No casts. Renal artery doppler: Normal.

Clinical Diagnosis: Chronic Kidney disease, most likely diabetic nephropathy with unusually rapid worsening to rule out superadded non-diabetic renal disease.

Differential diagnoses: Diabetic nephropathy with renal artery stenosis /associated paraproteinemia/ Infection related GN.

Light microscopy:

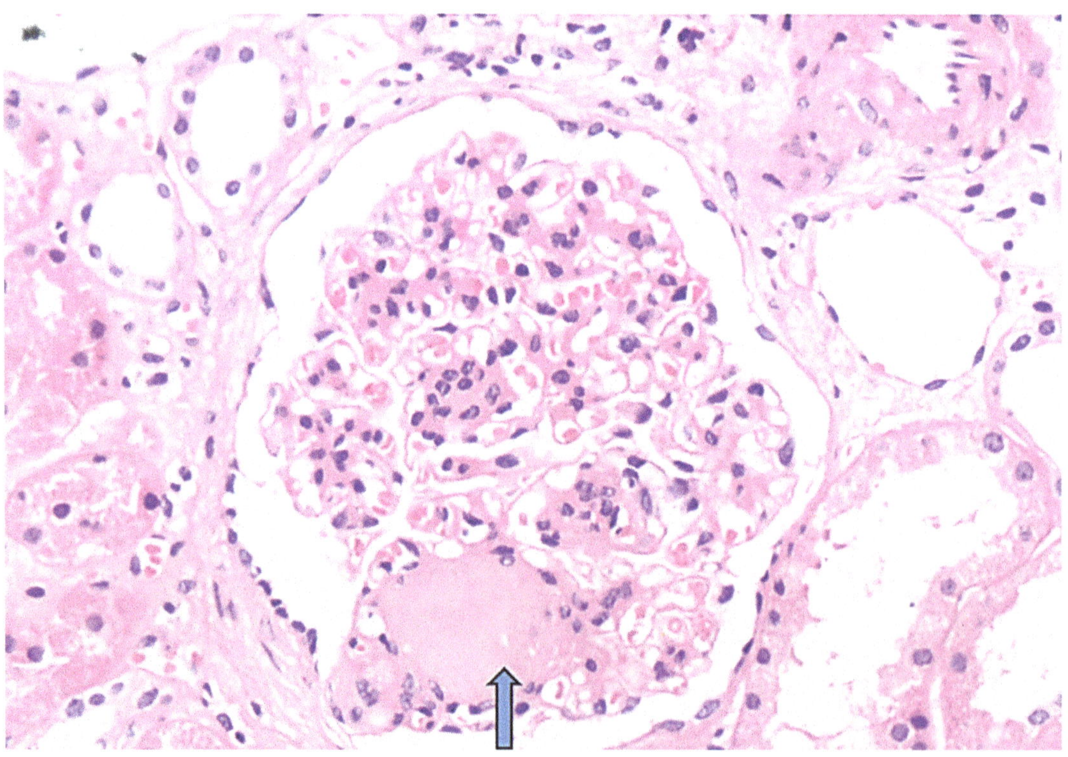

Figure 2:22.1: H&E Stain: 20x: Glomerulus: KW (Kimmelstiel-Wilson) lesion

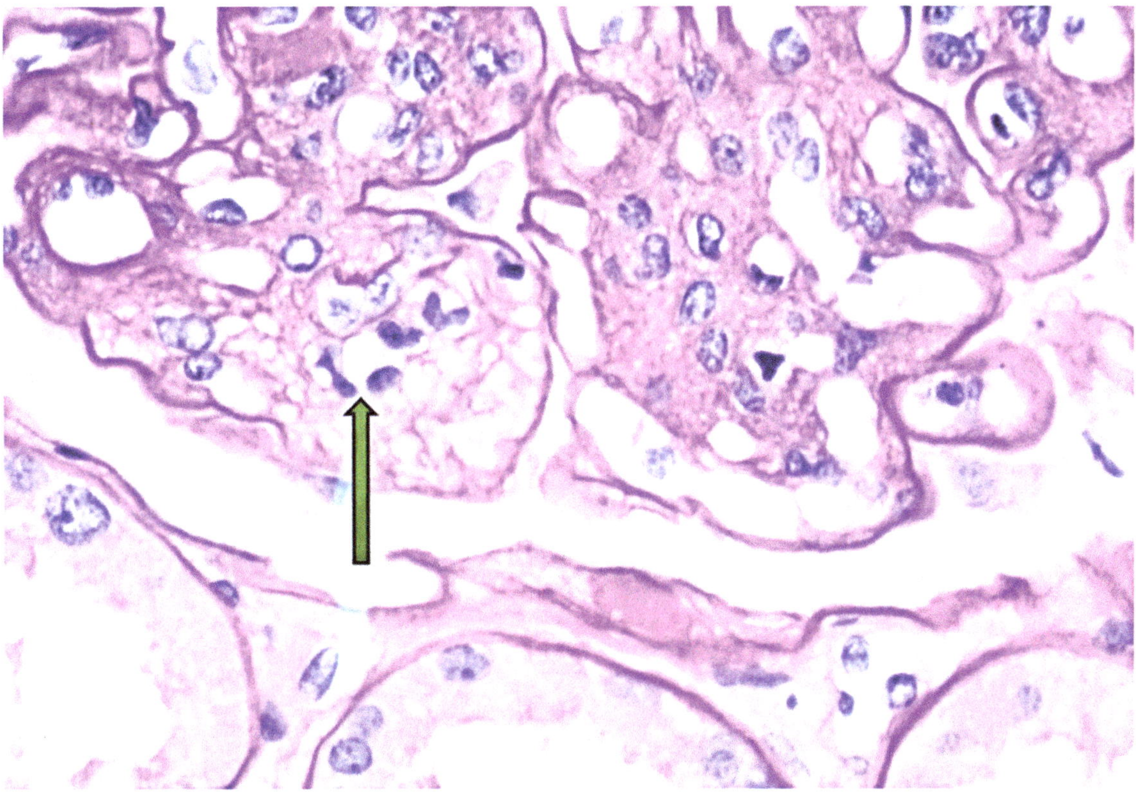

Figure 2:22.2: PAS Stain: 40x: Glomerulus: Microaneurysm: Cystic dilatation of capillary containing blood elements. It precedes the development of KW lesions.

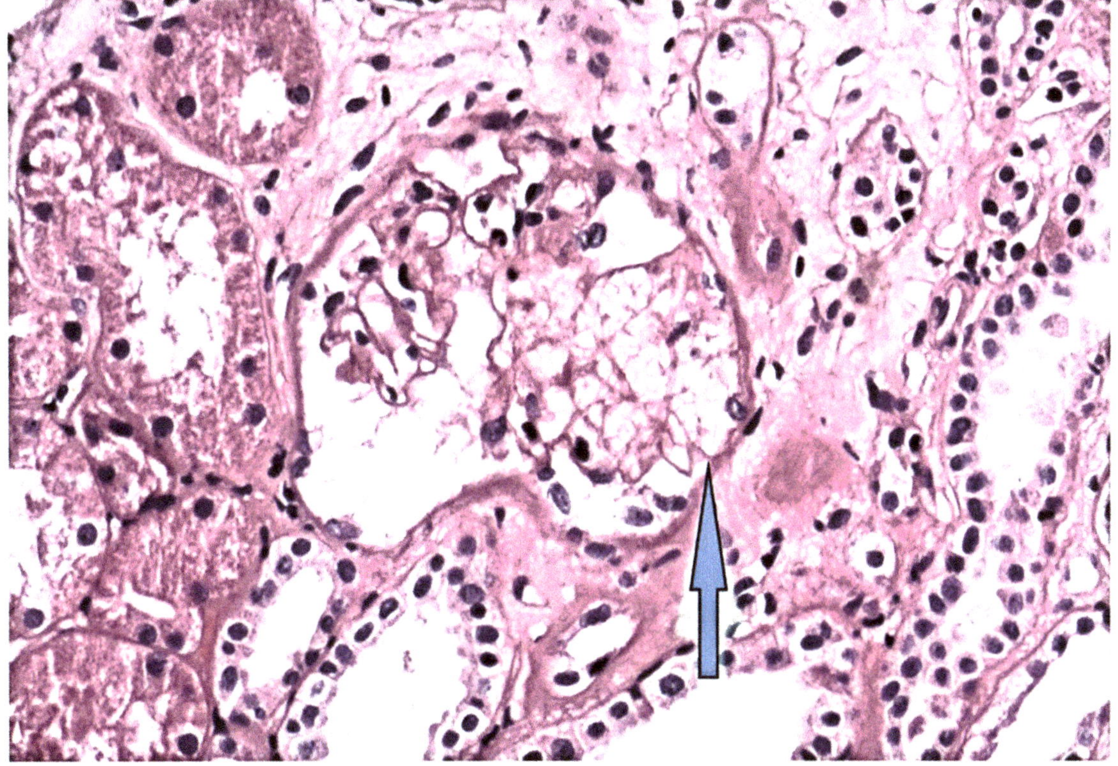

Figure 2:22.3: H&E Stain: 20x: Glomerulus: Segmental mesangiolysis with the fibrillary appearance of mesangium.

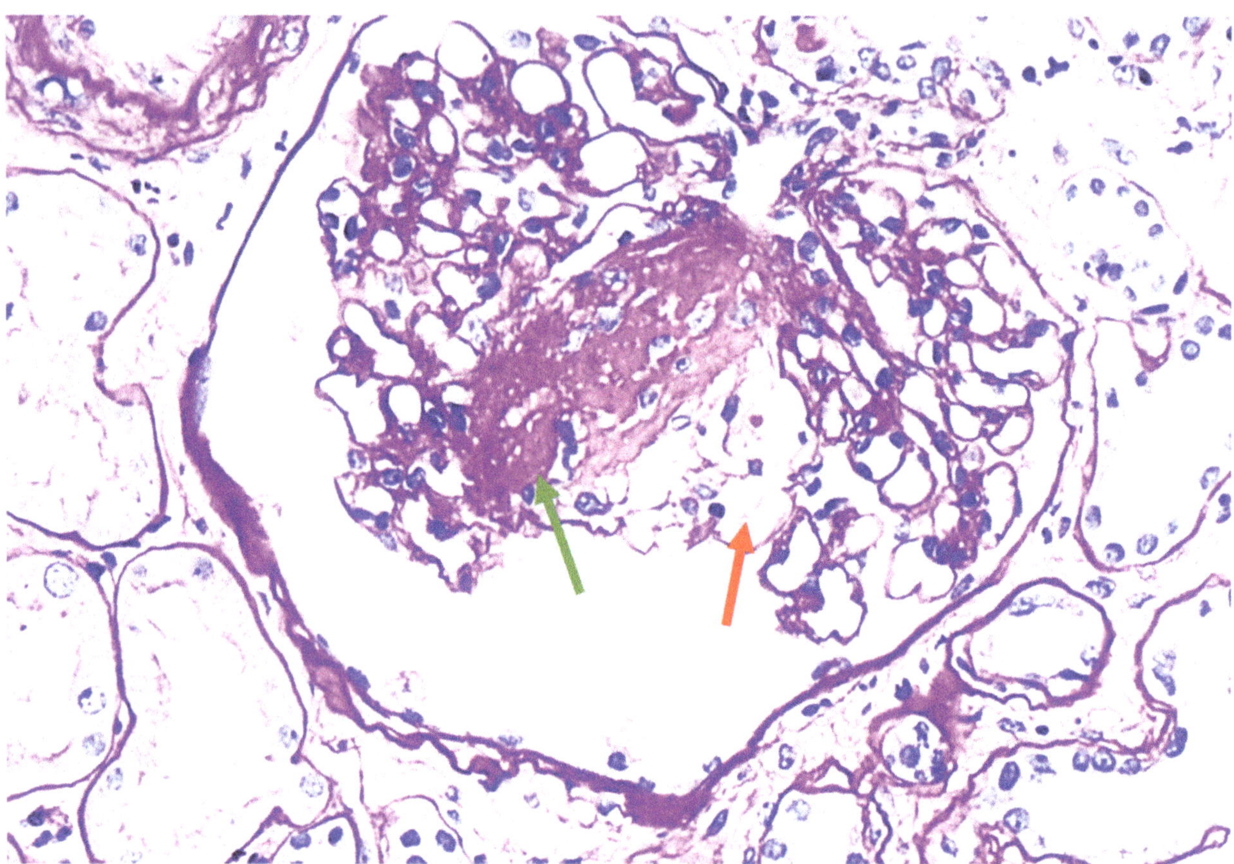

Figure 2:22.4: PAS Stain:20x: The same glomerulus shows prominent PAS-positive mesangial widening focally exceeding the diameter of adjacent capillary lumina and segmental fibrillar appearance of mesangium (mesangiolysis-shown by red arrow) forming a large Kimmelstiel-Wilson (KW) nodule* and mild thickening of basement membranes.

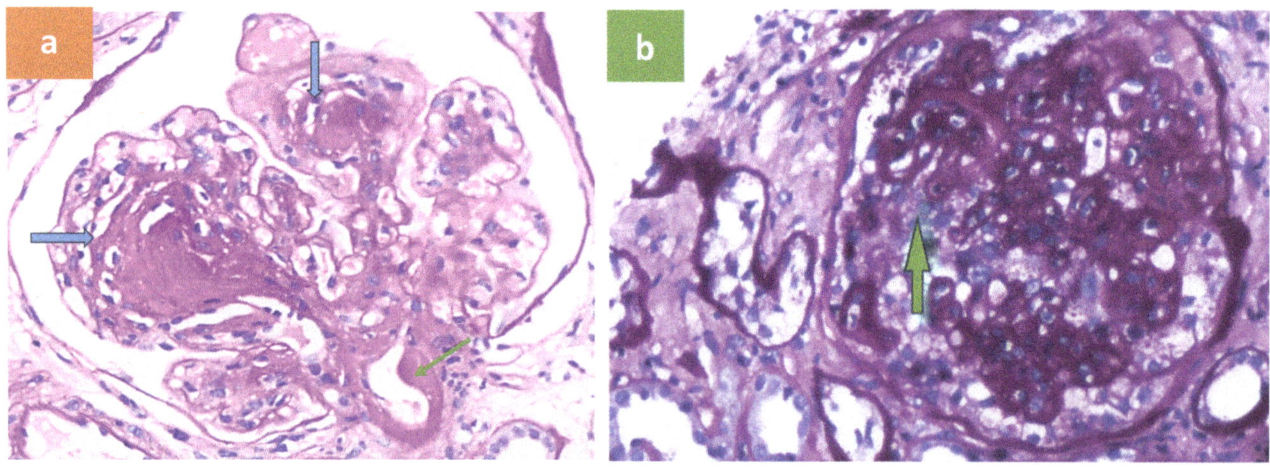

Figure 2:22.5: (a) PAS Stain: 20x: Glomerulus with KW nodules of uneven sizes (blue arrows) and hilar (afferent) arteriolar hyalinosis (green arrow).
(b) PAS Stain: Glomerulus: 20x: Segmental collapse of the tuft with hypertrophy and hyperplasia of overlying podocytes with the presence of protein resorption droplets. *Reference: Collapsing glomerulopathy in diabetic nephropathy with advanced vascular hyalinosis is presumably due to ischemic podocyte injury and is of prognostic significance. Salvatore SP et al. Nephrol Dial Transplant. 2014 Feb;29(2):392-399.

Immunofluorescence:

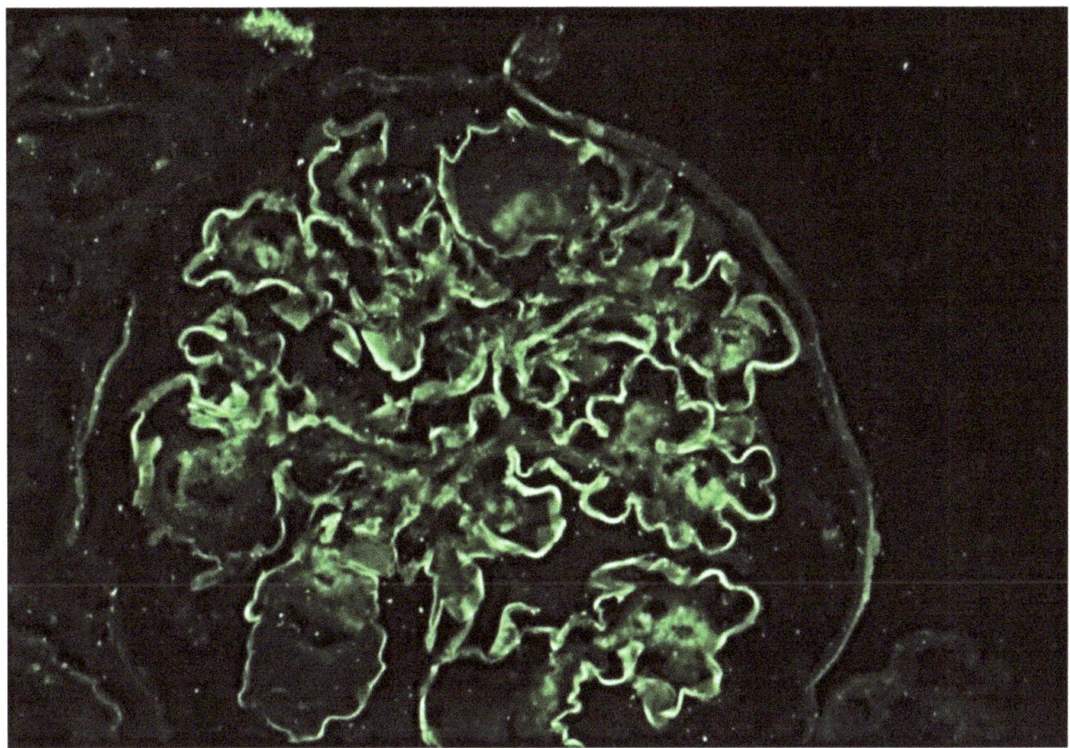

Figure 2:22.6: IF: IgG: 20x: Glomerulus: Minimal pseudo linear capillary wall deposits.

Interpretation: Nodular Diabetic Nephropathy with Collapsing Glomerulopathy, moderate IF/TA (40%), arteriolar hyalinosis, and arteriosclerosis.

Glomeruli: class III

IF/TA: 2/3

Interstitial inflammation: 1/2

Arteriolar hyalinosis: 2/2

Arteriosclerosis: 1/2

Additional investigations:

1. ANA: negative, ANCA: negative, serum immunofixation electrophoresis: negative
2. Viral screening: CMV, EBV Parvovirus B-19: Negative
3. Peipheral smear: normal with no hematologic abnormalities.

Electron microscopy:

Diffuse thickening of GBM

Absence of any electron dense deposits.

Final diagnosis: Diabetic Nephropathy with Collapsing Glomerulopathy

***Suggested reading:**

Table 2:22.1: Glomerular pathologic classification in DN.

Class	Criteria
I	GBM thickening: under EM: >395nm in females & >430nm in males in >9years of age
II(a)	Mild mesangial expansion *(smaller than diameter of a capillary lumen) in >25% of the observed mesangium
II(b)	Severe mesangial expansion (larger than diameter of a capillary lumen) in >25% of the observed mesangium
III	At least one KW nodule & ≤50% globally sclerotic glomeruli
IV	Advanced diabetic glomerulosclerosis >50% globally sclerotic glomeruli

Table 2:22.2: Scoring system for Interstitial and vascular lesions in DN.

Lesion	Criteria	Score
Interstitial lesions:		
IF/TA	No IF/TA	0
	<25%	1
	25-50%	2
	>50%	3
Interstitial inflammation	Absent	0
	Only relation to IF/TA	1
	In relation to areas without IF/TA	2
Vascular lesions:		
Arteriolar hyalinosis	Absent	0
	At least one area of arteriolar hyalinosis	1
	>one area of arteriolar hyalinosis	2
Large vessels		Present/absent
Worst artery affected: arteriosclerosis	No intimal thickening	0
	Intimal thickening<thickness of the media	1
	Intimal thickening >thickness of the media	2

Reference:

Tervaert TW et. al., Pathologic classification of diabetic nephropathy. J Am Soc Nephrol 2010;21(4):556-563. *Mesangial expansion means the width of more than two mesangial nuclei.

Pathology Pearls

Table 2:22.3: Differentiating Diabetic Nephropathy from MIDD/LCDD.

Sr. No.	Features	Diabetic Nephropathy	MIDD/LCDD:
1.	Size of Nodules	Asymmetrical	Symmetrical
2.	Silver stain	Strongly positive	Weak positive/negative
3.	IF Study: Light chain restriction	Absent	Present
4.	IF Study: Albumin	Present	Absent
5.	EM study: Randall Deposits	Absent	Present

***Randall deposits in LCDD/MIDD:** These are granular, punctate and powdery electron dense deposits on the inner aspect of glomerular basement membranes and the outer aspect of the tubular basement membranes.

*** Table 2:22.4:** Differentiating Diabetic Nephropathy from nodular MPGN.

Sr. No.	Features	Diabetic Nephropathy	MPGN
1.	Nodular formation	All glomeruli may not be uniformly affected	Usually, all glomeruli are uniformly affected
2.	Cellularity	± Mild mesangial hypercellularity around the periphery of the nodule	Mesangial hypercellularity
3.	Silver stain: GBM duplication & mesangial cell interposition	Absent	Present

CASE 23

History: 56-year-old male, diabetic for 15 years and Hypertensive for 10 years. Pedal oedema for last 6 months with numbness in feet. He was detected to have diabetic retinopathy 6 months back and was also found to have renal dysfunction, presumed diabetic nephropathy based on clinical presentation. Now presenting with shortness of breath and diminution of vision. He has basal crepitations in lungs, pedal oedema and BP is 200/110 mm of Hg.

Previous baseline investigations: 4 months back: Serum creatinine 1.5mg/dl, UPCR :0.8 g/g.

Current Investigations: Serum creatinine:6.03mg/dl, Urine analysis: Protein:4+, RBCs: 8-10 /HPF and Pus cells:4 to 5/HPF, UPCR: 6 g/g. Renal artery doppler: Normal. USG abdomen: Normal size kidney with no hydroureteronephrosis.

Clinical diagnosis: Malignant Hypertension with nephrotic range proteinuria due to diabetic nephropathy, to rule out superadded nondiabetic renal disease.

Differential diagnoses: TMA/ Renal artery stenosis/ paraproteinemia.

Light microscopy:

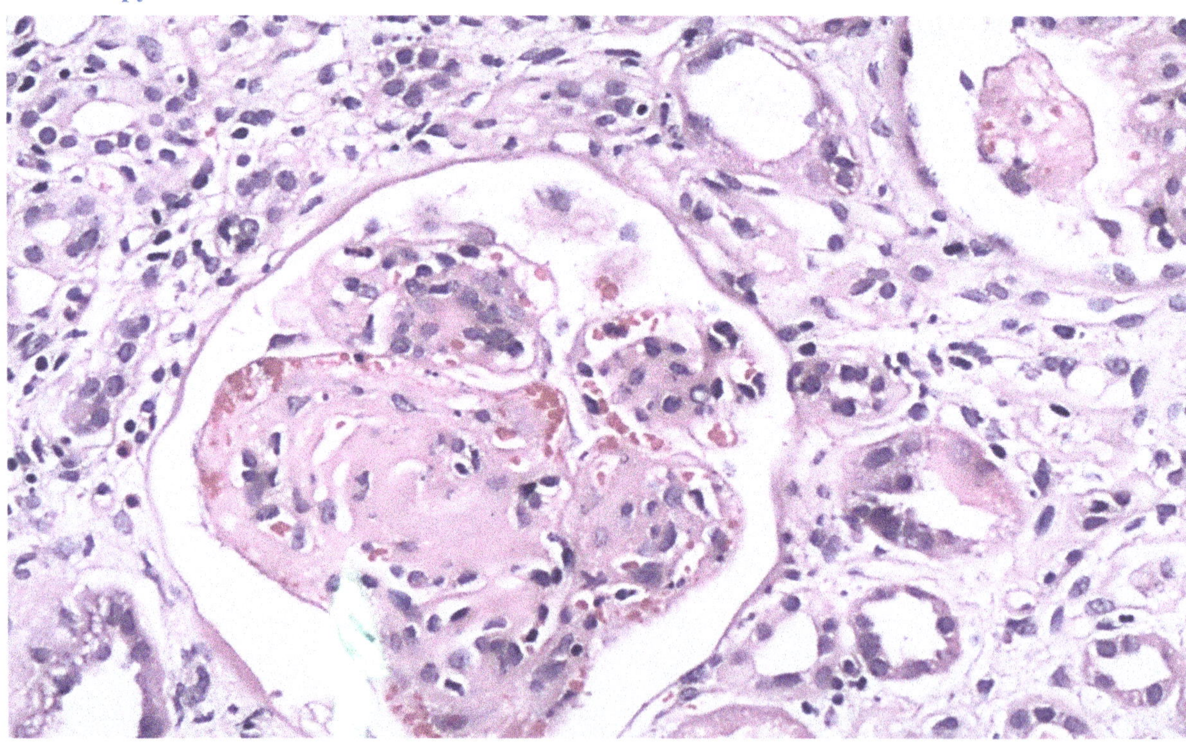

Figure 2:23.1: H&E Stain: 20x: Complicated nodule with red blood cells.

Plasminogen activator inhibitor -1 (PAI-1) is increased in such lesions with fragmented red blood cells, indicating microvascular injury.

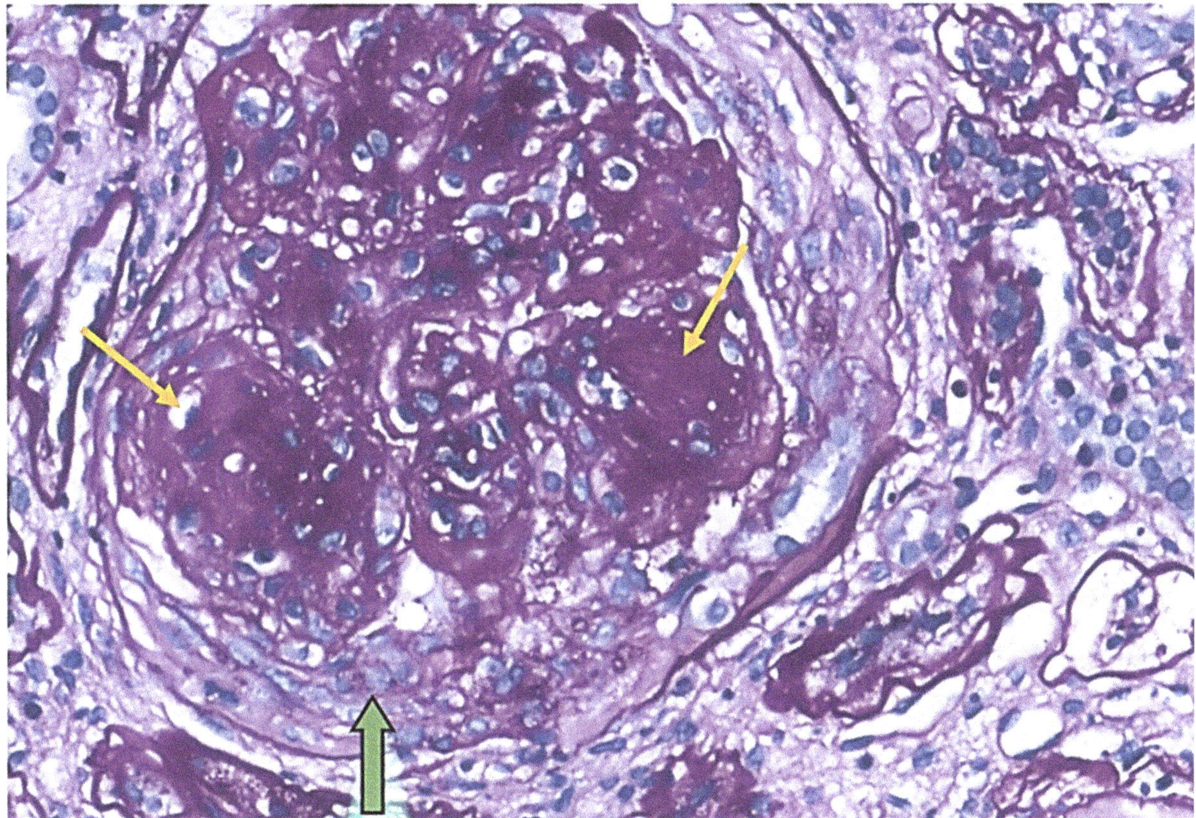

Figure 2:23.2: PAS Stain:20x: Circumferential cellular crescent** and PAS positive KW nodules (yellow arrows).

Immunofluorescence: No immune deposits.

Interpretation: Diabetic Nephropathy with focal crescents.

Additional investigations:

Viral markers: Negative, Serum C3& C4: normal, ANA: negative, ANCA: negative, ANTI-GBM: negative, Serum Protein electrophoresis negative for M-Band, ASO Normal.

Final Diagnosis: Diabetic Nephropathy with Focal crescents.

Pathology Pearls

*Crescents in diabetic nephropathy possibly result from rupture of microaneurysms and usually fibrinoid necrosis is not observed.

**Crescents in diabetic nephropathy are due to an unusual response to heavy proteinuria.

References

*Diagnostic Atlas of Renal Pathology:3rd edition: Agnes B. Fogo: Chapter 4: Vascular Diseases-Diabetic Nephropathy page no.296.
**Diagnostic Pathology Kidney Diseases, 2nd edition: Colvin/Chang: Diabetic Nephropathy: page no.276.

CASE 24

History: 58 years old male, non-diabetic, hypertensive for 8 years, chronic smoker for 20 years. Presented with progressive pedal edema, facial puffiness, and distension of abdomen with gross anasarca over a span of 2 months. No history of indigenous medication or NSAIDs use. No history of any preceding or on-going chronic infection. No history of weight loss. BP 150/90 mm of Hg.

Investigations: Serum creatinine: 1.1 mg/dl, Urine analysis: Protein: 4+, RBCs: 8-10/ HPF, RBC Casts: 1-2 / HPF, UPCR: 8.9 g/g, HIV: Non-reactive, HBSAg: Non-reactive, HCV: Non-reactive.

Clinical diagnosis: Nephrotic syndrome with microscopic hematuria with hypertension without renal dysfunction.

Differential diagnoses: Membranous nephropathy/FSGS/ MCD/IgA N.

Light microscopy:

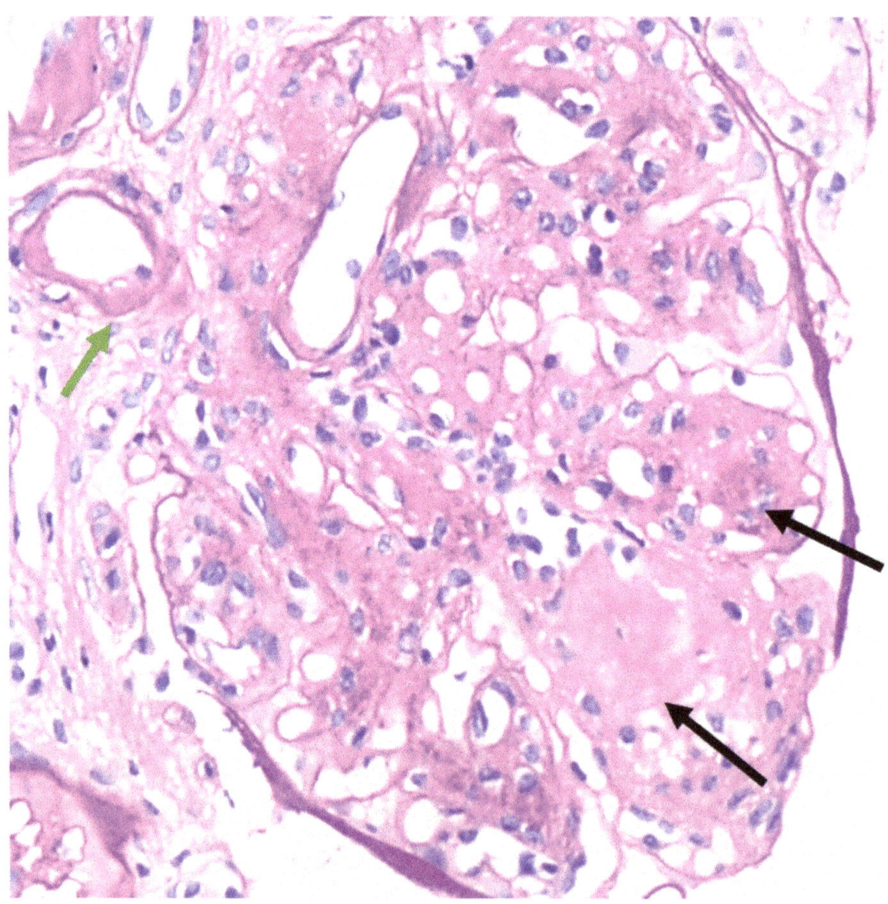

Figure 2:24.1: PAS Stain:20x: PAS positive nodular lesions (**black** arrow) and arteriolar hyalinosis (**green** arrow).

Congo red stain: Negative for amyloid.

Immunofluorescence: No immune deposits.

Interpretation: Idiopathic Nodular Glomerulosclerosis

Additional investigations:

C3, C4 Normal, ANA Profile Negative, Serum protein electrophoresis: No M band.

Final diagnosis: Idiopathic Nodular glomerulosclerosis possibly due to chronic smoking/hypertension.

Pathology Pearls

Table 2:24.1: Special stains in Nodular glomerular Lesions.

Sr. No.	Nodular glomerulosclerosis	PAS stain	PASM (Silver)	Masson trichrome	Congo red	DNA JB9
1.	Idiopathic nodular glomerulosclerosis	++	Black	Blue	-	-
2.	Diabetes mellitus	+++	Black	Blue	-	-
3.	Amyloidosis	-	-	Blue	+++	-
4.	Light/heavy chain deposition disease	++	-	Blue	-	-
5.	Fibrillary glomerulonephritis (FGN) / immunotactoid glomerulopathy	+++	-	Blue	-	+ in Fibrillary GN
6.	Fibronectin nephropathy	++	-	Red	-	-
7.	Collagenofibrotic glomerulopathy	-	-	Blue	-	-

CASE 25

History: 48 years female known hypertensive for 10 years (uncontrolled for 2years), Nondiabetic, came in ER with generalized tonic-clonic convulsions. There is no history of fever. No past history of seizures. There is the history of loss of appetite for the last 1 to 2 months with on-and-off symptoms of nausea and vomiting. Edema feet on and off for the last 2 months. No history of fever or any preceding infection. Nonsmoker and non-alcoholic. No skin rash or arthritis. No oral ulcers. BP is 190/100. No neck stiffness. No asymmetric pupils. No focal neurological deficits.

Investigations: Hemoglobin: 5.4 g/dl, Platelets count: 1 Lakh/cu mm, Total Leucocyte Count: 5000 /cu mm. Peripheral smear: Normochromic and normocytic anemia. Serum Creatinine: 10 mg/dl. Urine analysis: Protein:4+, RBCs: 20-30/HPF, RBC Casts: 3-4 /HPF. Urine Protein to creatinine ratio: 4.5 g/g.

Clinical Diagnosis: Uremic/Hypertensive encephalopathy. CKD vs RPGN. Anemia and thrombocytopenia? part of collagen vascular disease or CKD related.

Differential diagnoses: Immune complex mediated GN/ Pauci-immune crescentic GN/Paraproteinemia.

Light microscopy:

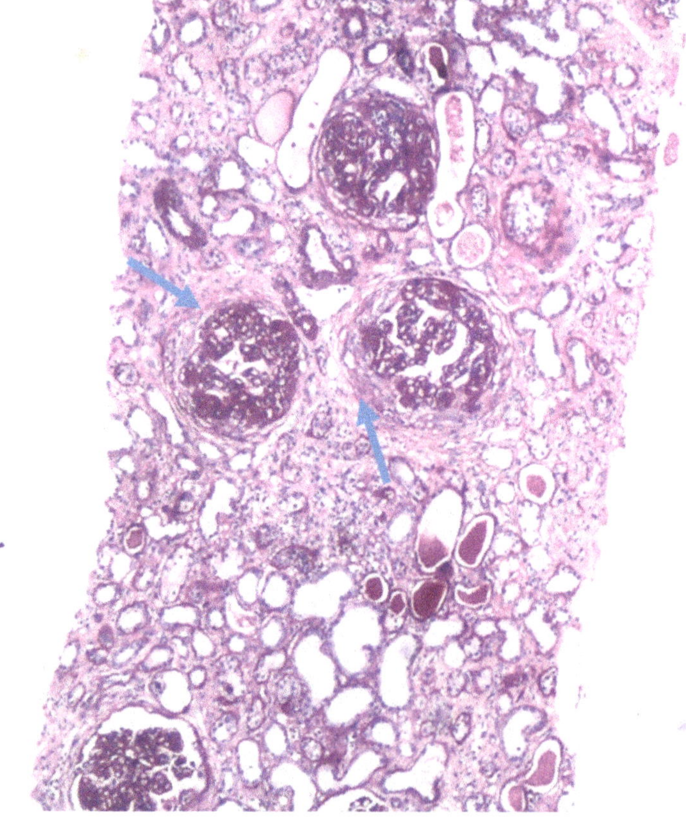

Figure 2:25.1: PAS Stain: 4x: Glomeruli showing circumferential crescents (blue arrows) and moderate IF/TA.

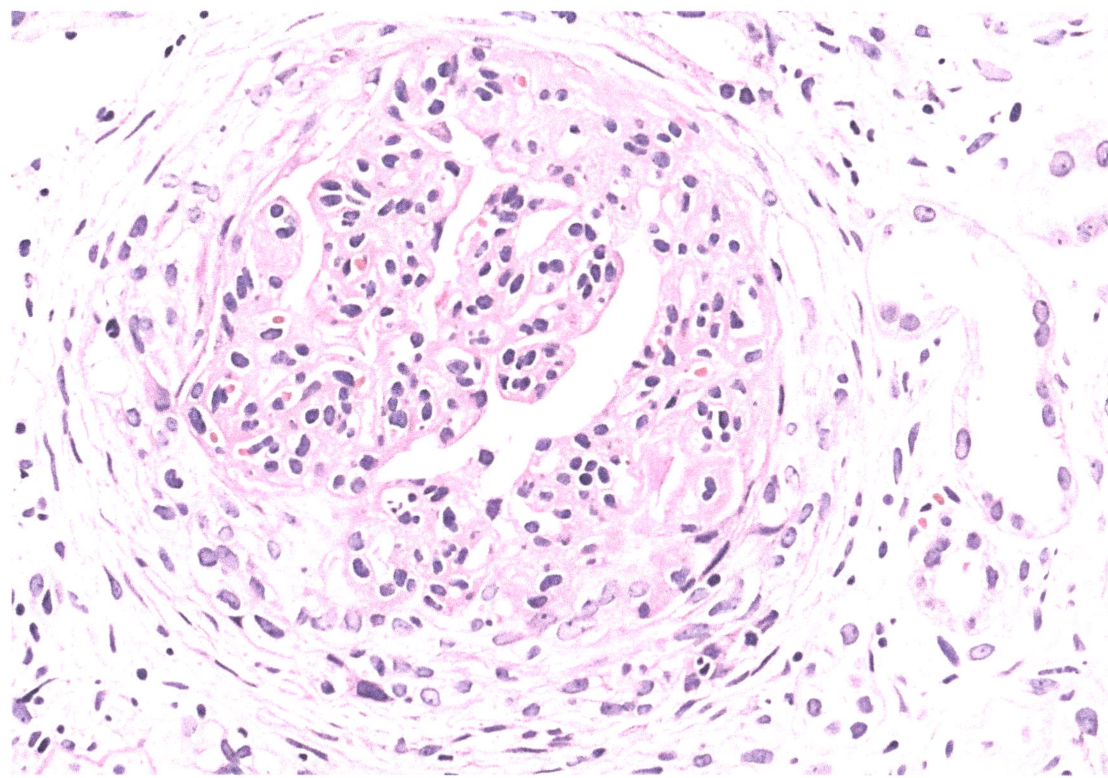

Figure 2:25.2: H&E Stain: (20x): Hypercellular glomerulus with diffuse mesangial and endocapillary hypercellularity and circumferential cellular crescent.

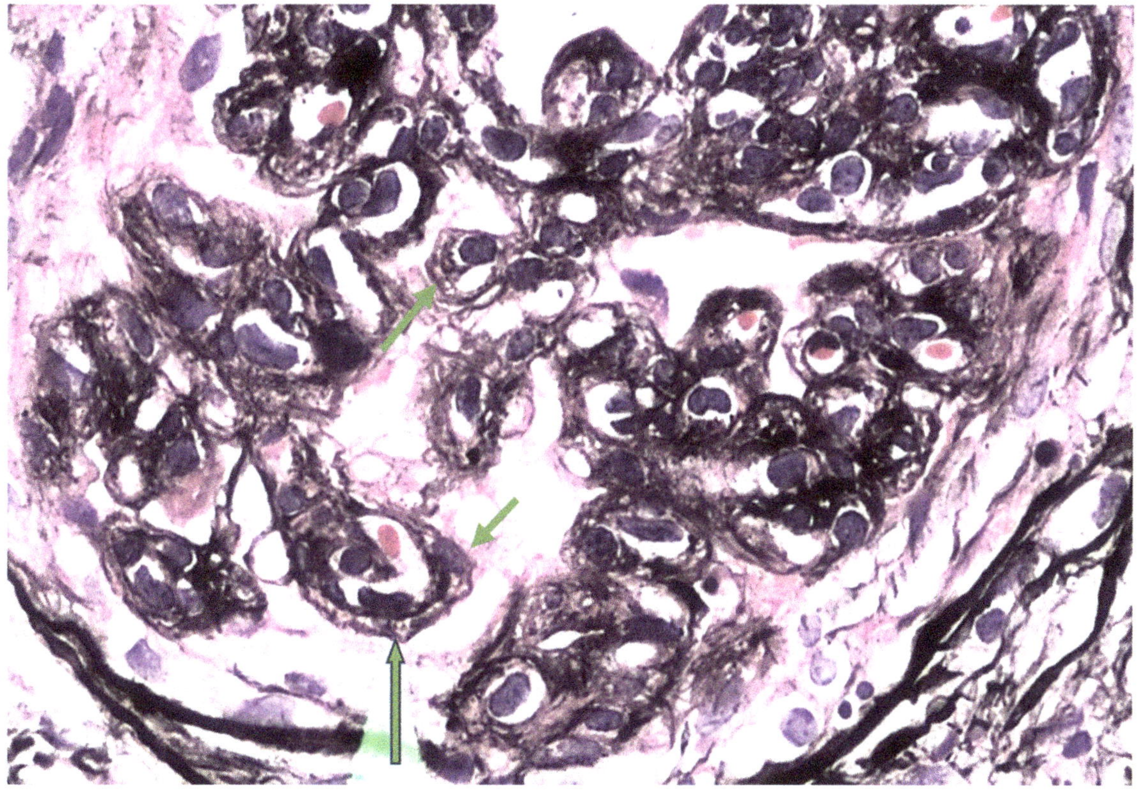

Figure 2:25.3: Periodic Acid Silver Methenamine (PASM) stain 40x: Glomerulus: (**green** arrows) showing tram track appearance with mesangial cell interposition.

Immunofluorescence:

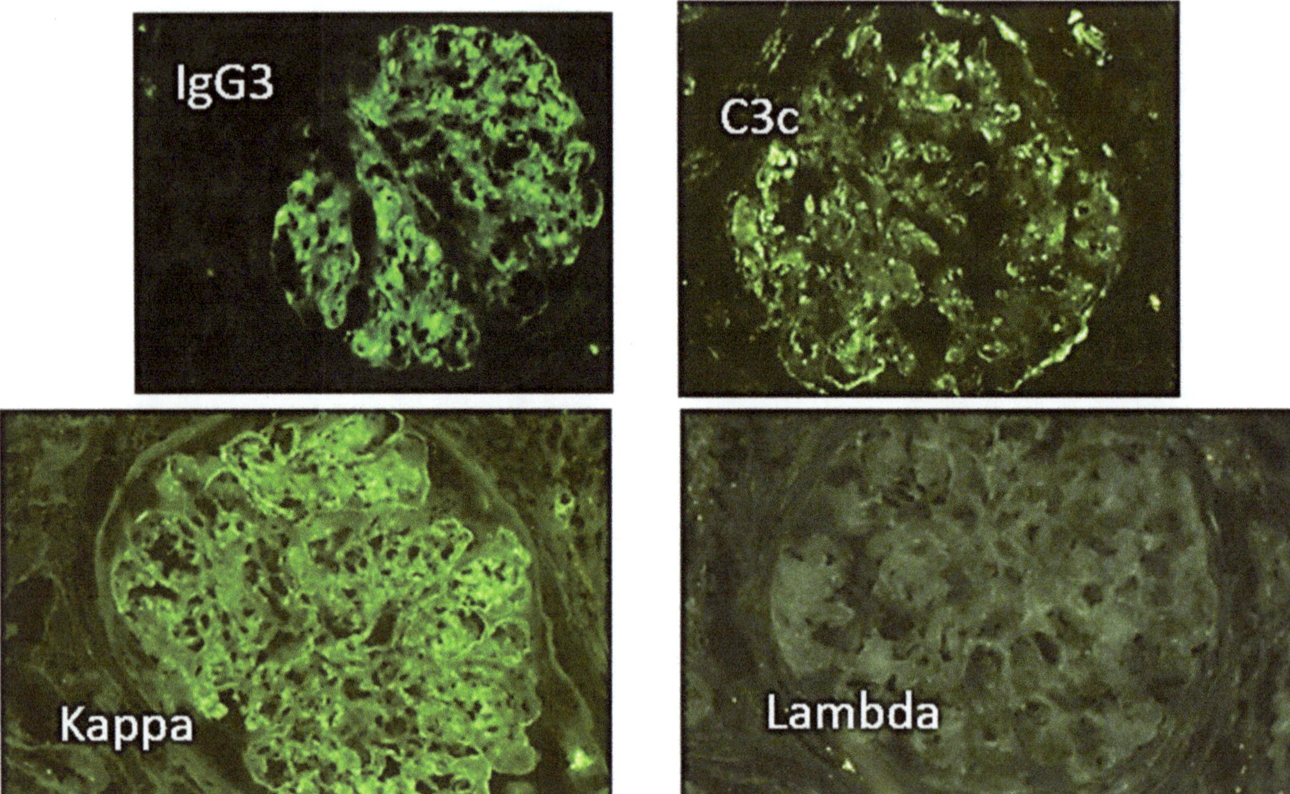

Figure 2:25.4: Immunofluorescence: Significant peripheral (capillary wall) and mesangial coarse granular deposits of IgG (IgG3) and C3c, with minimal deposits of C1q. There is Kappa light chain restriction seen in the glomeruli. There is no light chain restriction along the tubular casts or cytoplasm of tubular epithelial cells. IgG3 subtype was strongly positive in glomeruli.

Paraffin Immunofluorescence: Confirmed negative Lambda light chain.

Interpretation:

Primary diagnosis: Proliferative glomerulonephritis with monoclonal IgG (Kappa) deposits (PGNMID).

Pattern of injury: Membranoproliferative pattern of glomerulonephritis (MPGN) with diffuse crescents (11/20).

Additional findings: Focal global glomerulosclerosis (03/20), focal ischemic changes (02/20), with moderate tubulointerstitial changes of chronicity (30%), mild acute tubular injury, and mild arteriosclerosis. Chronicity score: mild: 03/10.

Ancillary studies: Congo red stain is negative for Amyloid.

Comments: Serum protein electrophoresis: M Band seen. Serum Immunofixation electrophoresis (qualitative)– Monoclonal gammopathy seen in IgG and Kappa region. Serum free Kappa light chain =365 mg/l, free Lambda light chain = 77 mg/l, FLC Ratio = 4.7.

Dysmorphic RBCs:

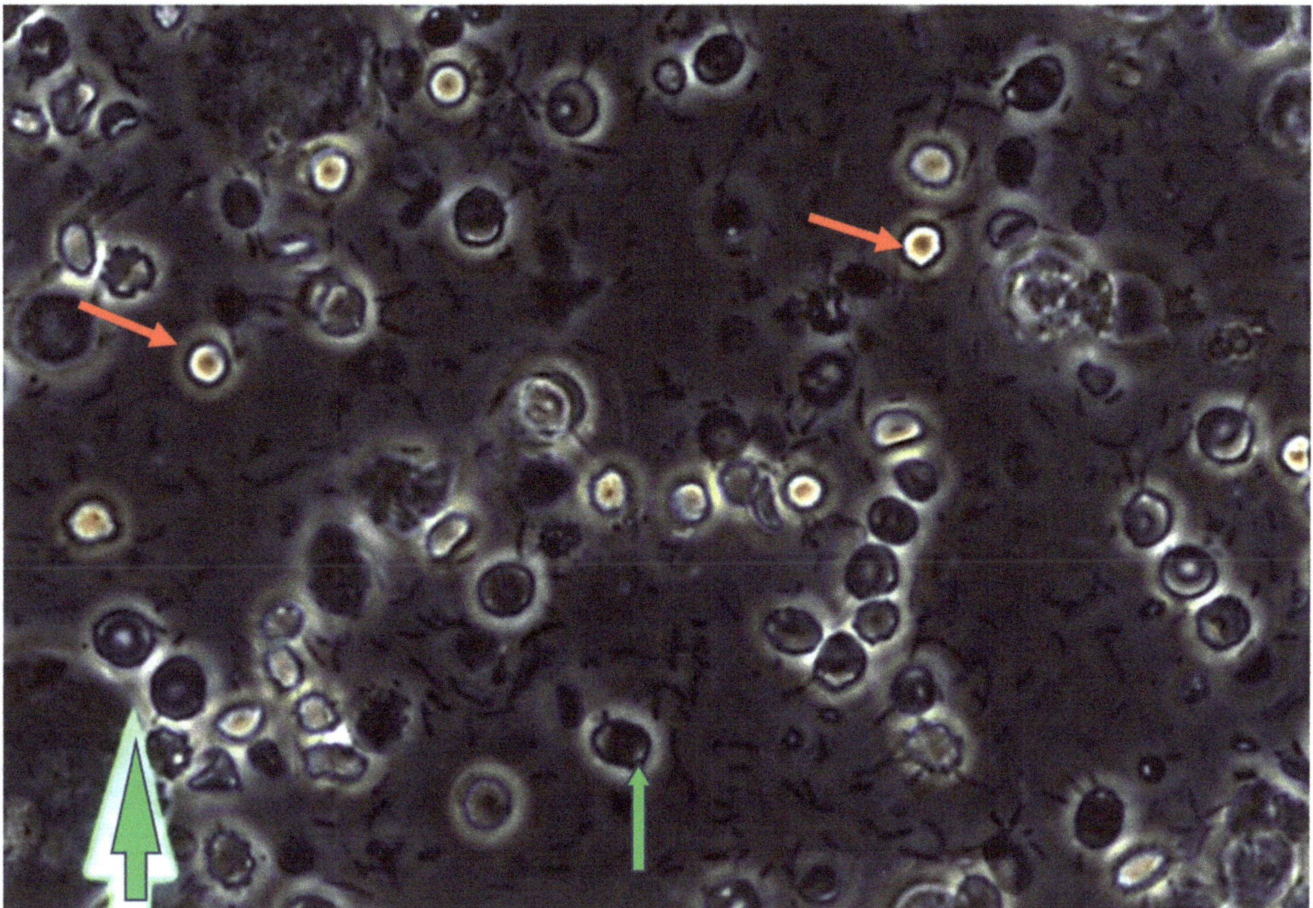

Figure 2:25.5: Phase contrast microscopy: Urine showed doughnut shaped dysmorphic RBCs >50% (green arrows) and normal RBCs (red arrows)

Final Diagnosis: Crescentic PGNMID.

* PGNMID-LC: PGNMID-Light Chain only:

PGNMID-LC is rare and is characterised by glomerular deposition of C3c + restriction of light chain only and no immunoglobulin deposits in the renal pathology.

Case 26

History: A 50-year-old male with a known case of diabetic mellitus and Hypertension for 5 years presented with pedal edema for the last week with shortness of breath on exertion and worsened Blood pressure (BP) control. For the last 2 days, he has had a drop in his urine output, and since morning, he has had a cough with fresh blood up to 2-3 spoons in sputum each time he is coughing. He now has come to the emergency room (ER) with worsened shortness of breath even at rest. BP 170/100mm of Hg. SPO2 85% on room air. Crepitations audible in bilateral lung bases.

Investigations: Hb: 7 g/dl. Serum creatinine: 6 mg/dl. Urine: Protein: 3+, RBCs: Plenty/HPF, Pus cells: 8-10/HPF. Urine Protein to creatinine ratio: 4. USG showed normal size kidneys.

Clinical diagnosis: Rapidly progressive GN/ Pulmonary renal syndrome.

Differential diagnoses: ANCA Vasculitis/ anti-GBM Disease/ IgA Nephropathy with crescents.

Light Microscopy:

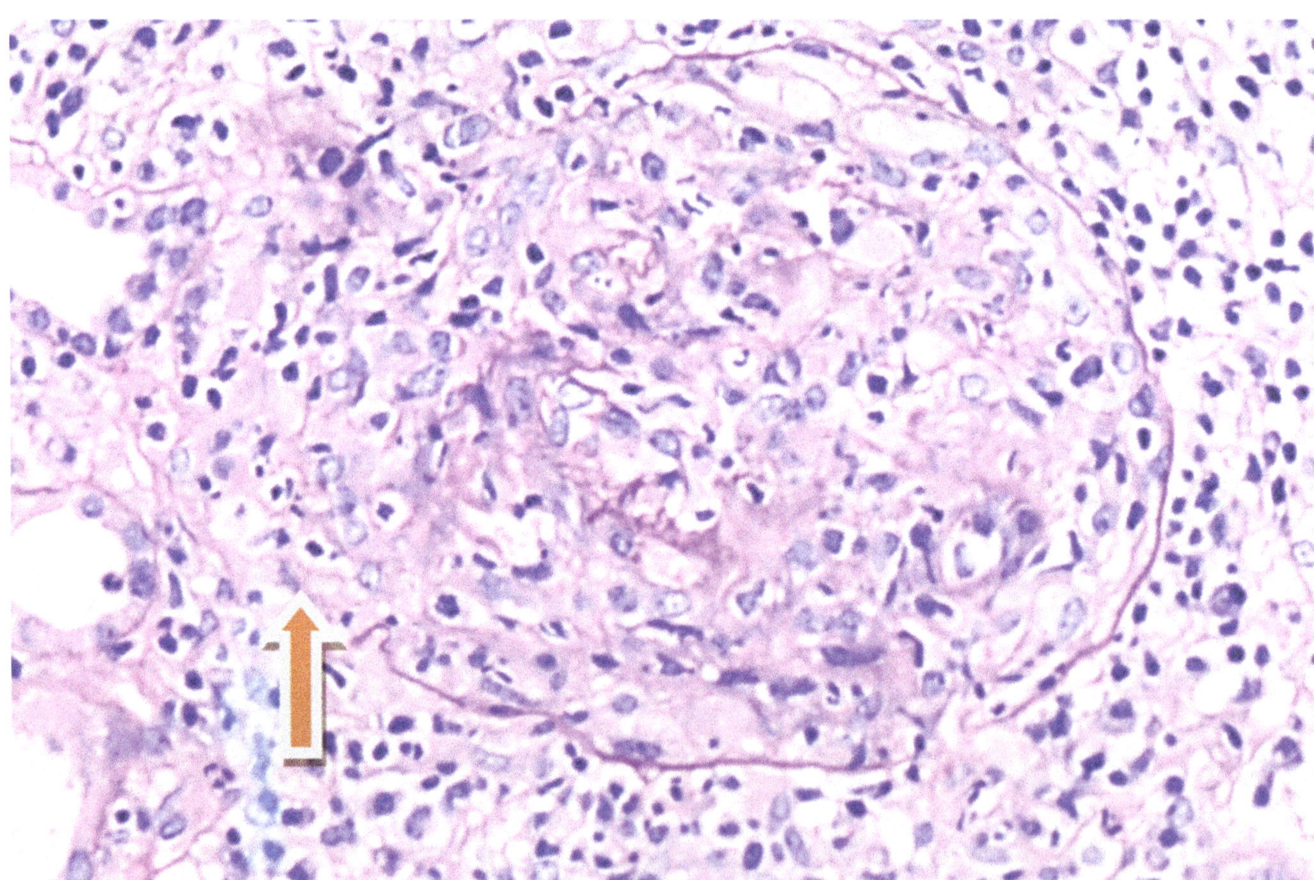

Figure: 2:26.1: PAS Stain: 20 x: Breach in Bowman capsule: circumferential cellular crescent.

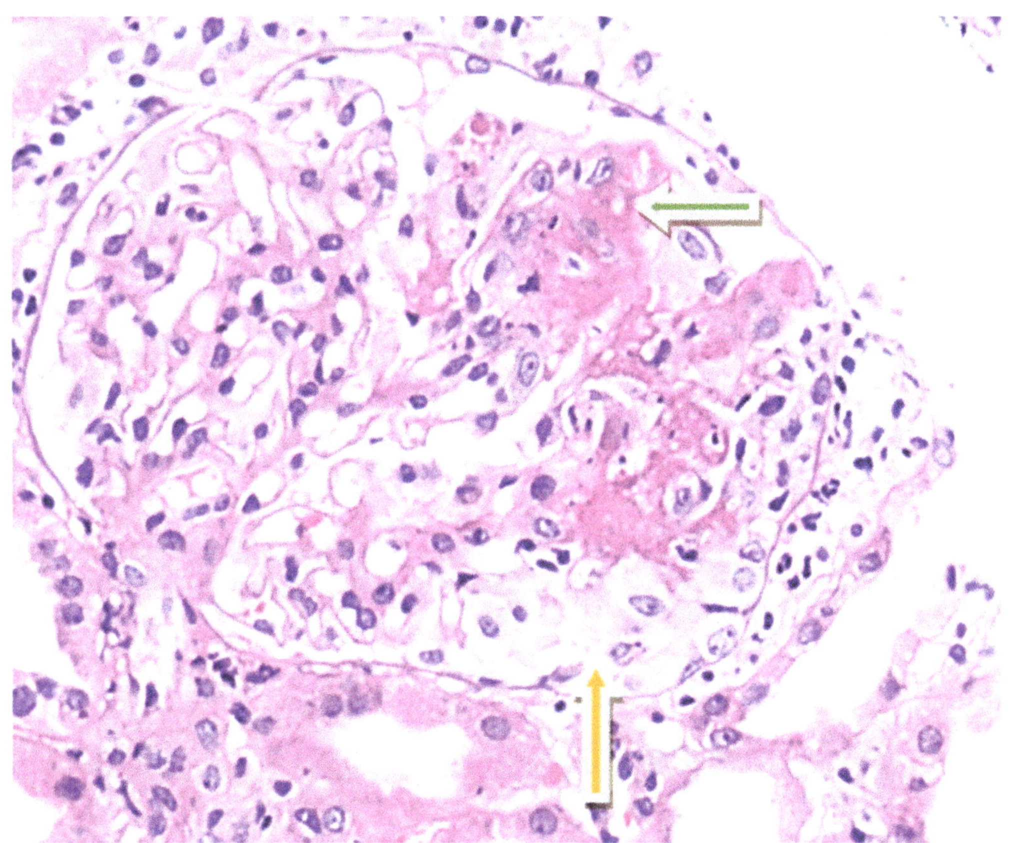

Figure: 2:26.2: H&E Stain: Segmental Fibrinoid necrosis (green arrow) and early cellular crescent formation (yellow arrow).

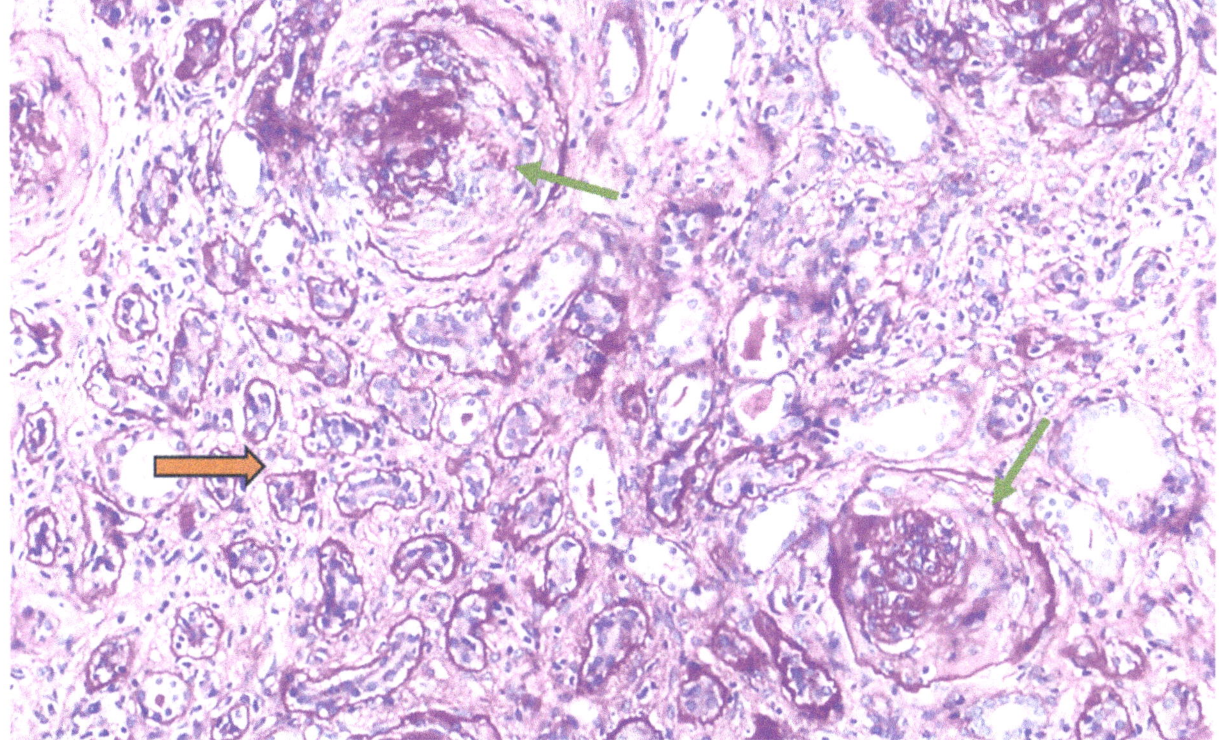

Figure 2:26.3: PAS Stain 10x: Fibrocellular crescents (red arrows) with moderate tubulointerstitial changes of chronicity (orange arrow).

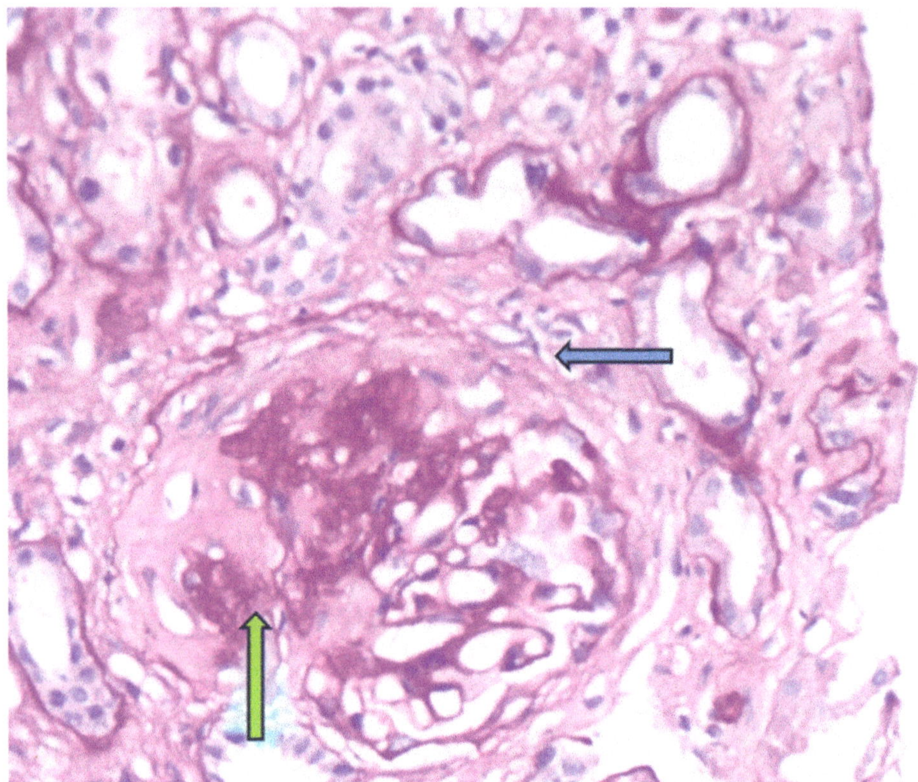

Figure 2:26.4: PAS Stain: 20x: Fibrous crescent: PAS -positive tuft (green arrow) and PAS-negative fibrous material in Bowman capsule and breach in Bowman capsule (blue arrow)

Immunofluorescence: Negative.

Interpretation: ANCA (antineutrophil cytoplasmic associated) mediated crescentic GN.

Additional investigations:

C3 & C4: Normal, anti-nuclear antibody (ANA): Negative, c-ANCA: cytoplasmic antineutrophil cytoplasmic autoantibody: Positive, p-ANCA: perinuclear antineutrophil cytoplasmic autoantibody: negative, Anti- GBM: Negative.

Final Diagnosis: c-ANCA mediated pauci-immune crescentic Glomerulonephritis

Suggested Reading

Berden (European Vasculitis Study Group) classification of ANCA Vasculitis:
4 classes:
1. Focal (> 50% normal glomeruli),
2. Crescentic (> 50% cellular crescents),
3. Sclerotic (> 50% sclerotic glomeruli),
4. Mixed (any other combination).

CASE 27

History: 42 years old male, a chronic smoker for 10 years, diabetic & hypertensive for 4 years, came with a history of decreased urine output for the last 2 days, with edema feet and shortness of breath. He is now also complaining of blood in sputum. He has no skin rash or joint pains. He has no fever. No past h/o Pulmonary TB or any lung disease. No history of using NSAIDs or any indigenous medication. BP is 160/90 mm of Hg, SPO2 :88% on room air. Crepitations in both lung bases and pedal edema.

Investigations: Serum creatinine: 4 mg/dl. Urine analysis: Protein:4+, RBCs: Plenty/HPF, RBC Casts: 3-4/HPF. Oliguric Urine with UPCR:8 g/g. USG: Normal sized kidneys. X-ray chest: Bilateral lungs haziness all over.

Clinical Diagnosis: RPGN/ Pulmonary renal syndrome

Differential diagnoses: ANCA Vasculitis/ anti-GBM Disease/ IgA Nephropathy with crescents.

Light Microscopy:

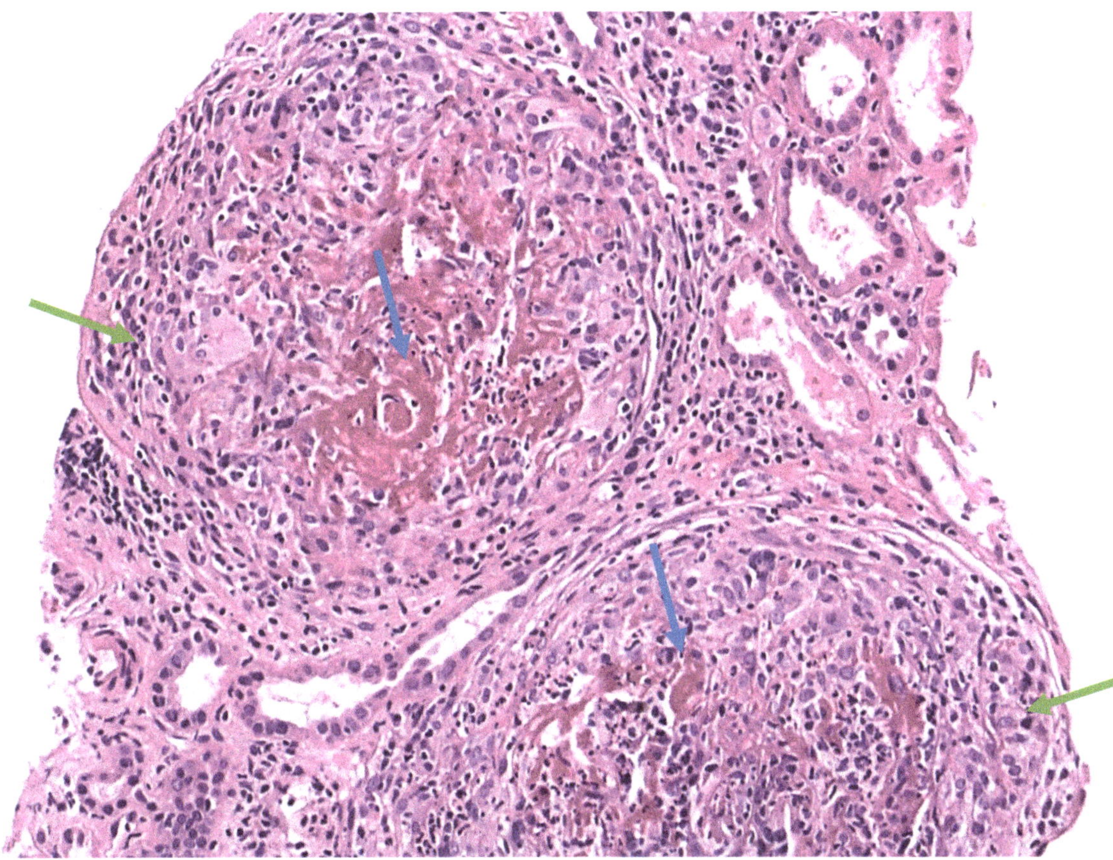

Figure: 2:27.1: H&E Stain: 20x: Glomerulus showing fibrinoid necrosis (blue arrow) with circumferential cellular crescents (green arrows).

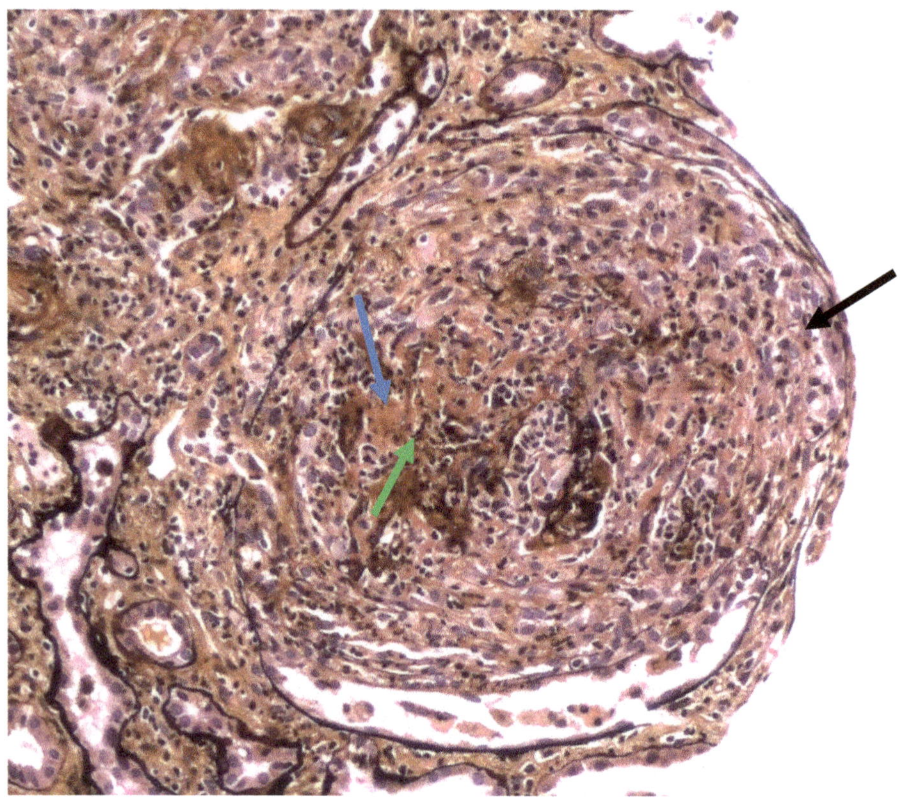

Figure: 2:27.2: Silver stain:20x: Glomerulus: Necrosis (blue arrow) of the tuft, breaks in glomerular basement membrane (green arrow) with a circumferential cellular crescent (**black** arrow).

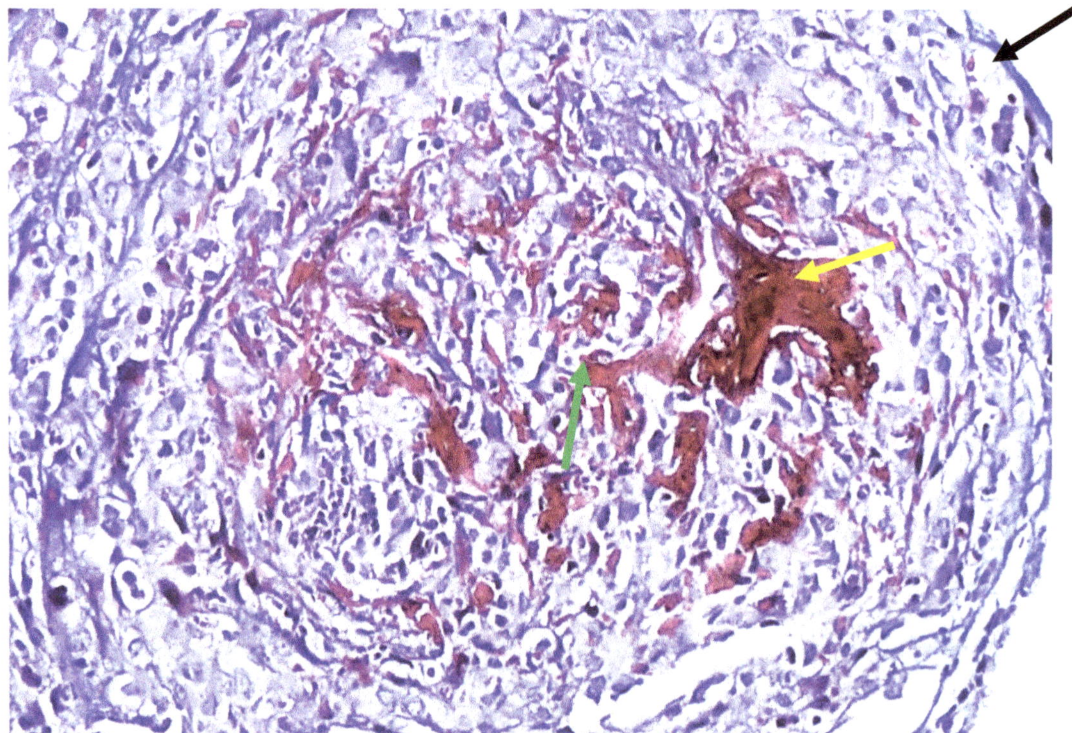

Figure: 2:27.3: MT stain: 40x: Glomerulus: Necrosis (yellow arrow) of the tuft, breaks in glomerular basement membrane (green arrow)with a circumferential cellular crescent (**black** arrow).

Immunofluorescence

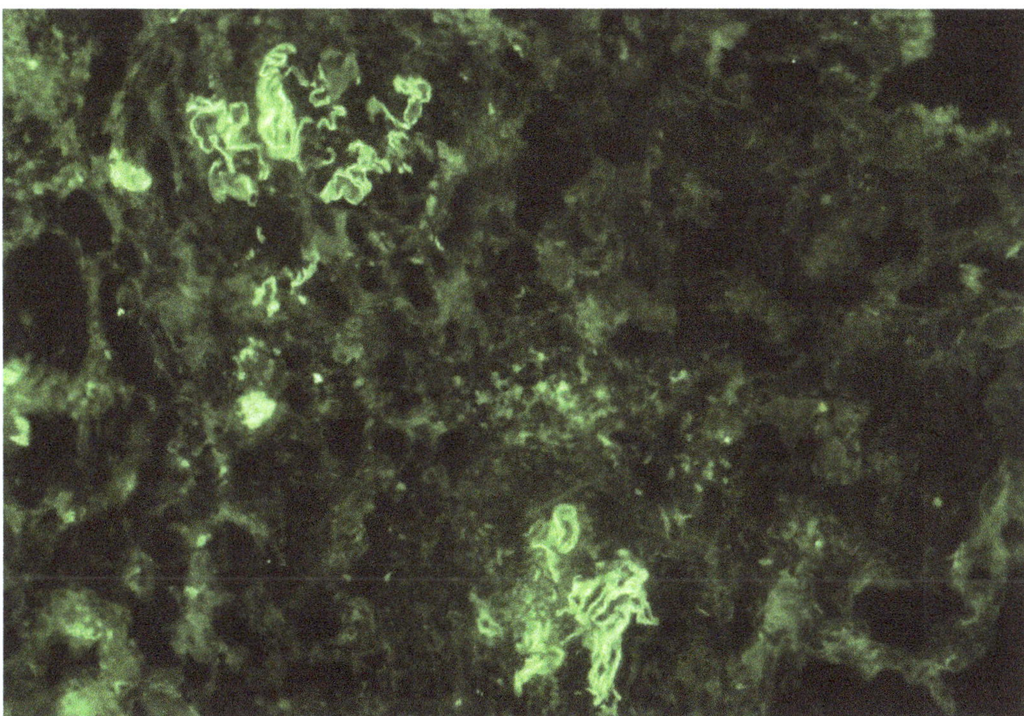

Figure: 2:27.4: Immunofluorescence: IgG:10x: Glomerul with circumferential crescents: significant diffuse capillary wall linear continuous deposits.

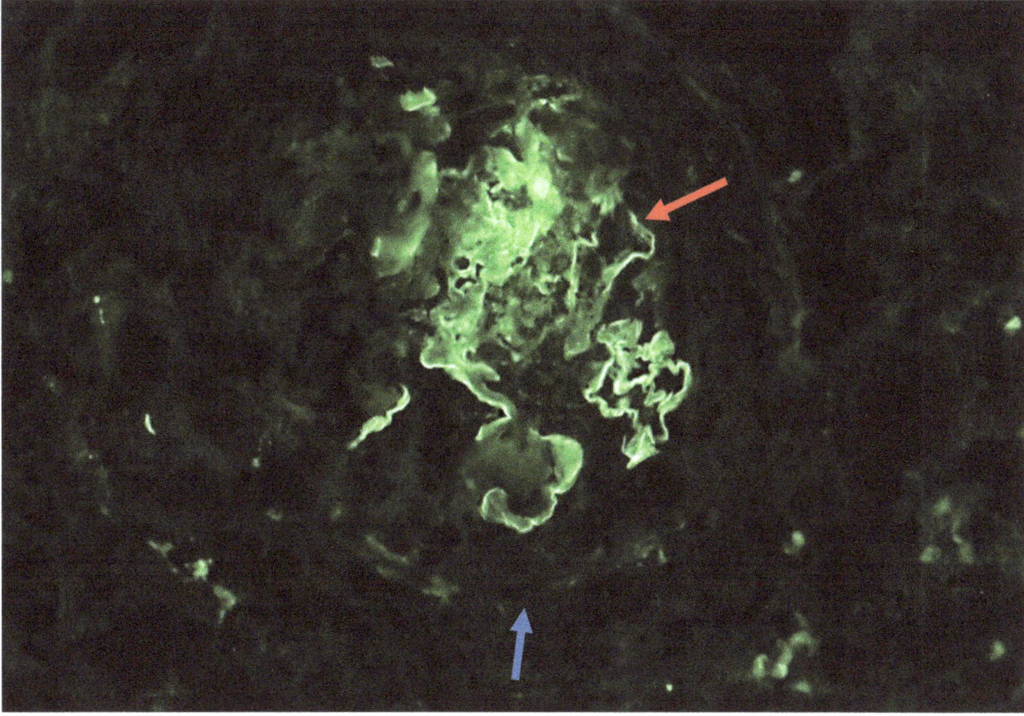

Figure: 2:27.5: Immunofluorescence: IgG:20x: Glomerulus with circumferential crescent: significant diffuse capillary wall linear continuous deposits (red arrow) with destruction of GBMs, look at the breach in Bowman space (blue arrow), the crescentic cells not positive for IgG.

Interpretation: Necrotizing crescentic GN with significant linear IgG deposits.

Additional investigations: C3 and C4: normal, Viral screen: negative. ANA Profile negative. ANCA Negative. Anti GBM antibody: Elevated.

Final Diagnosis: Anti Glomerular basement membrane disease.

Pathology Pearls

Variants of anti-GBM Disease:

1. **Anti-GBM disease: Post renal transplant in a case of Alport syndrome:** There are IgG antibodies formed against alpha 5(IV) collagen. So serologic testing may be falsely negative despite of histological anti-GBM disease.

2. **Anti-GBM disease in case of Membranous nephropathy:** It can precede, coincide with or follow the membranous nephropathy: In Immunofluorescence study two layers of deposits can be appreciated. An inner layer of linear continuous IgG deposits along the capillary wall and an outer layer of fine granular IgG deposits.

3. **Atypical anti-GBM nephritis:** Patients present with mild renal dysfunction with proteinuria & hematuria without pulmonary involvement. In kidney biopsy bright linear capillary wall IgG immune deposits along the GBM are noted without crescentic transformation. It has indolent course rather than RPGN. Anti-GBM antibodies are not detected in serum.

4. **Double antibody positive: Anti-GBM disease & ANCA associated disease:** Initial outcome is similar to anti-GBM disease but long-term outcomes are like ANCA vasculitis and they have chances of relapse unlike the anti-GBM disease alone.

5. **Rarely IgA & IgM antibodies** may be directed against the GBM instead of IgG1, IgG3 that are common in anti-GBM disease.

Table 2:27.1: Differentials for the linear IgG deposits on Immunofluorescence (IF) study:

Features	Diabetic nephropathy	Fibrillary GN	Anti-GBM disease
IgG Staining	Non specifically absorbed on highly permeable GBM	Non-specifically absorbed on fibrils	Specifically IgG1 or IgG3 against NC-1domain of alpha-3 chain of type IV collagen of GBM
IgG location, pattern, and intensity on Immunofluorescence (IF)	Capillary wall pseudolinear minimal	Capillary wall ± mesangial Smudgy Significant	Capillary wall Linear continuous Significant
Linear deposition albumin on IF	+	-	-
Circulating anti-GBM antibodies in serum	-	-	+
Electron microscopy: Characteristic fibrils seen	-	+	-

CASE 28

History: 42-year-old female, non-diabetic, non-hypertensive, nonsmoker, presented with pedal edema for the last week and decreased urine output for the last few days. No h/o NSAIDs/ indigenous medicine use. No systemic features were suggestive of collagen vascular disease. BP 170/90 mm of Hg.

Investigations: Serum creatinine: 16 mg/dl. Urine analysis: protein:2+, blood: 3+, UPCR:5 g/g, USG findings: normal sized kidneys.

Clinical diagnosis: AKI/RPGN.

Differential diagnoses: IgA Nephropathy with crescents/ANCA Vasculitis/Anti-GBM disease

Light Microscopy:

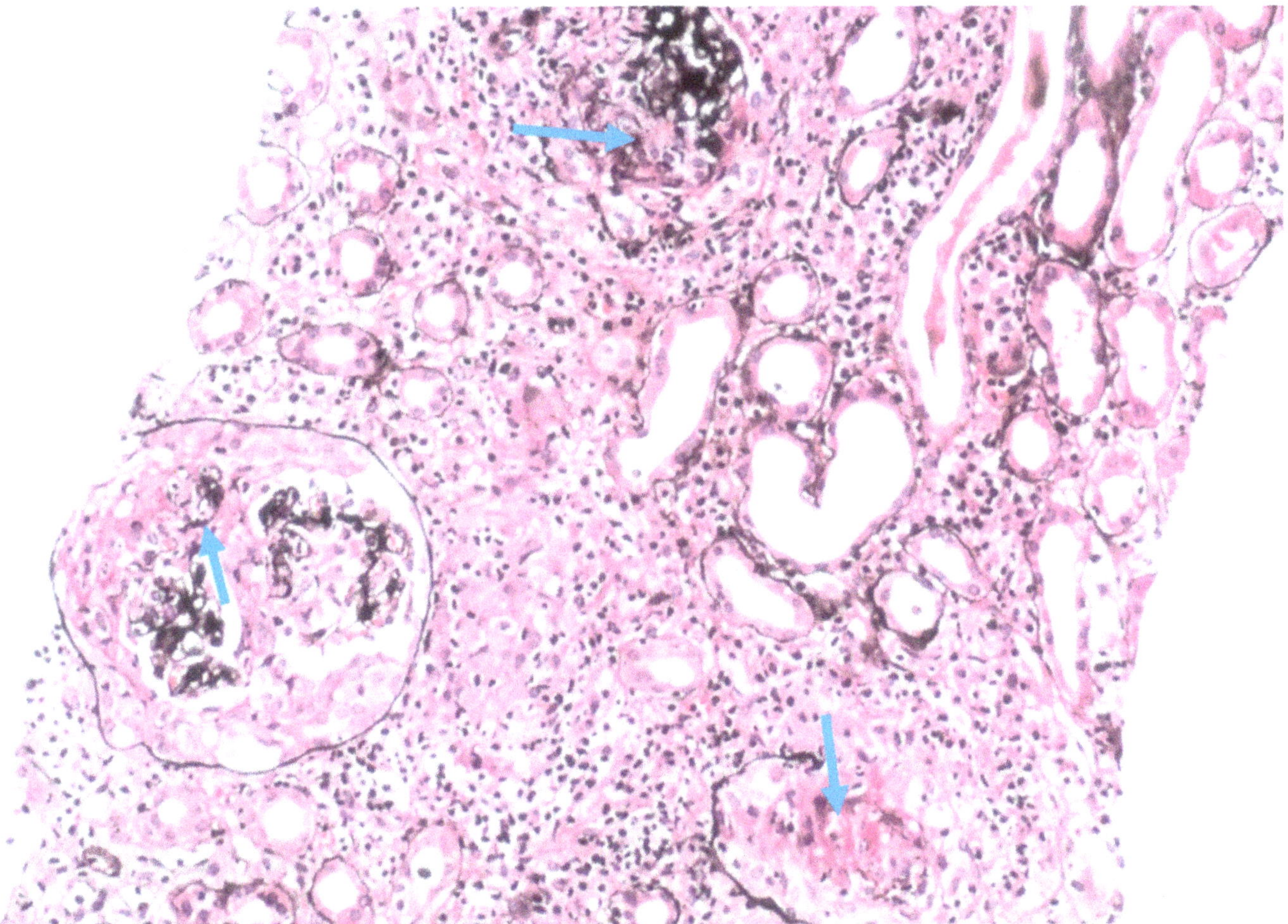

Figure 2:28.1: PASM Stain:10x: Glomeruli: Necrotizing and crescentic GN. There are moderate tubulointerstitial changes of chronicity.

Immunofluorescence:

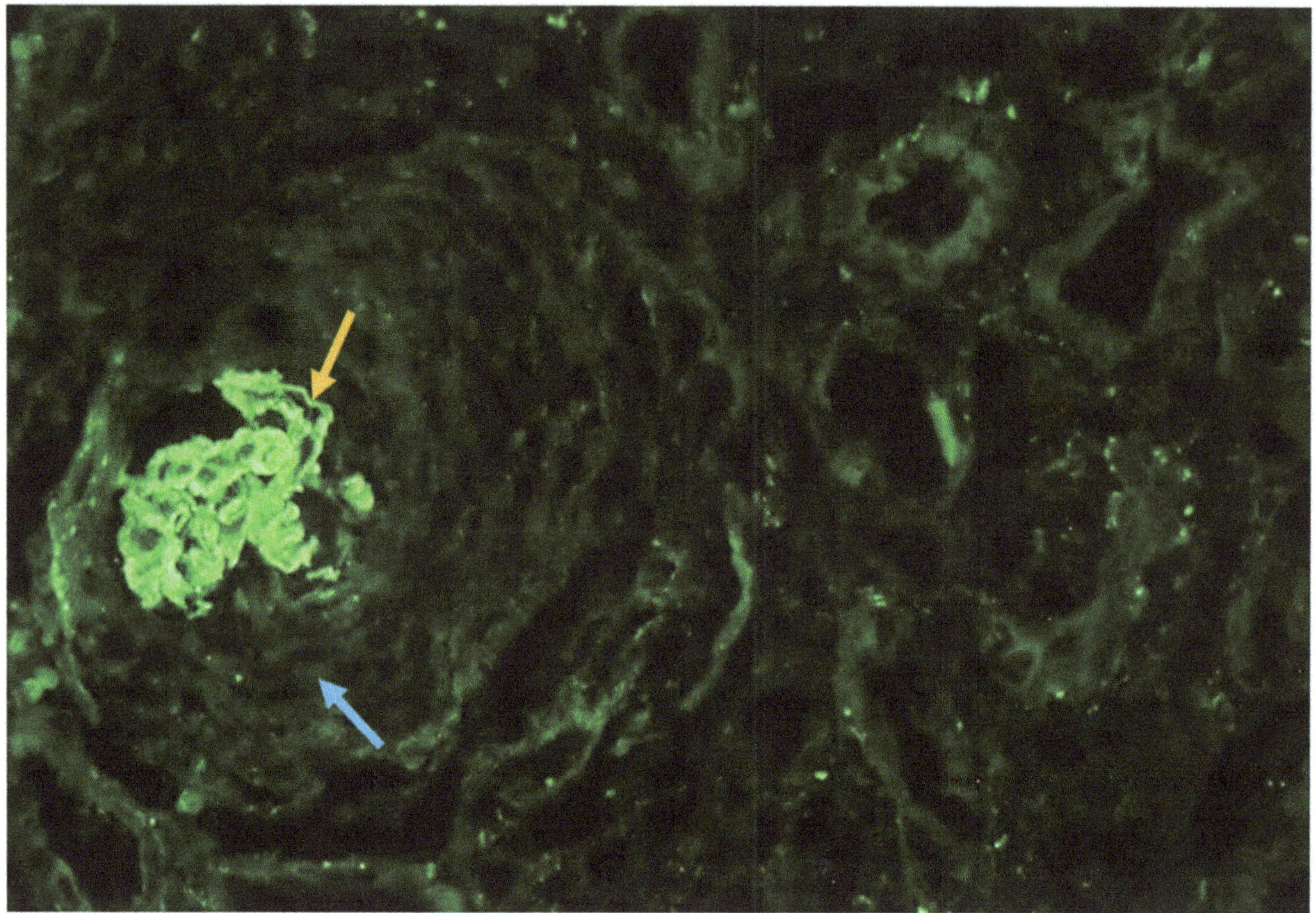

Figure 2:28.2: Immunofluorescence: IgG: 20x: glomerulus with circumferential crescents which don't take up stains (blue arrow) but the capillary walls (orange arrow) with significant linear continuous immune deposits of IgG.

Interpretation: Anti-GBM mediated crescentic GN.

Additional investigations: C3 & C4 Normal, p-ANCA: positive ANA: Negative. Anti GBM antibody: Elevated.

Final diagnosis: Double antibody positive disease: Anti Glomerular basement membrane disease with concurrent ANCA mediated crescentic GN.

CASE 29

History: 60 years old male, nondiabetic, non-hypertensive, chronic smoker, known case of COPD, a farmer by occupation. Presented with cough, shortness of breath, occasional streaks of blood in sputum, decreased urine output for 3 days, and anuric at presentation to hospital. Edema feet for last 2 days. There is no past history of any lower urinary tract symptoms like – hesitancy, increased urinary frequency, or nocturnal frequency. No h/o fever or weight loss. B.P.:160/90 mm of Hg. SPO2: 90% on room air.

Investigations: serum creatinine: 9 mg/dl. Viral screen: Negative

Clinical Diagnosis: Anuric AKI with pulmonary edema/RPGN with pulmonary renal syndrome.

Differential diagnoses: ANCA Vasculitis/anti-GBM disease/Cryoglobulinemic GN/IgA Nephropathy with crescents.

Light Microscopy:

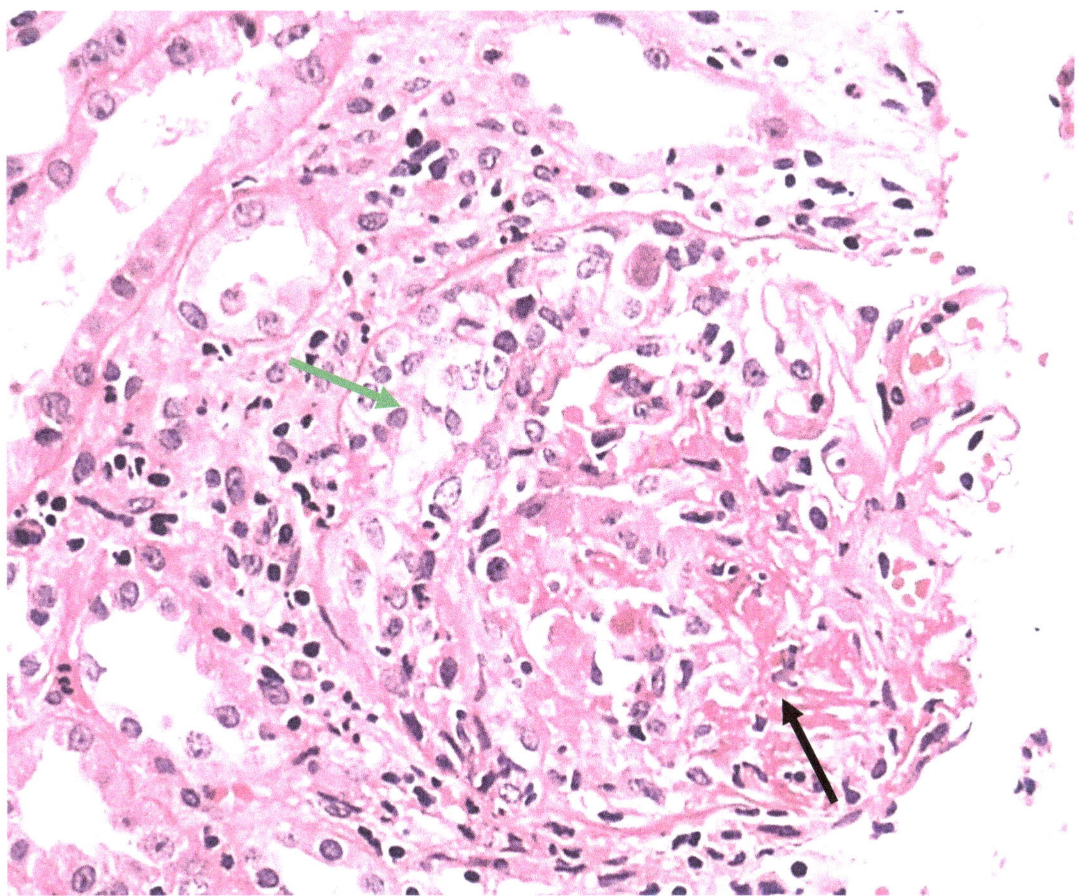

Figure 2:29.1: H&E Stain: 20x: Glomerulus with fibrinoid necrosis (**black** arrow) with circumferential cellular crescent (green arrow).Periglomerular inflammation is seen.

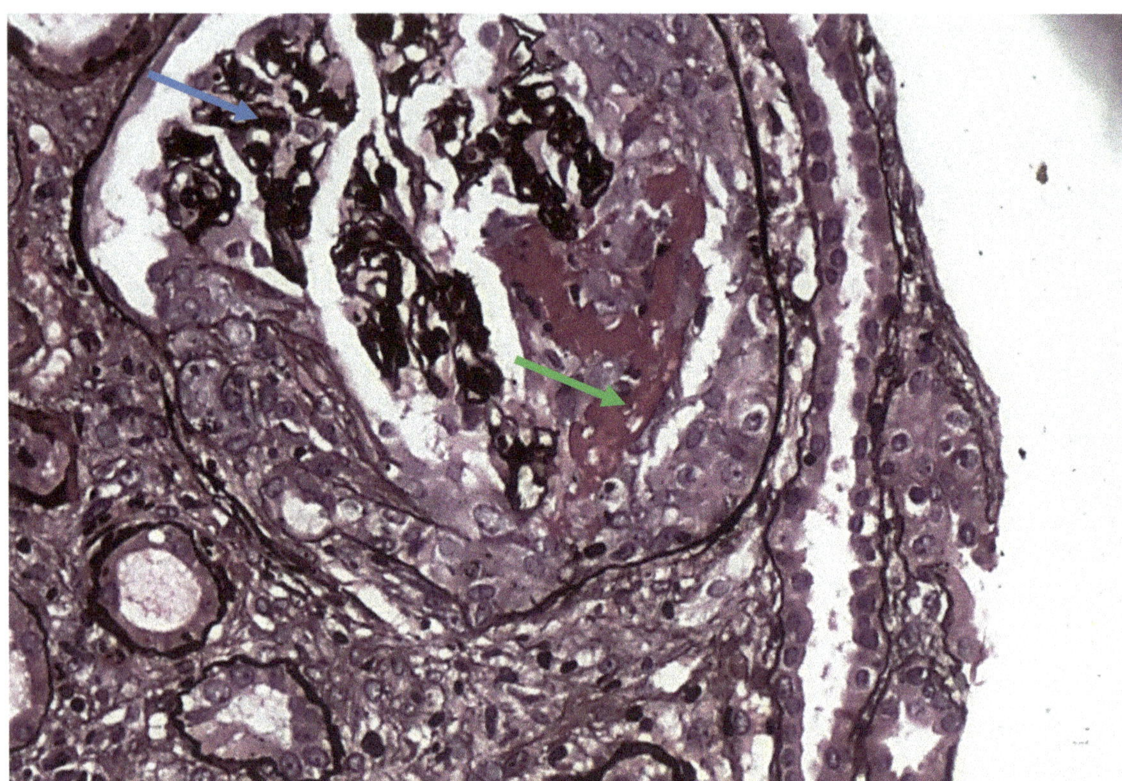

Figure 2:29.2: PASM Stain: 20x: Silver negative fibrin strands (**green** arrow) admixed with cells of crescent. The tuft (**blue** arrow) appears normal and does not show significant increase in mesangial/endocapillary cellularity.

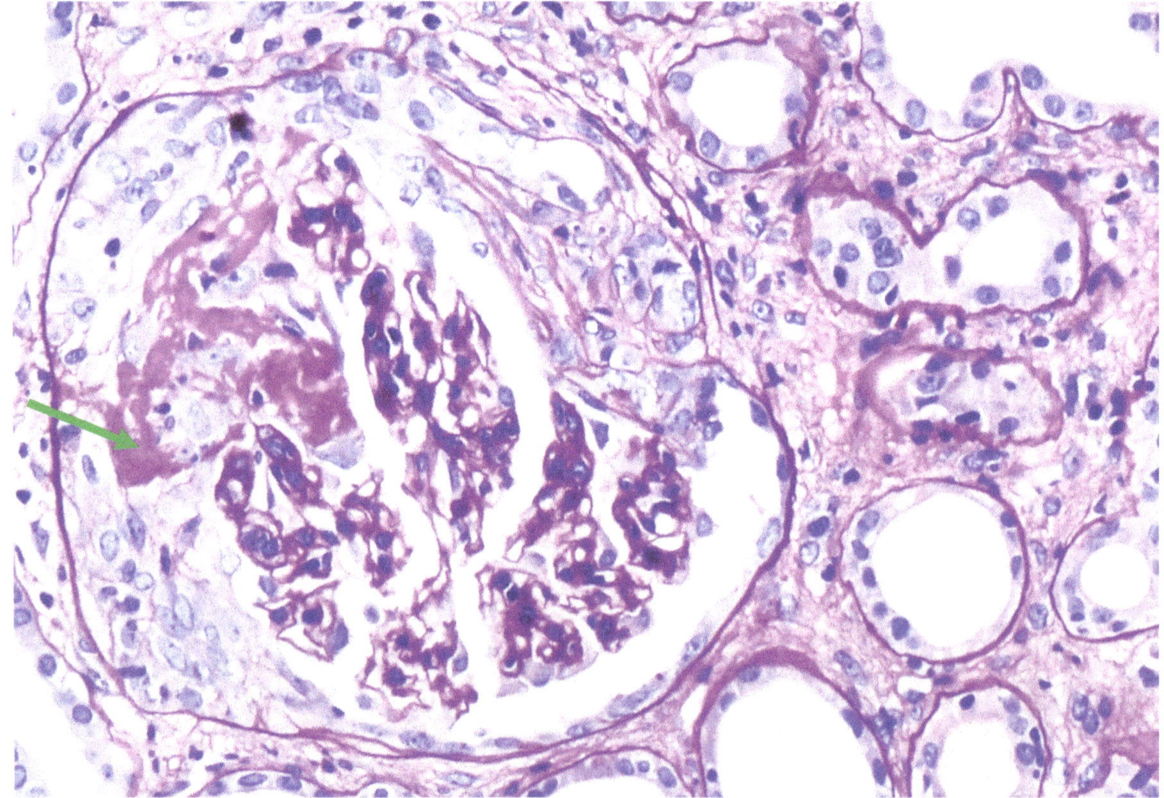

Figure 2:29.3: PAS Stain: 20x: Fuchsinophilic fibrin strands (**green** arrow) admixed with cells of crescent.

Immunofluorescence:

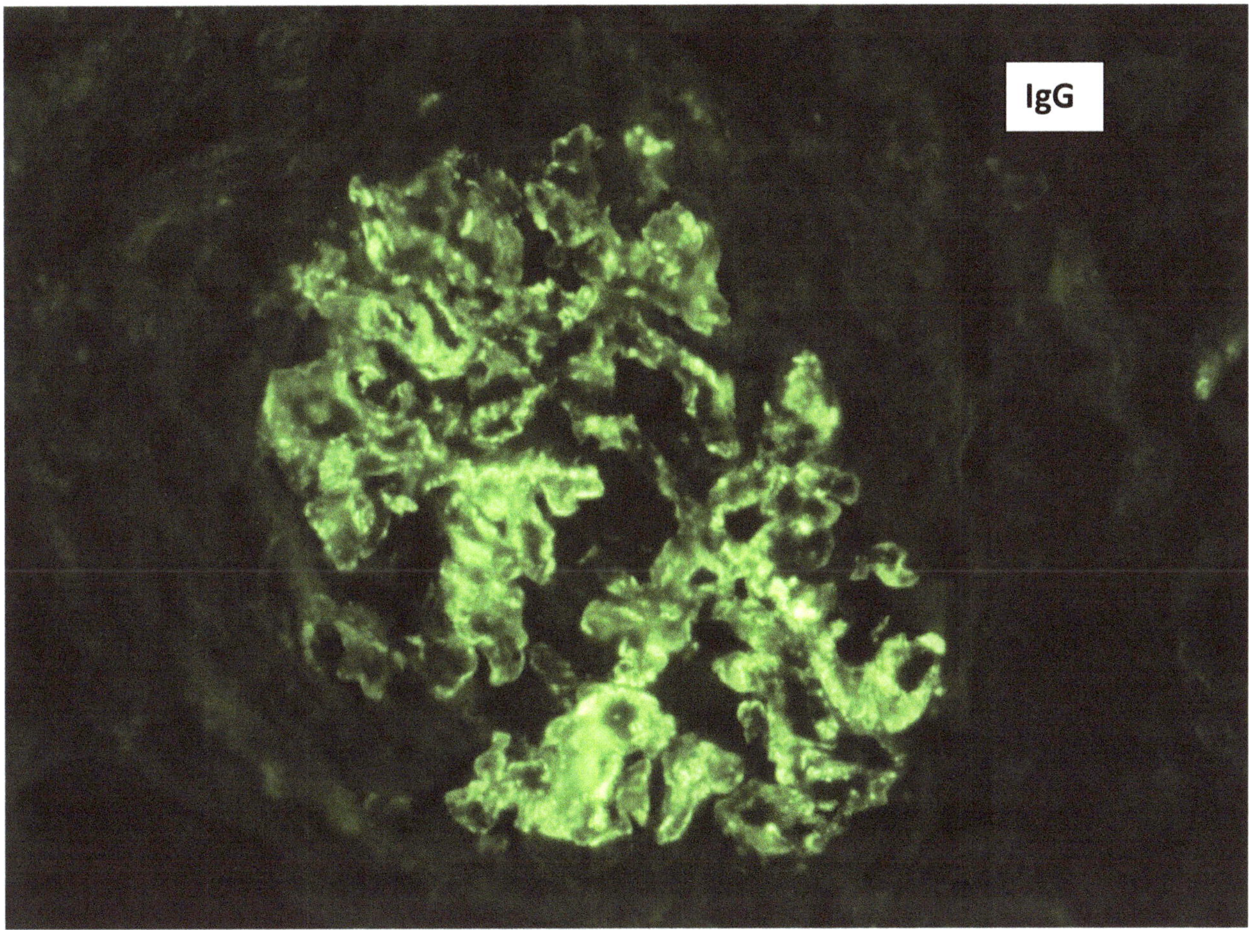

Figure 2:29.4: Immunofluorescence IgG: 20x: Significant capillary wall coarse granular immune deposits.

Interpretation: Anti - GBM disease (Granular IgG deposits).

Additional Investigations: ASO titer: Normal, C3 & C4: Normal, ANA Profile: Negative. ANCA Negative. Anti-GBM serology: Strongly positive.

***Reference:**

Granular Immunofluorescence deposition of IgG in anti-GBM antibody disease, Syed Amer et.al, Pan Afr Med J.2014:17:296.

CASE 30

History: 17-year-old female came with a history of non-pruritic erythematous palpable rash over limbs and trunk a month back associated with polyarthralgia involving large and small joints of upper and lower limbs. She was treated with analgesics and oral steroids with improvement in symptoms. Last 2 weeks she is having frothyuria and pedal edema. No dysuria. She came to ER with headache and bilateral eyes: blurring of vision. No other neurological deficit. Her BP is 160/90 mm of Hg. Fundus examination: papilledema +.

Investigations: CUE: albumin:2+, RBCs: 4 to 5/HPF, WBCs:100 to 110/HPF, 24 hour Urine protein: 804.76mg, spot UPCR:1333 mg/g, serum creatinine:0.61mg/dl, serum albumin:3.32g/dl. Hb 8.5 g/dl, Platelet 1.2 lakhs/cu mm, total leucocyte count: 4,500/cu mm, reticulocyte proliferation index 2.5 %.

Clinical diagnosis: Sub nephrotic proteinuria with active urinary sediment with hypertension and multisystemic involvement: cutaneous, musculoskeletal, hematological and renal. Likely SLE.

Differential diagnoses: Lupus nephritis /HSP Nephritis/ANCA Vasculitis.

Light microscopy:

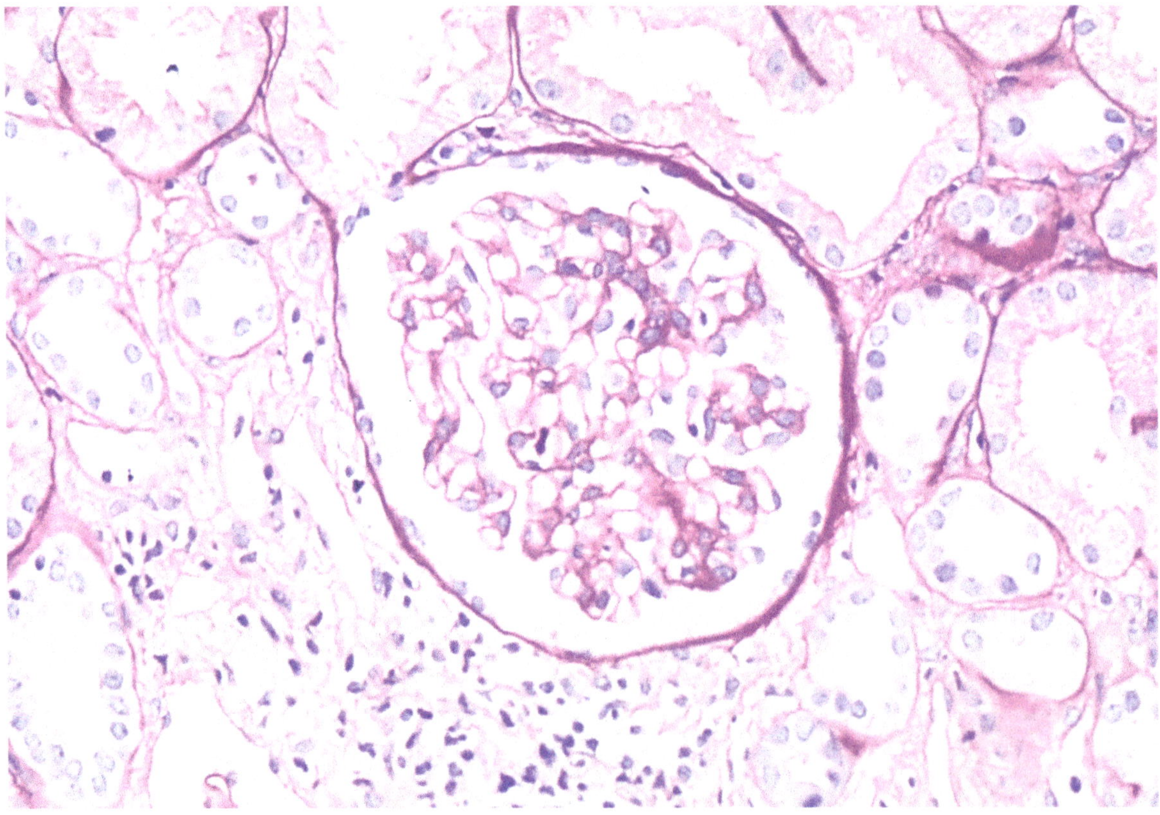

Figure: 2:30.1: PAS Stain: 20x: Normal glomerulus with no evidence of increase in cellularity, basement membrane thickening, segment of sclerosis/necrosis or crescents with surrounding mild interstitial inflammation.

Immunofluorescence:

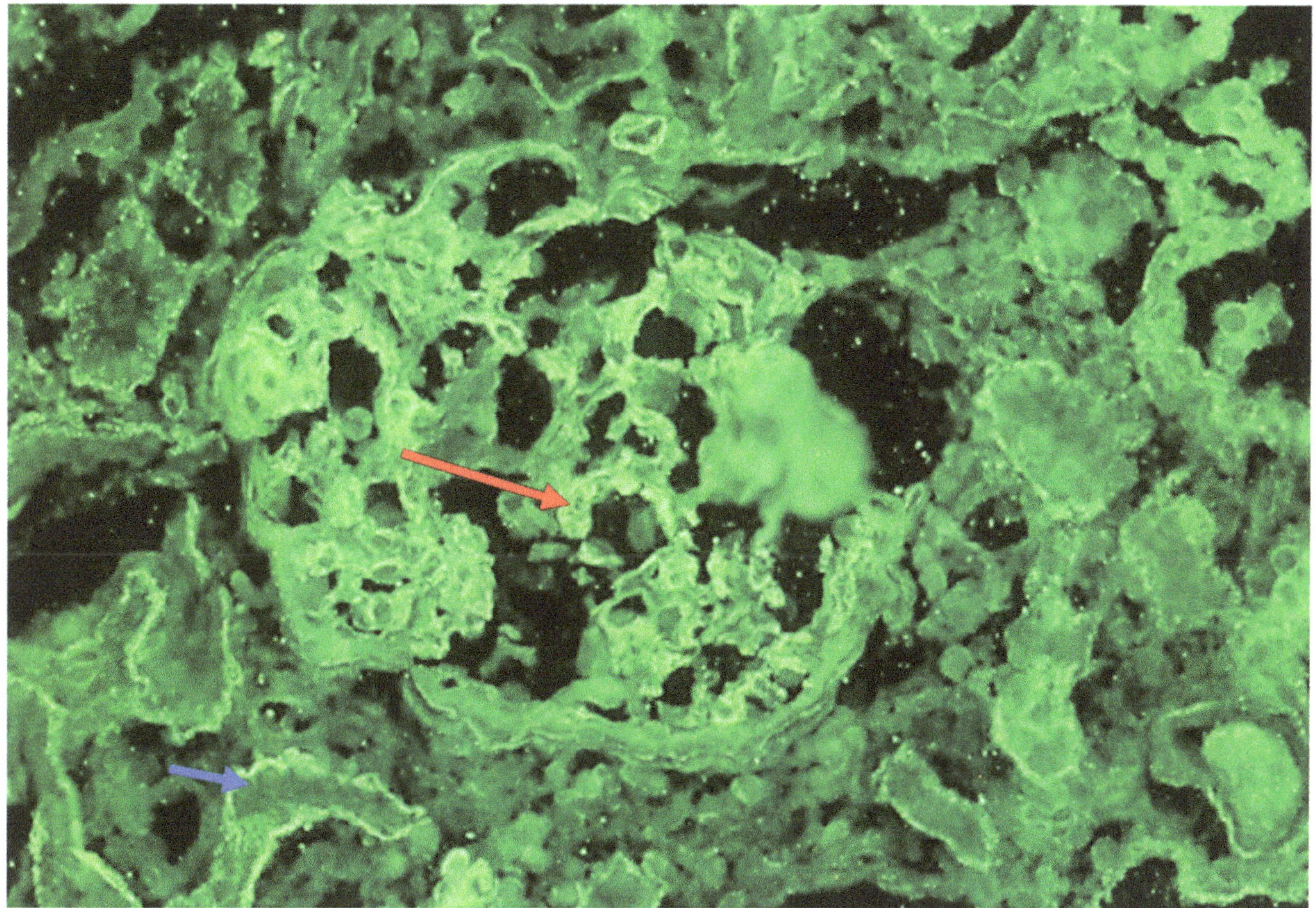

Figure: 2:30.2: Immunofluorescence: IgG:20x: Significant paramesangial and mesangial (red arrow) coarse granular immune deposits of IgG, IgM, C3c, C1q and insignificant IgA. The deposits are seen along the TBMs (tubular basement membranes: blue arrow).

Interpretation:

Pattern of injury: Normal histology on light microscopy and significant Paramesangial and mesangial coarse granular immune deposits on the IF study.

Additional Investigations: ANA: 4+, C3 & C4: both low, anti-histone: +, anti-Sm: +, viral markers: negative.

Final Diagnosis: Lupus nephritis ISN/RPS classification 2004: Class I- Minimal Mesangial LN with minimal activity (activity index:01/24) and no chronicity (chronicity index:00/12)

CASE 31

History: 28 years old female came with one week history of pain and swelling of small and large joints of upper and lower limbs with malar rash on face with painless oral ulcers. She has fever for last one month and generalized weakness for 2 months. No urinary complaints. No cough. No pedal edema. BP is mildly elevated :150/90 mm of Hg.

Investigations: CUE: albumin: 1+, RBCs: 6 to 8 /HPF, WBCs:0 to 1/HPF, 24 hours urine protein:927mg, serum creatinine:0.83mg/dl, serum albumin:3.11gm/dl, HIV: non-reactive, Hep.B: non-reactive, Hep. C: non-reactive.

Clinical diagnosis: Subnephrotic proteinuria and microscopic hematuria with hypertension without renal dysfunction and systemic features of collagen vascular disease likely SLE -Lupus Nephritis: Class II.

Light microscopy:

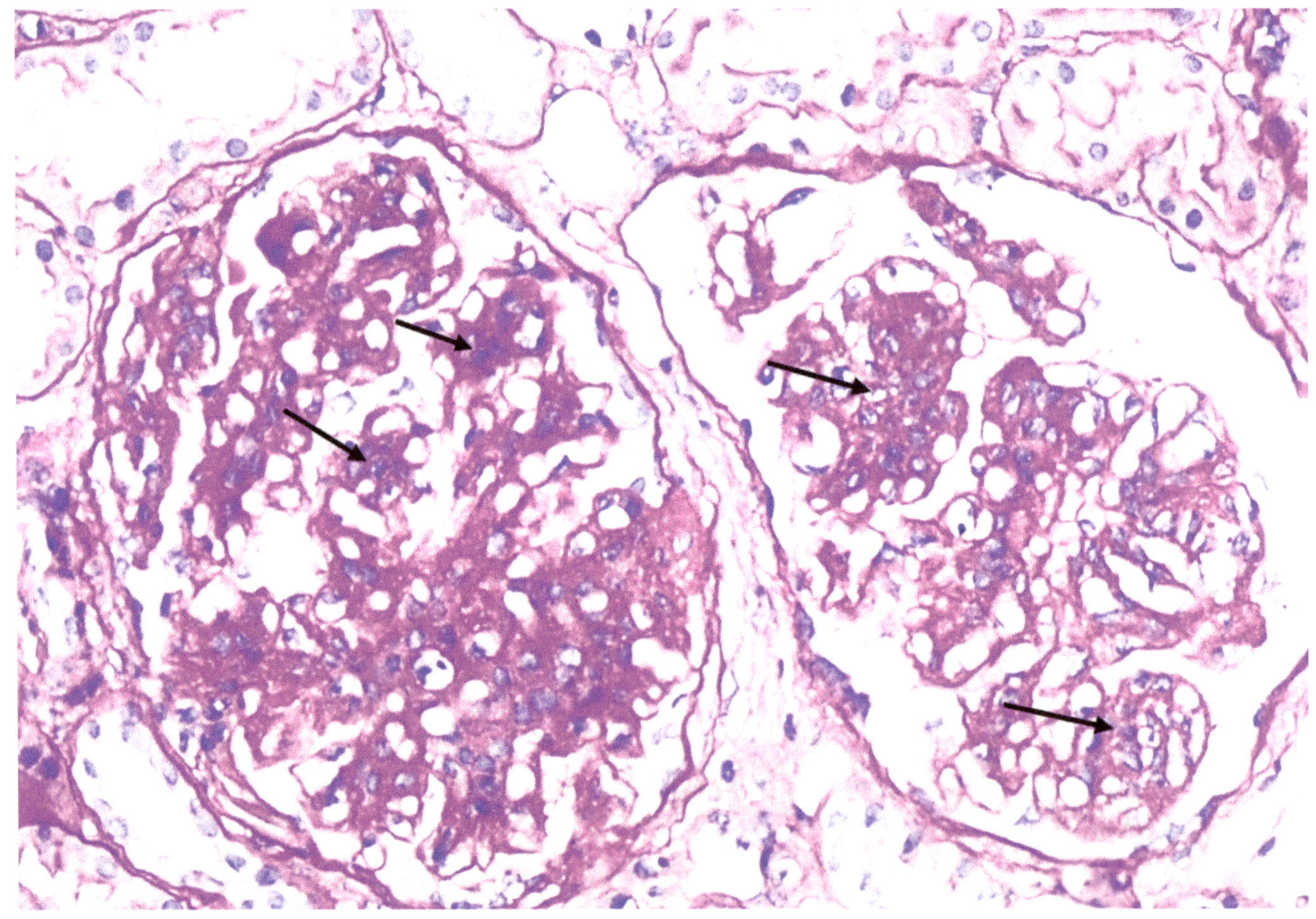

Figure 2:31.1: PAS Stain:20x: Glomeruli: Moderate to marked mesangial hypercellularity. There is no evidence of endocapillary hypercellularity, segment of sclerosis/necrosis, basement membrane thickening or crescents.

Immunofluorescence:

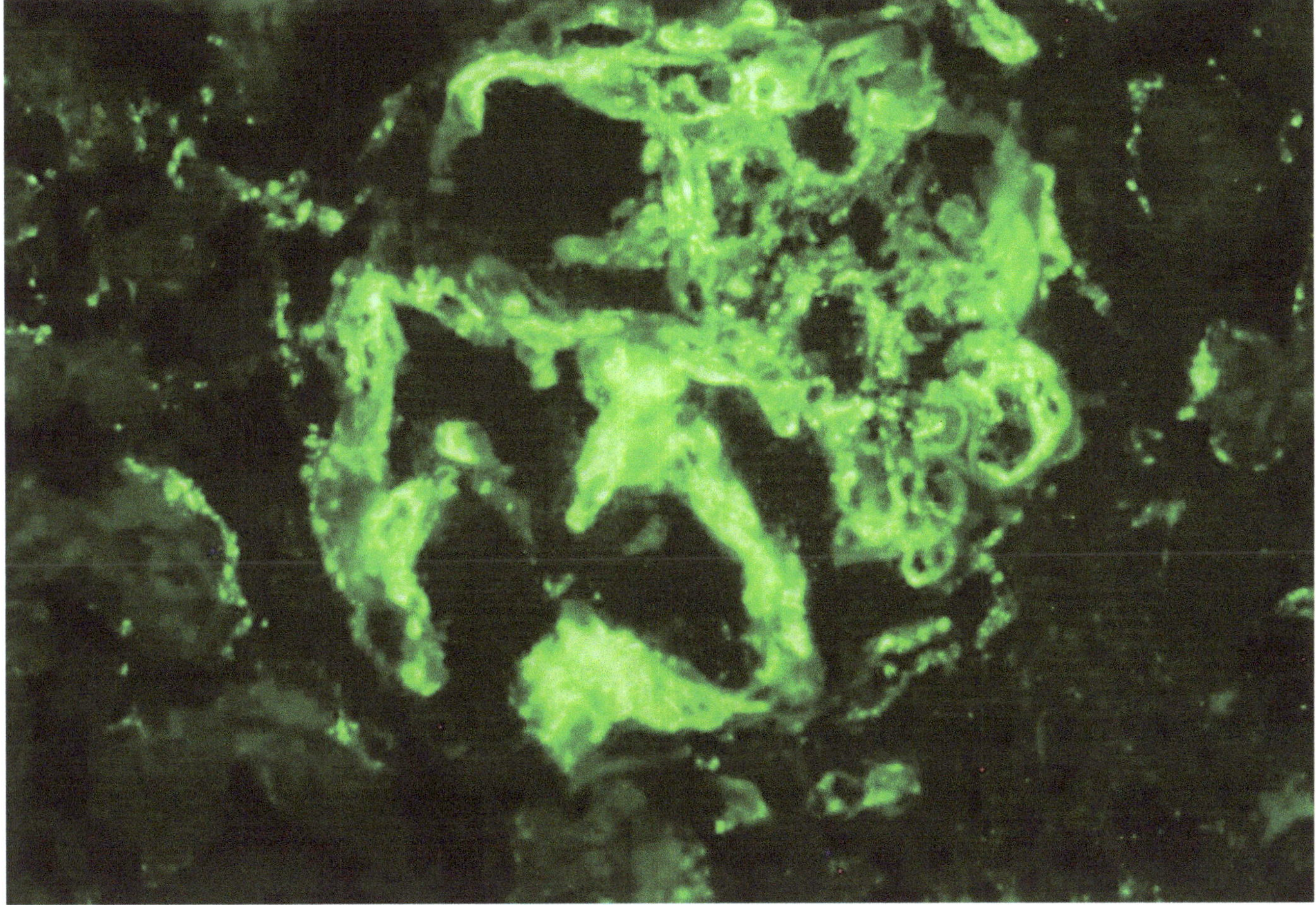

Figure 2:31.2: Immunofluorescence: Glomerulus: Significant Paramesangial and mesangial coarse granular immune deposits of IgG, C3c, C1q. These deposits are seen along the Tubular Basement membranes (TBMs).

Interpretation: Mesangial proliferative GN with IgG, C3c & C1q deposits.

Additional investigations: ANA: 3+, speckled pattern on IF, anti-ds-DNA: positive, C3 and C4: both low.

Final diagnosis: Lupus nephritis

Pattern of injury: Diffuse mesangial hypercellularity

ISN/RPS classification 2004: Class II-Mesangial Proliferative Lupus Nephritis.

CASE 32

History: 20 years old female, non-hypertensive, non-diabetic, no family history of renal disease, presented with malar rash/polyarthralgia in the last 6 months, anasarca since 2 months.

Investigations: ANA: positive, Anti-ds-DNA: positive, 24 hour urine protein: 3 gm/24hrs, CUE: protein:3+, RBCs: plenty/HPF, WBCs:15to 20/HPF, RBC casts: 2-3/HPF, serum albumin:2.9gm/dl. Serum creatinine :2 mg/dl, B.P.:160/90mm of Hg.

Clinical diagnosis: Nephrotic range proteinuria with active urinary sediment with hypertension, renal dysfunction accompanied by systemic features suggestive of collagen vascular disease most likely SLE.

Differential diagnoses: Lupus Nephritis Class III/IV.

Light microscopy:

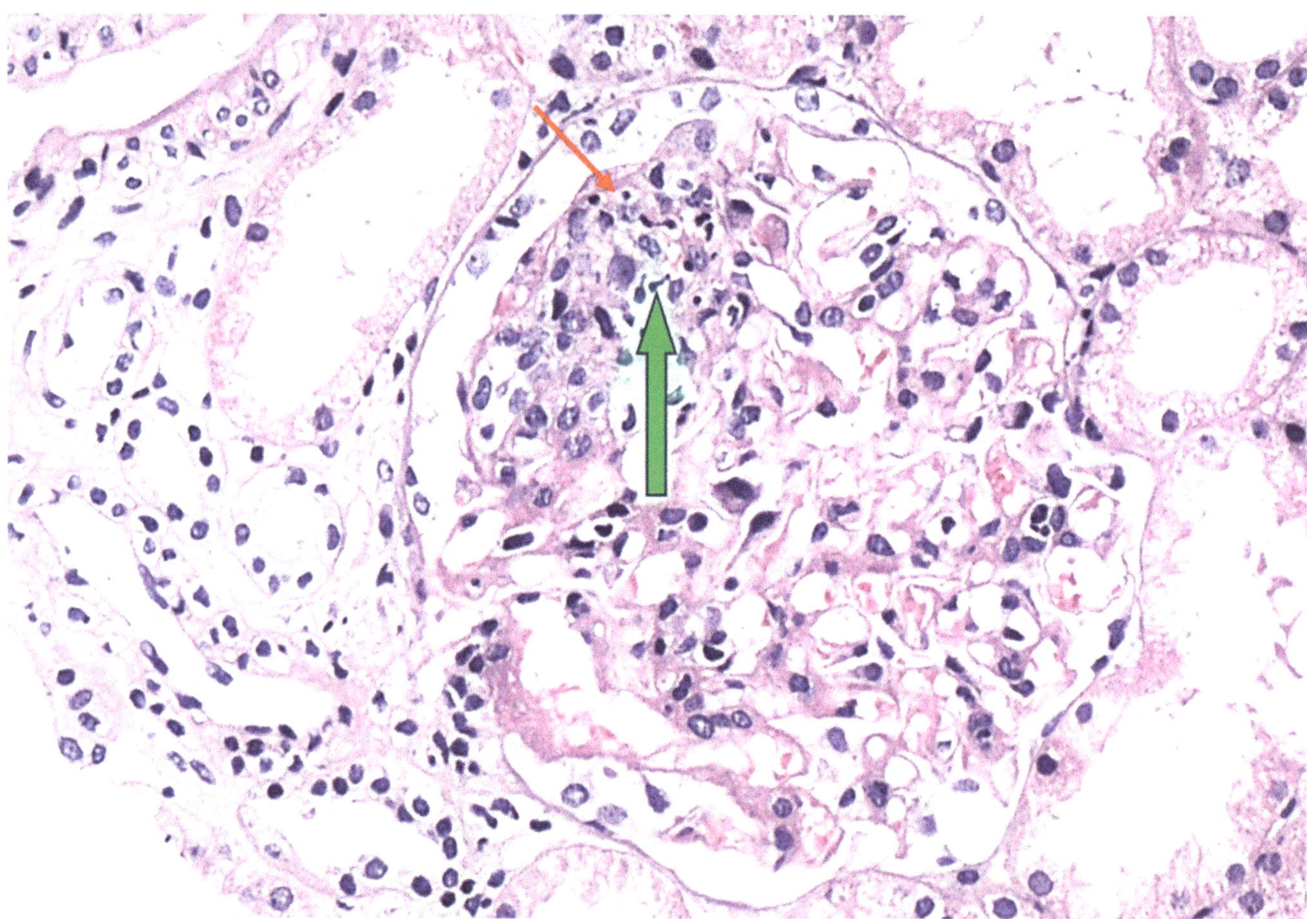

Figure 2:32.1: H&E Stain: 20x: Glomerulus: Segmental endocapillary hypercellularity obliterating the capillary lumina with neutrophilic infiltrate (green arrow) and karyorrhectic debris (red arrow).

Immunofluorescence:

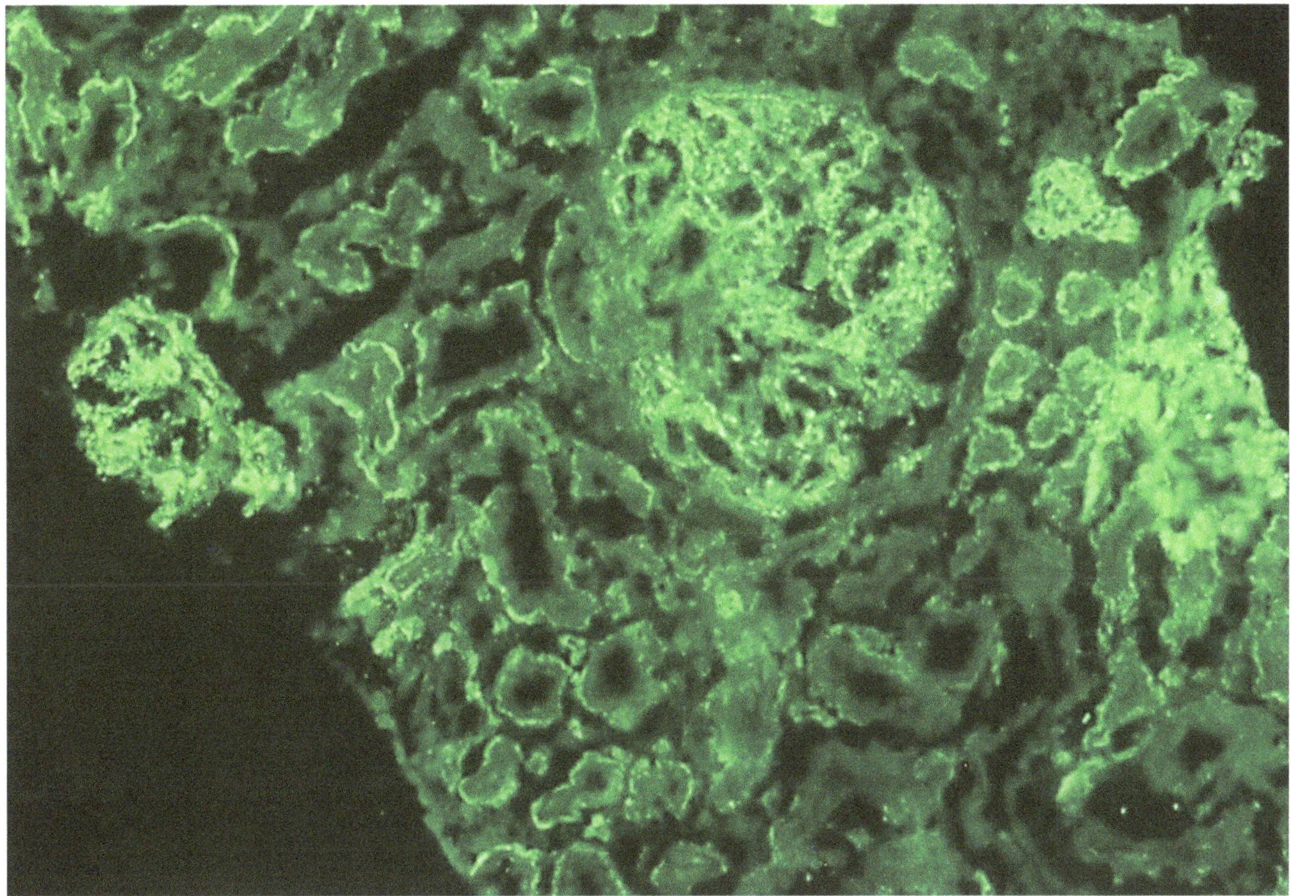

Figure 2:32.2: Immunofluorescence study: IgG 10x: Glomeruli: Significant Paramesangial and mesangial and some capillary wall coarse granular immune deposits of IgG, C3c, C1q, IgM and insignificant IgA. The deposits are seen along the TBMs (tubular basement membranes).

Interpretation:

Primary diagnosis: Lupus nephritis

Pattern of injury: Focal endocapillary hypercellularity

ISN/RPS classification 2004: Class III Focal LN

Additional findings: Uncomplicated vascular immune deposits.

CASE 33

History: 21 years old Female, presented with h/o arthralgias, skin rash and pedal edema. She has elevated BP: 150/90 mm of Hg. She has pedal and periorbital edema. She had a h/o spontaneous first trimester abortion 6 months back. No h/o any episode of DVT.

Investigations: Serum creatinine: 1.3mg/dl. Urine analysis: Protein: 3+, RBCs:15 to 20/HPF, UPCR: 15, ANA: positive, anti-ds-DNA: positive.

Clinical diagnosis: Nephrotic range proteinuria with active urinary sediment with hypertension and renal dysfunction with cutaneous & musculoskeletal involvement and first trimester abortion, most likely SLE.

Differential diagnoses: Class III/IV Lupus Nephritis.

Light microscopy:

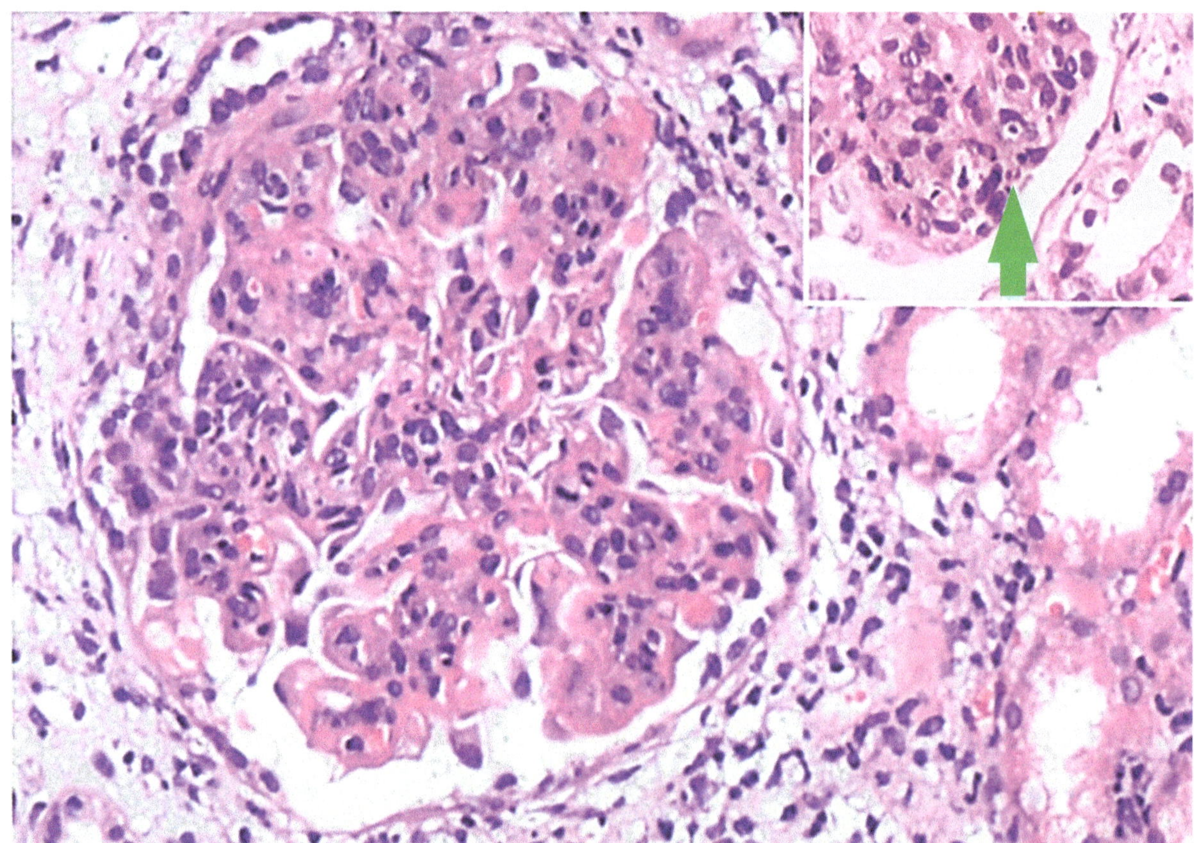

Figure 2:33.1: H&E Stain: 20x: Glomerulus: Diffuse proliferative glomerulonephritis: >50% of glomeruli in this case were hypercellular with diffuse mesangial and endocapillary hypercellularity obliterating the capillary lumina with neutrophilic infiltrate and karyorrhectic debris. **(inset image)** H&E Stain: 40x: Glomerulus: Diffuse proliferative GN, **(green** arrow) karyorrhectic debris.

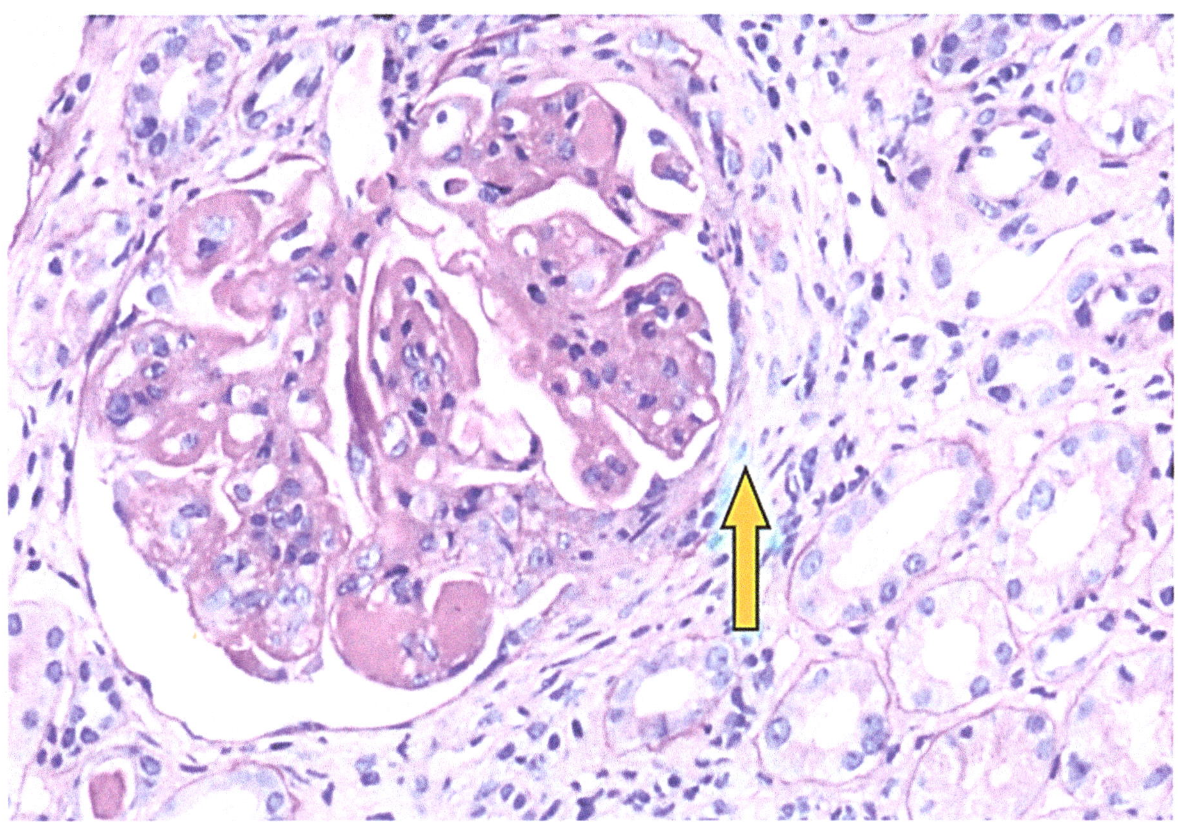

Figure 2:33.2: PAS Stain: 20x: Glomerulus: Segmental cellular crescent: arrow is showing breach in Bowman capsule.

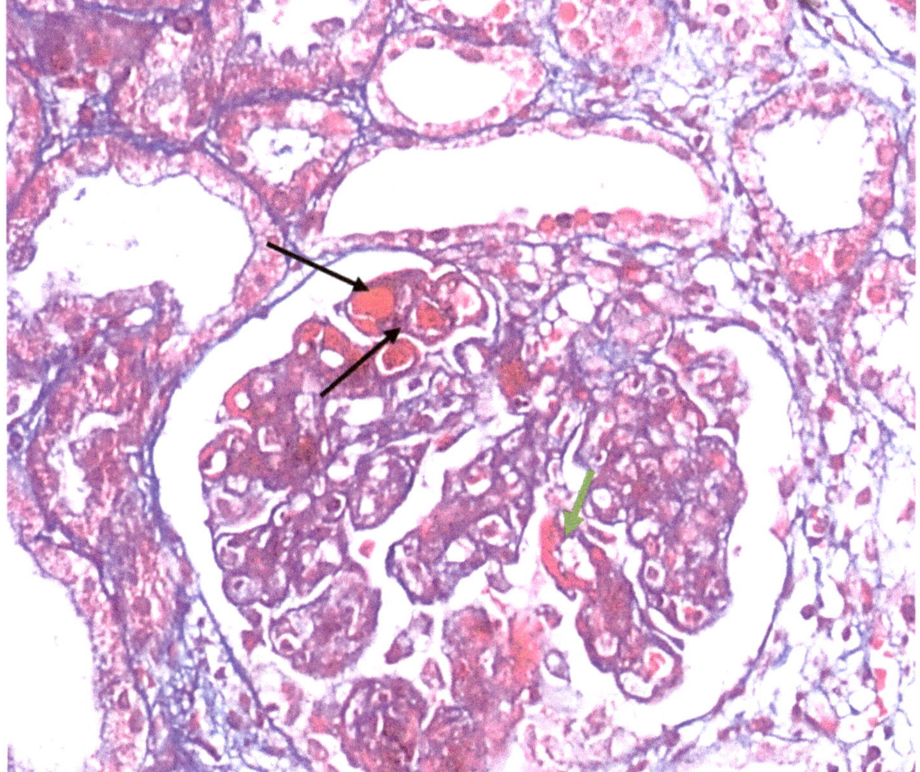

Figure 2:33.3: Masson Trichrome Stain: 20x: Glomerulus: Hyaline thrombi (**black** arrows) and wire-loop lesions (green arrow).

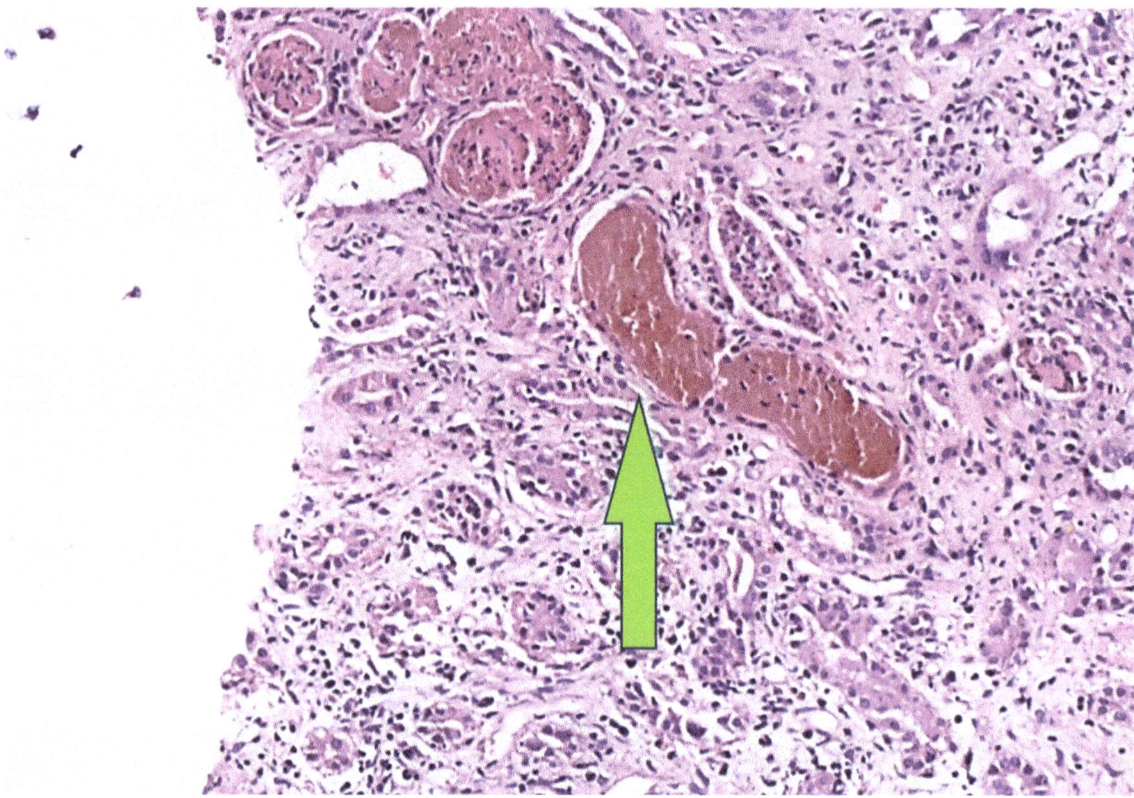

Figure 2:33.4: H&E Stain-10x: Tubules with red cells casts (green arrow).

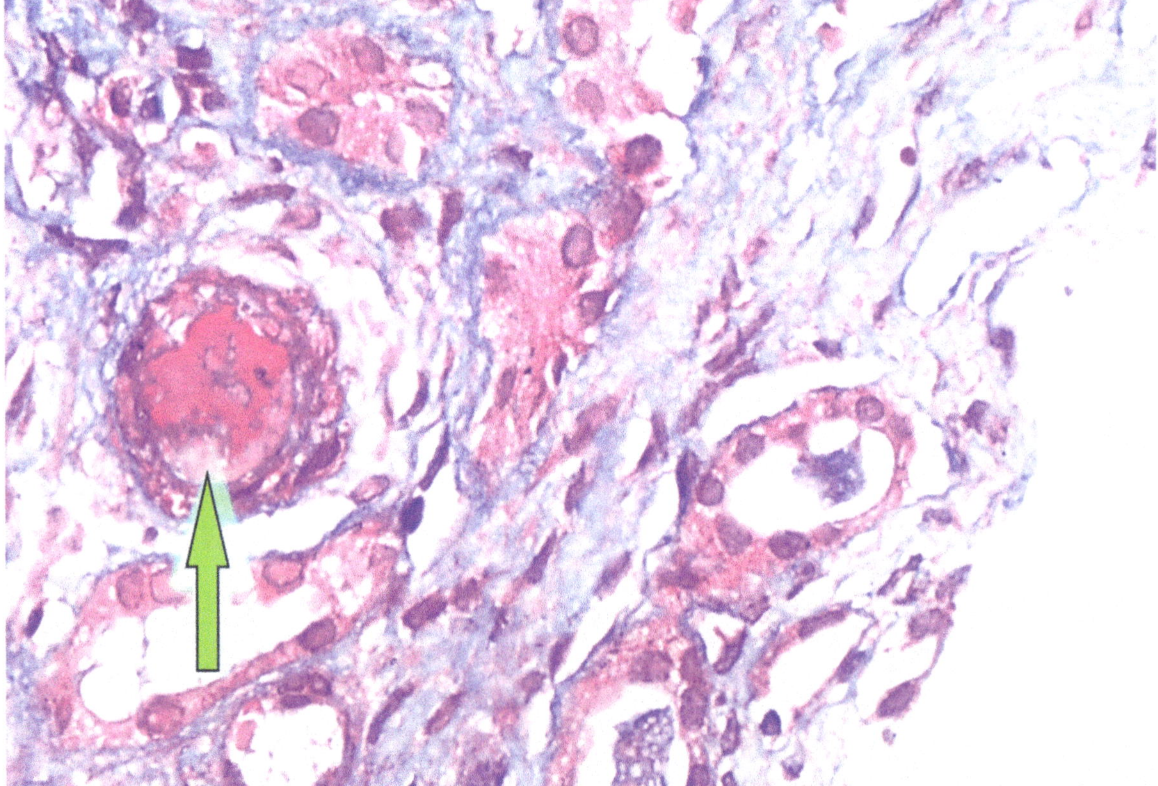

Figure 2:33.5: Masson Trichrome Stain: 40x: Fuchsionphilic fibrin thrombus occluding the arteriole: necrotizing non-inflammatory vascular lesion: Lupus vasculopathy.

Immunofluorescence:

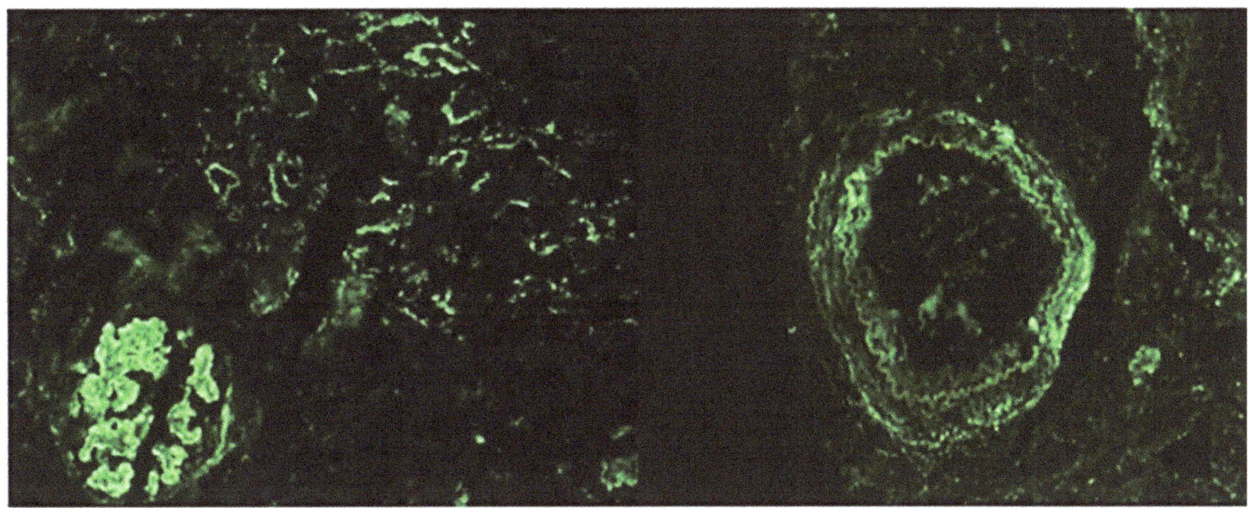

Figure 2:33.6: C1q: Significant capillary wall and mesangial coarse granular immune deposits of IgG, C3c, C1q, IgM and insignificant IgA. glomeruli, tubular basement membranes and vessel wall.

Interpretation: Diffuse proliferative glomerulonephritis (DPGN) with diffuse crescents.

Primary diagnosis: Lupus nephritis

Pattern of injury: Diffuse proliferative GN with crescents (10/18)

ISN/RPS classification 2004: Class IV Diffuse LN with moderate activity (activity index:13/24) and mild chronicity (chronicity index:04/12)

Additional findings: Lupus Vasculopathy

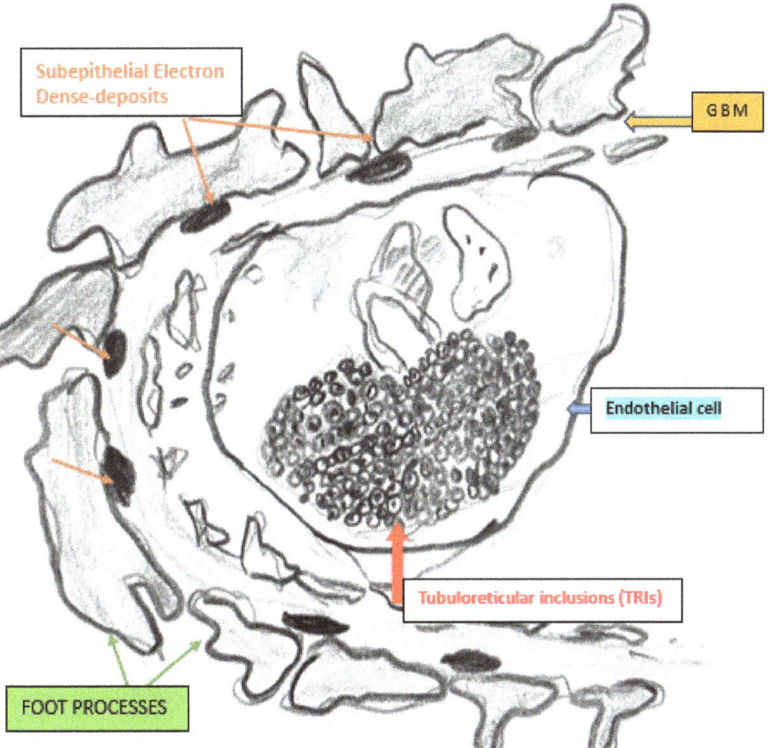

Figure 2:33.7: Diagrammatic representation of Electron Microscopy of tubuloreticular inclusions (TRIs).

Pathology Pearls

Electron microscopy: Lupus Nephritis:

1. **Tubuloreticular inclusions (TRIs):** Detected in: endothelial cells of glomerulus, peritubular capillaries, arteries.

   Located in: dilated cisternae of endoplasmic reticulum.

   Not specific for SLE. Seen in other conditions: HIV infected patients, exposure of excess Interferon, few healthy individuals.

2. **Fingerprint pattern substructure:** Subendothelial electron dense deposit with a fingerprint-whorled, lamellated substructure.

***Vascular lesions in Lupus Nephritis:**

1. **Uncomplicated vascular immune deposits:** Usually clinically silent and most common vascular lesion in Lupus nephritis.

   Light microscopy: The vessels appear normal.

   Immunofluorescence study: Granular immune deposits of IgG, IgM , IgA, C3c & C1q, Kappa, Lambda within intima and media of the vessels.

2. **Lupus vasculopathy (Noninflammatory necrotizing vasculopathy):** Preglomerular arterioles and interlobular arteries are affected.

   Light microscopy: Partial or near total occlusion of vessels by fibrin thrombi may be extending into media and no inflammatory infiltration of the vessel walls.

   Immunofluorescence study: Granular immune deposits into intima of the vessel: IgG, IgM, IgA, C3c & C1q, Kappa, Lambda within intima and media of the vessels.

3. **TMA (Thrombotic microangiopathy):** Difficult to differentiate from Lupus vasculopathy.

Features	TMA	Lupus vasculopathy
Preglomerular arterioles &interlobular arteries affected	+	+
Glomerular fibrin thrombi, mesangiolysis	+	-
Myointimal proliferation (onion skinning)	+	-
IF: IgG	-	+
C4d stain	+	-

4. Lupus necrotizing vasculitis.

5. SLE with Anti phospholipid antibody syndrome.

6. SLE with scleroderma/ mixed connective tissue disorder.

***Reference**

Heptinstall's Pathology of Kidney, Seventh edition, Chapter 14: Connective tissue diseases: Page no.572-576.

CASE 34

History: 27-year-old female, non-hypertensive, non-diabetic, no family H/O renal disease, presented with mild fever of 2 months duration without cough or dysuria. She was treated with multiple antibiotics for last few weeks with no significant relief. No significant weight loss. She has started having excessive hair loss and noticed worsening pedal edema over last 3 weeks, B.P.:140/90 mm of Hg.

Investigations: serum creatinine: 1.18mg/dl, UPCR: 4.84, serum albumin: 1.2gm/dl, urine protein: 4+, RBCs: 8 to 10/HPF, pus cells: 2 to 3/HPF. ANA: positive. C3& C4: both low, anti-Smith antibodies: +, anti-nucleosome antibodies: 3+, anti-histone antibodies: 2+.

Clinical Diagnosis: Nephrotic range proteinuria with microscopic hematuria without renal dysfunction.

Differential diagnoses: Lupus Nephritis Class V.

Light microscopy:

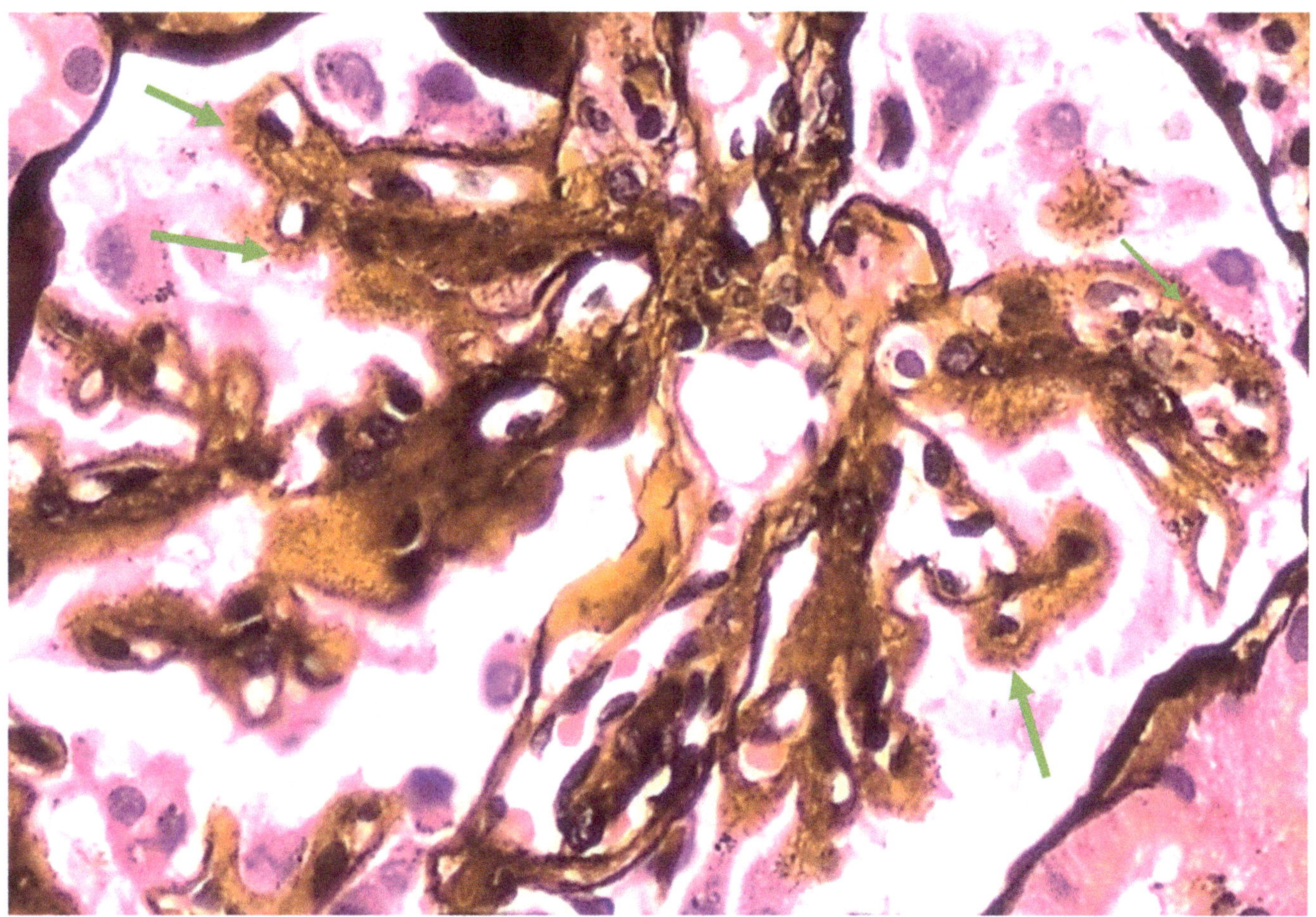

Figure 2:34.1: PASM Stain: 40x: Glomerulus: Diffuse subepithelial spikes.

Immunofluorescence:

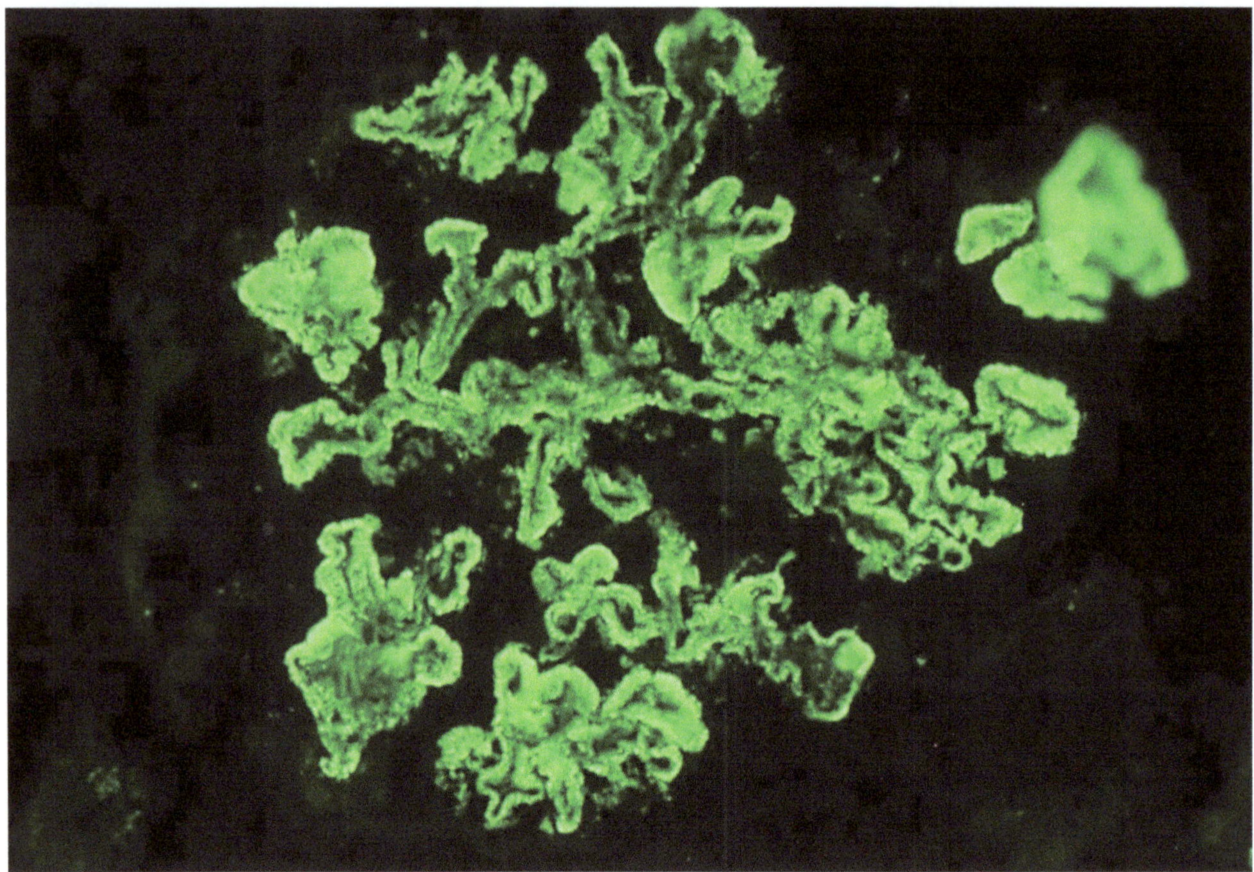

Figure 2:34.2: Immunofluorescence: IgG, C3c, C1q: 20x: Significant diffuse capillary wall fine granular immune deposits.

Interpretation:

Kidney (needle) biopsy:

Primary diagnosis: Lupus nephritis.

Pattern of injury: Diffuse subepithelial spikes .

ISN/RPS classification 2004: Class V-Membranous Lupus Nephritis with minimal activity (activity index:01/24) and mild chronicity (chronicity index:02/12).

Additional findings: Uncomplicated vascular immune deposits.

History: 25 years old female, K/C/O SLE for last 2 years received treatment on and off for arthralgias and skin lesions, now on treatment for skin and early renal involvement with Mycophenolate and low dose steroids along with other supportive medicines for last 3 months. She stopped medication for last 1 month due to psychological issues. Now presented with accelerated hypertension, headache, and gross anasarca.

Investigations: ANA: positive, anti-ds-DNA: positive, spot UPCR:9 g/g, serum creatinine:3.8mg/dl.

Clinical diagnosis: RPGN-SLE/Lupus nephritis.

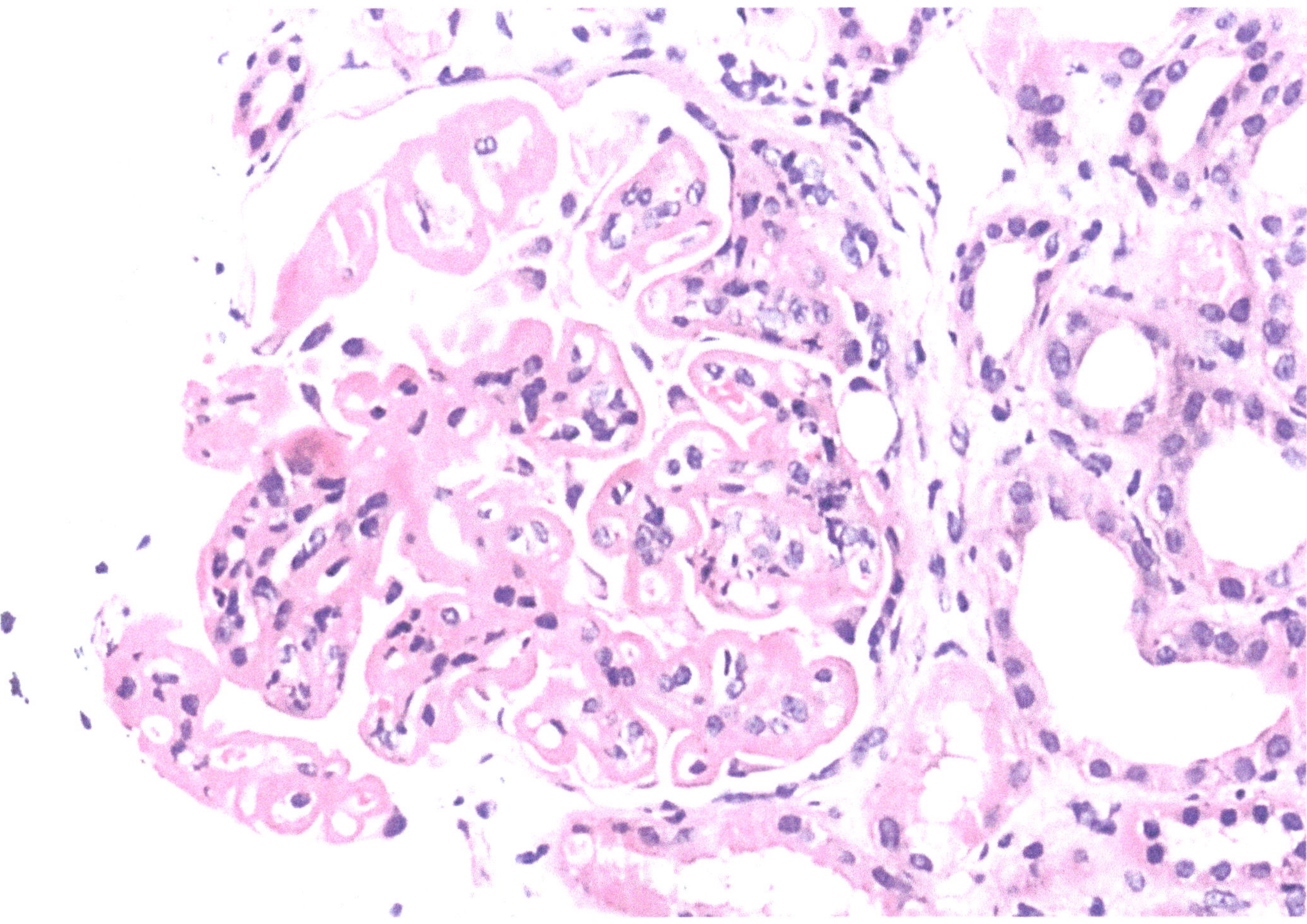

Figure 2:35.1: H& E Stain: Glomerulus: The basement membranes show diffuse uniform thickening and rigidity with diffuse endocapillary hypercellularity obliterating the capillary lumina with neutrophils, karyorrhectic debris is also seen.

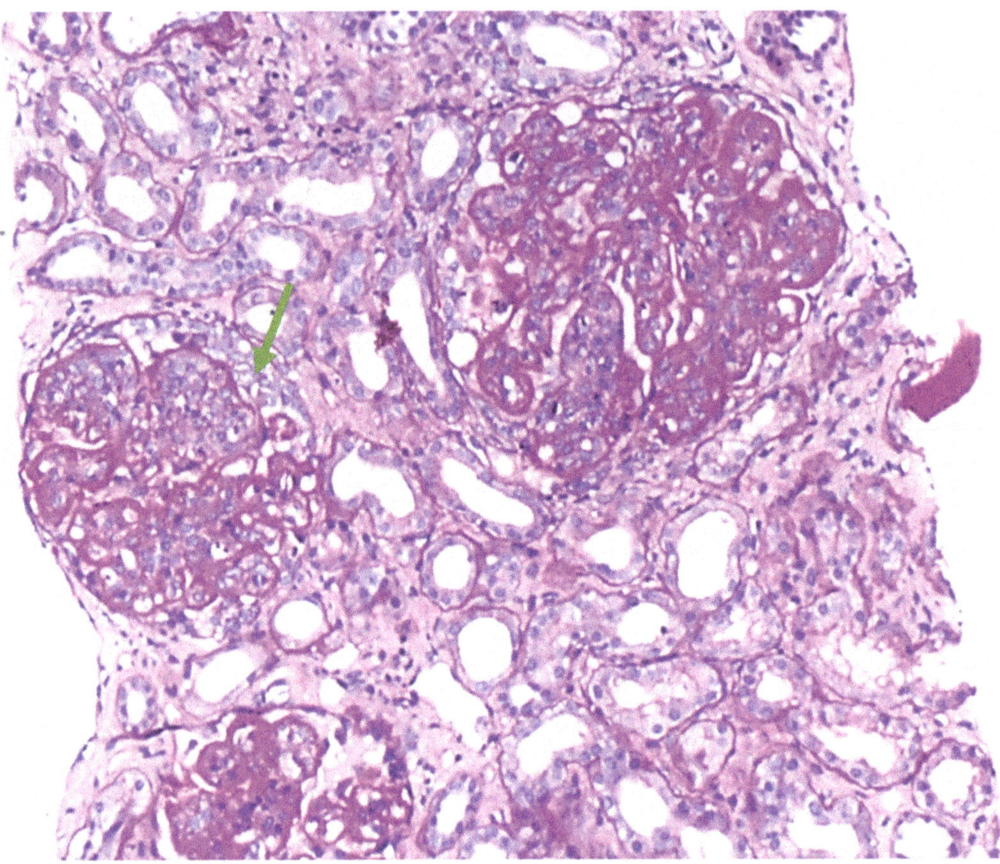

Figure 2:35.2: PAS Stain:10x: Glomeruli: diffuse proliferative GN with segmental cellular crescent (green arrow). The glomerular basement membranes are thickened.

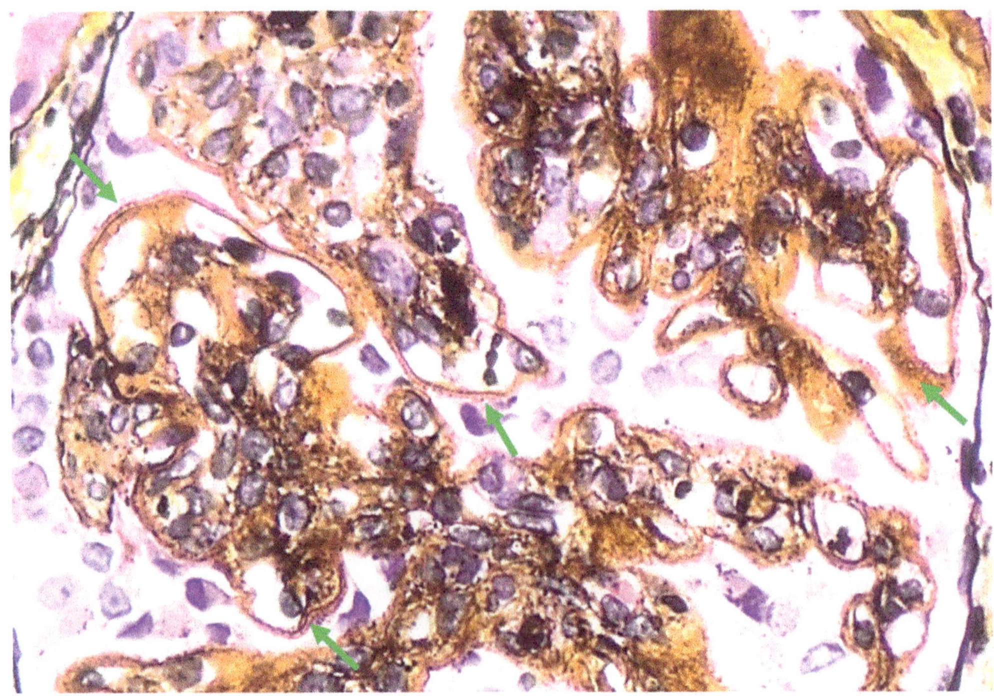

Figure 2:35.3: PASM Stain:40x: diffuse subepithelial spikes (green arrows).

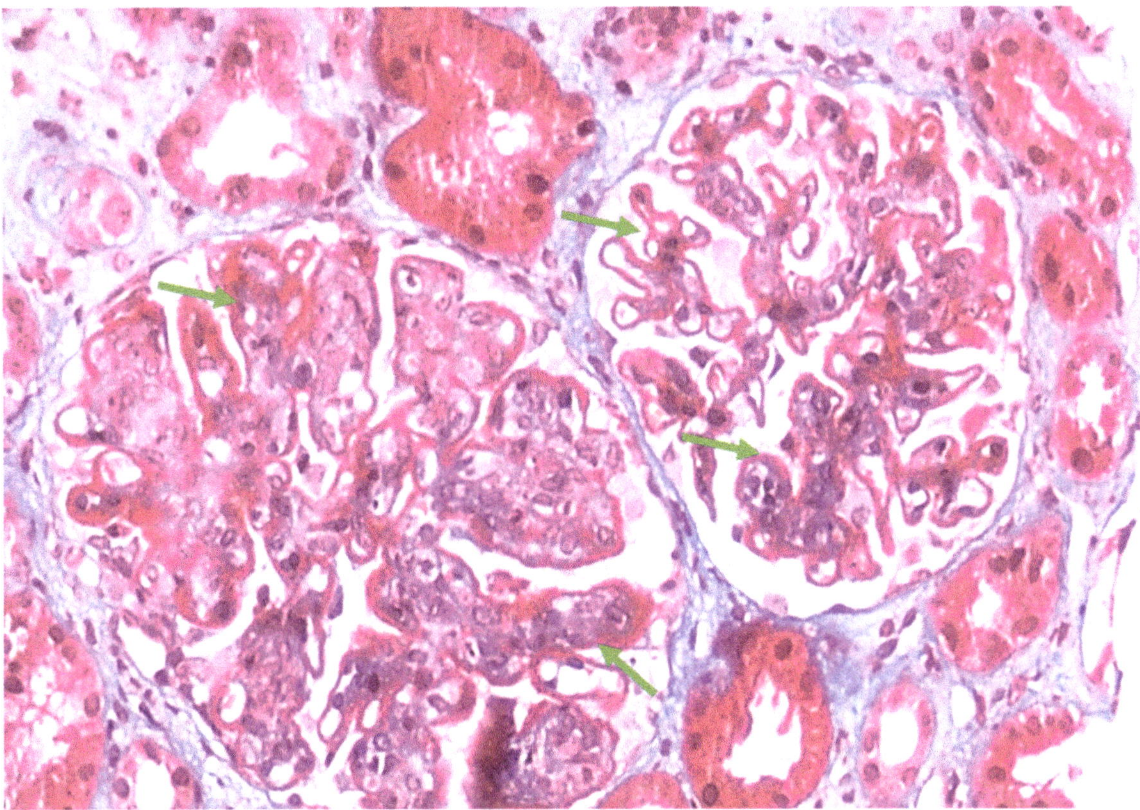

Figure 2:35.4: MT Stain:20x: Glomeruli with diffuse subepithelial fuchsinophilic deposits (green arrows).

Immunofluorescence:

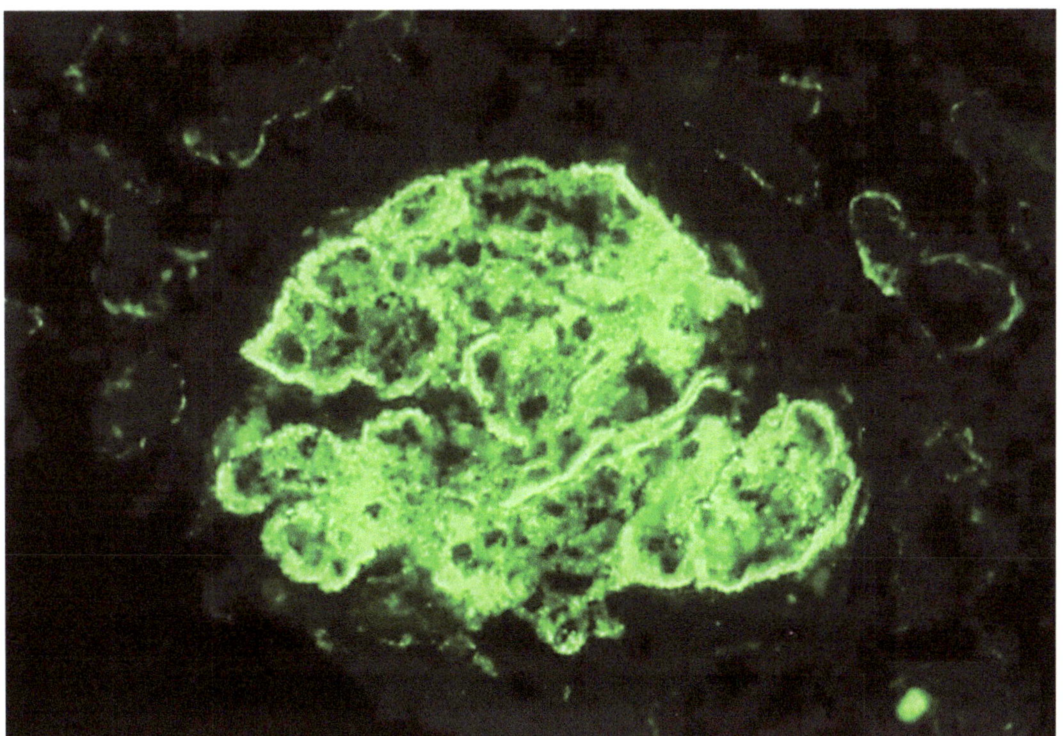

Figure 2:35.5: Immunofluorescence: Significant IgG, C3c, C1q: capillary wall and some mesangial granular immune deposits.

Interpretation:

Primary diagnosis: Lupus nephritis.

Pattern of injury: Diffuse subepithelial spikes and diffuse proliferative GN with focal crescents (04/11), focal wire-loop lesions & hyaline thrombi.

ISN/RPS classification 2004: Mixed Lupus Nephritis: Class V-Membranous LN + Class IV -Diffuse LN with moderate activity (activity index:13/24) and mild chronicity (chronicity index:04/12).

Pathology Pearls

The threshold for diagnosis of membranous lupus nephritis in a proliferative class is membranous involvement of > 50% of the tuft of > 50% of the glomeruli by light microscopy or immunofluorescence.

***Reference**

The classification of glomerulonephritis in systemic lupus erythematosus revisited, Weening JJ, et.al: J Am Soc Nephrol 2004;15(2):241-250.

History: 23 years old female, a diagnosed case of Lupus Nephritis class 3, on immunosuppression for more than 3 years duration. Progressive worsening BP control and renal function over last 6 months despite of optimal immunosuppression with MMF. Creatinine has risen from 3mg/dl last year to 6mg/dl now in last 1-2 months' time. No other extra renal symptoms except anemia.

Clinical diagnosis: Lupus Nephritis. Renal biopsy planned to confirm class change and chronicity to decide regarding treatment with cyclophosphamide versus stepping down immunosuppression.

Light microscopy:

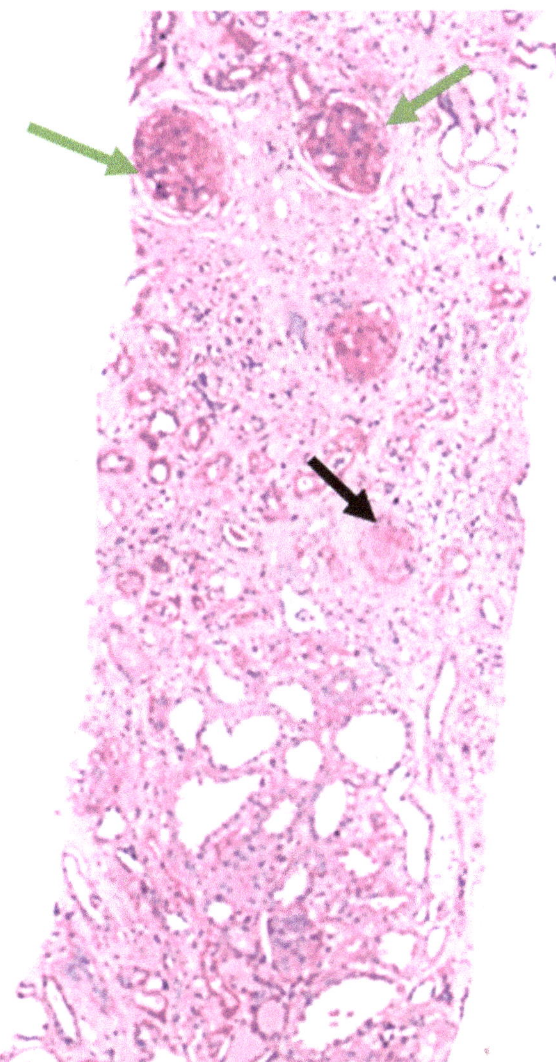

Figure 2:36.1: PAS Stain:10x: Dark PAS positive globally sclerosed glomeruli (green arrows), marked IF/TA and PAS negative fibrous crescent (**black** arrow).

Immunofluorescence:

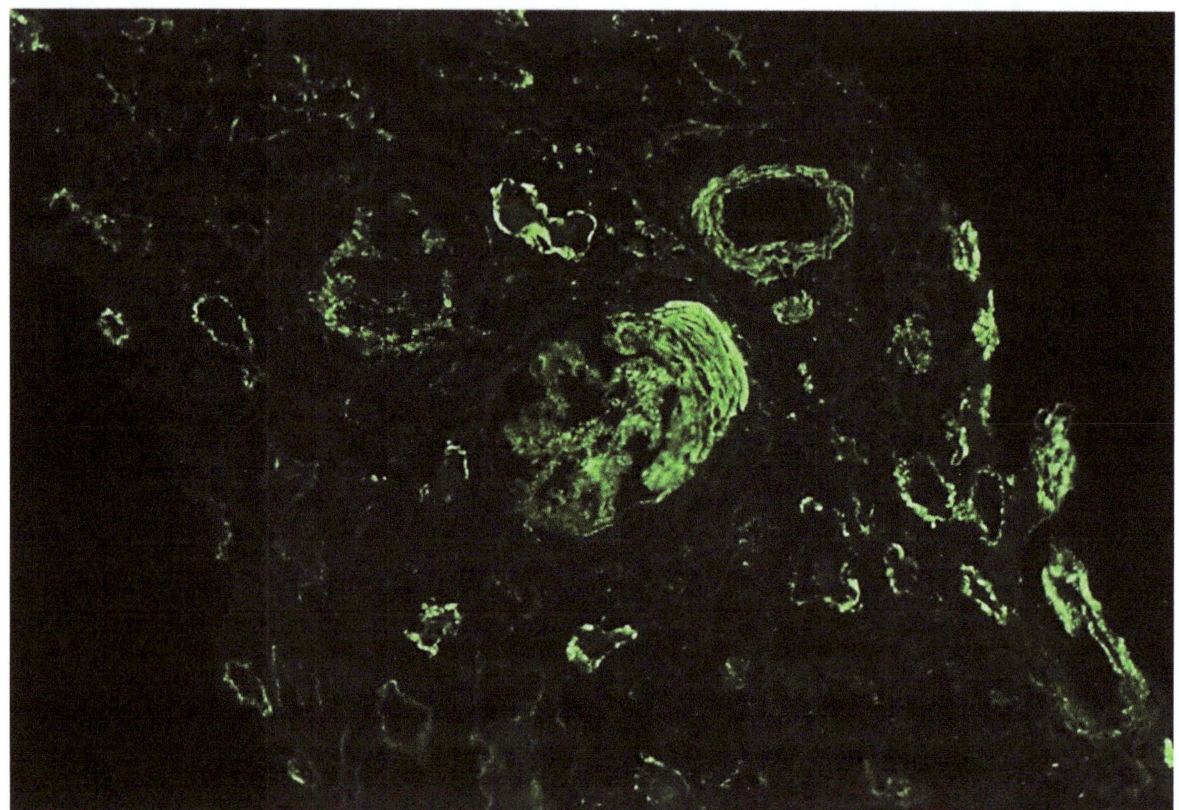

Figure 2:36.2: Immunofluorescence: 10x: Glomeruli, tubules and vessels with full-house immune deposits.

Interpretation: In view of K/C/O Lupus Nephritis, a diagnosis of ISN/RPS Classification 2004: Class VI: Advanced sclerosing lupus nephritis with mild activity (activity index:02/24) and marked chronicity (chronicity index:10/12) to be considered.

Pathology Pearls

Non-lupus Full House Nephropathy:

Glomerular "full-house" immunofluorescence: common in Lupus Nephritis.

Full house meaning (3 of a kind and 2 of a kind in poker parlance).

IF study: 03 immunoglobulins (IgG, IgM and IgA) and 02 complements: C3 and C1q are strongly positive.

Some non-lupus nephropathy also can present with a "full-house" immunofluorescence pattern, which are:

1. Membranous Nephropathy.

2. Membranoproliferative Glomerulonephritis.

3. IgA Nephropathy.

4. Infection Related Glomerulonephritis.

5. C1q Nephropathy.

6. Idiopathic Non-Lupus full-house nephropathy.

Lupus Nephritis /RPS Classification: 2004:

Class I: Minimal Mesangial Lupus Nephritis:

Normal glomeruli by LM, but mesangial immune deposits by IF

Class II: Mesangial Proliferative LN:

Purely mesangial hypercellularity of any degree or mesangial matrix expansion by LM with mesangial immune deposits.

There may be a few isolated subepithelial or subendothelial deposits visible by IF or EM but not by LM.

Class III: Focal LN:

Active or inactive focal, segmental and /or global endocapillary and /or extracapillary GN involving <50% of all glomeruli, typically with focal subendothelial immune deposits with or without mesangial alterations.

Class IV: Diffuse LN:

Active or inactive focal, segmental and /or global endocapillary and /or extracapillary GN involving ≥50% of all glomeruli, typically with focal subendothelial immune deposits with or without mesangial alterations.

Class V: Membranous LN:

Global or segmental subepithelial immune deposits or their morphological sequelae by LM and by IF or EM, with or without mesangial alterations.

Class VI: Advanced Sclerosing LN:

90% or more of glomeruli globally sclerosed without residual activity.

Table 2:36.1: Modified NIH lupus nephritis activity scoring system.

Modified NIH activity index	Definition	Score
Endocapillary hypercellularity	In <25% (1+),25%–50% (2+), or >50% (3+) of glomeruli	0-3
Neutrophils/karyorrhexis	In <25% (1+),25%–50% (2+), or >50% (3+) of glomeruli	0-3
Fibrinoid necrosis	In <25% (1+),25%–50% (2+), or >50% (3+) of glomeruli	(0-3)x2
Hyaline deposits	In <25% (1+),25%–50% (2+), or >50% (3+) of glomeruli	0-3
Cellular/fibrocellular crescents	In <25% (1+),25%–50% (2+), or >50% (3+) of glomeruli	(0-3)x2
Interstitial Inflammation	Interstitial leukocytes in <25% (1+),25%–50% (2+), or >50% (3+) in the cortex	0-3
Total		0-24

Table 2:36.2: Modified NIH lupus nephritis chronicity scoring system.

Modified NIH chronicity index	Definition	Score
Total glomerulosclerosis score	Global and/or segmental sclerosis in <25% (1+), 25%–50% (2+), or >50% (3+) of glomeruli	0-3
Fibrous crescents	In <25% (1+),25%–50% (2+), or >50% (3+) of glomeruli	0-3
Tubular atrophy	in <25% (1+),25%–50% (2+), or >50% (3+)of the cortical tubules	0-3
Interstitial fibrosis	in <25% (1+),25%–50% (2+), or >50% (3+) in the cortex	0-3
Total		0-12

***Reference:**

Revision of the International Society of Nephrology/Renal Pathology Society classification for lupus nephritis: clarification of definitions and modified National Institutes of Health activity and chronicity indices: Kidney Int 2018 Apr;93(4):789-796.

CASE 37

History: 51-year-old female, non-diabetic, hypertensive for last 2 years, has numbness in both feet for last 6 months; she is non-alcoholic & had a normal vitamin B12 level when last checked. Now presented with worsening edema feet and feeling lightheaded/giddy on standing for last one month. She has stopped taking her BP medicines for last one week. There has been generalized weakness and loss of appetite for the last 2 weeks. There is no h/o of using any indigenous medicines or NSAIDs or skin lightening creams. No h/o suggestive of any chronic infection or inflammatory condition like arthritis. BP: 90/60 mm of Hg, Pedal edema, skin showing bruises suggesting capillary fragility.

Investigations: Viral screening: Negative. Urine protein 4+, Urine glucose: 2+, HBA1c: 5.4 %, 24 hrs urine protein: 4.7 gm, serum creatinine: 0.5 mg/dl, Serum Potassium :3.4 mEq/L, Serum Sodium: 138 mEq/L, Serum Chloride: 111 mEq/L, Serum Bicarbonate: 14 mEq/L, serum albumin:3.4g/dl.

Clinical Diagnosis: Nephrotic range proteinuria with normal anion gap hyperchloremic metabolic acidosis with glucosuria without hypertension or renal dysfunction with sensory neuropathy and autoimmune symptoms

Differential diagnoses: (1) Membranous nephropathy -autoimmune etiology with RTA (2) Paraproteinemia-Amyloidosis with type 2 Renal Tubular Acidosis (RTA).

Light microscopy:

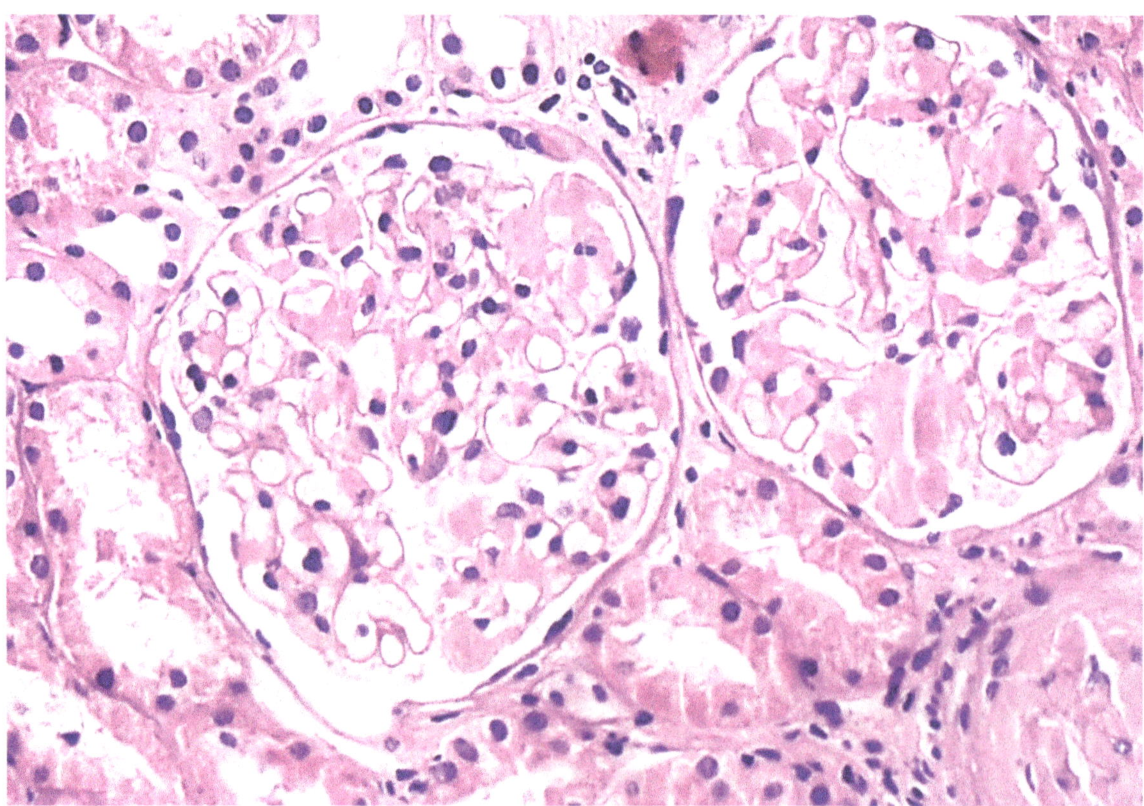

Figure 2:37.1: H&E Stain: 20x: Glomerulus: Eosinophilic, waxy material in mesangium.

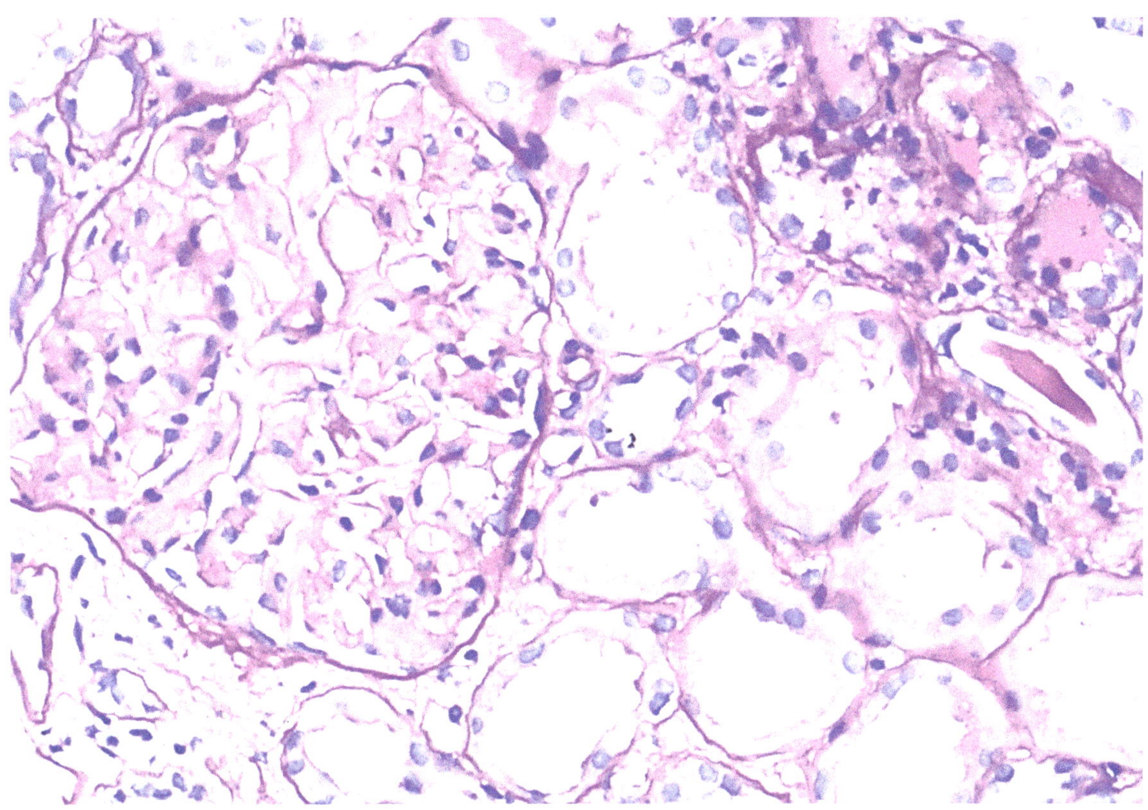

Figure 2:37.2: PAS Stain: 20x: Glomerulus: PAS-negative material in mesangium, look at GBM &TBM, tubular cast and Bowman capsule are PAS positive.

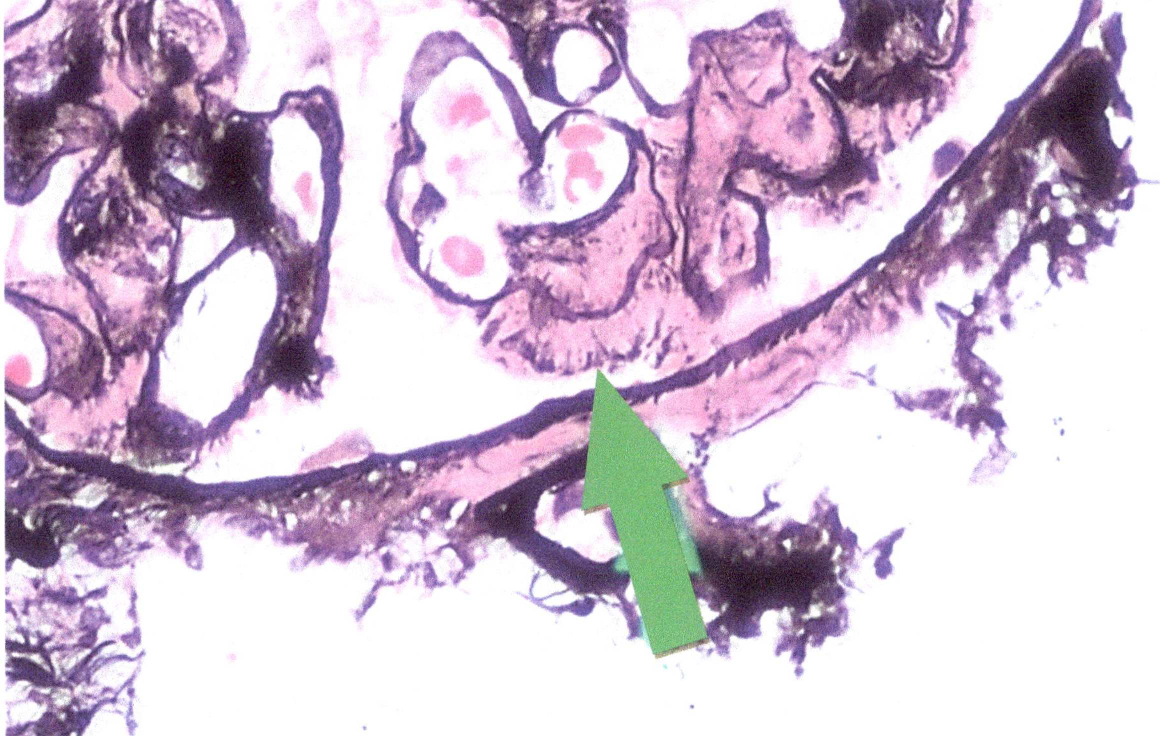

Figure 2:37.3: PASM Stain: 40x: Glomerulus: Silver negative material in Mesangium and Silver positive Amyloid spicules/eye lash sign.

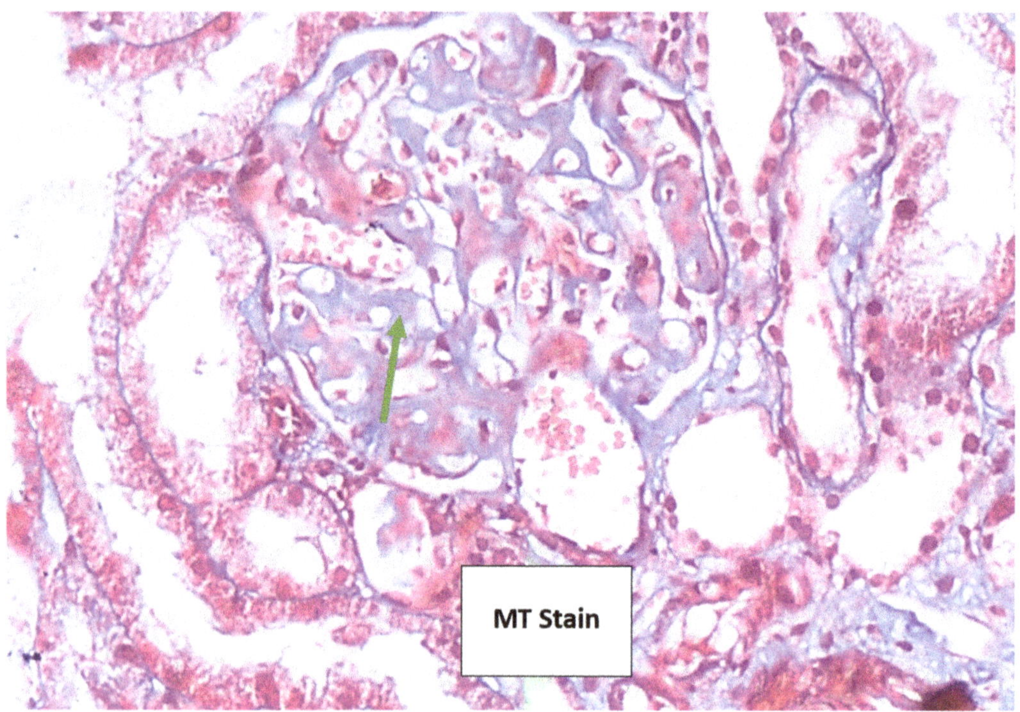

Figure 2:37.4: MT Stain: 20x: Glomerulus: Bluish material in mesangium (green arrow).

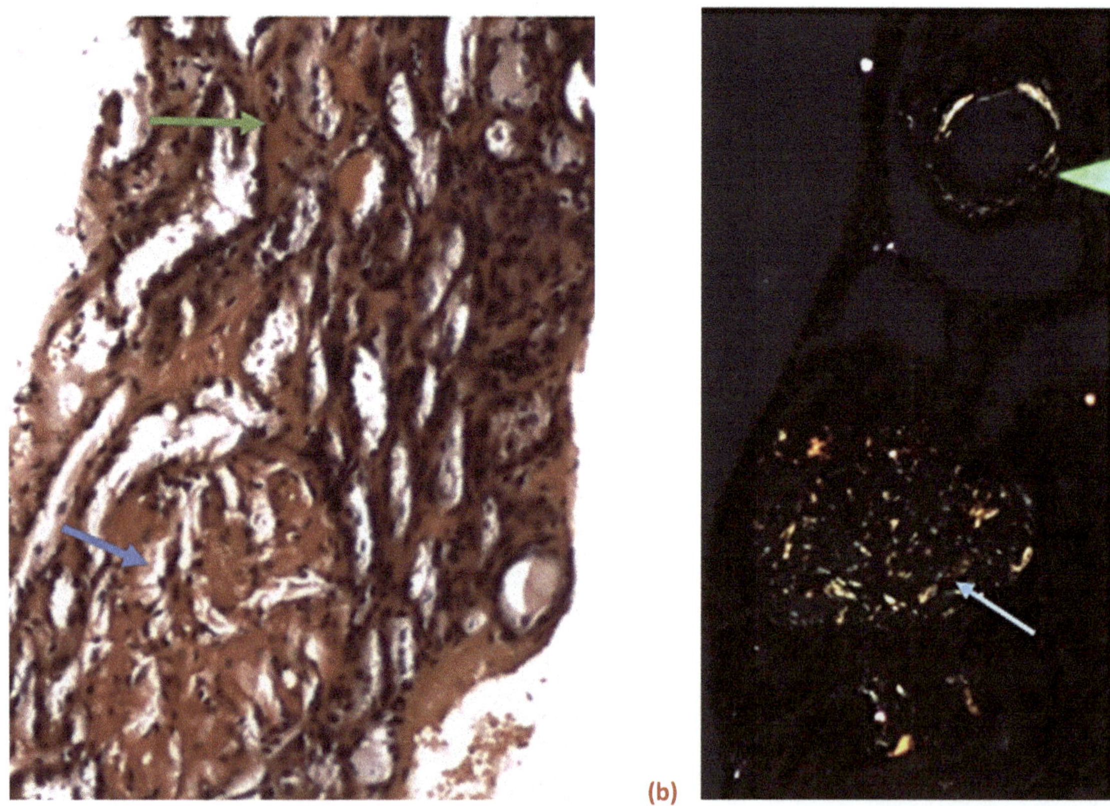

Figure 2:37.5: (a) Congo Red Stain: Congophilc Amyloid in glomerulus (blue arrow) &
arteriole (green arrow) **(b)** Amyloid under polarization-glomerulus (blue arrow) and the arteriole (green arrowhead):10x:
Apple-green birefringence.

IF:20x:Lambda Light Chain restriction

Kappa : 1+

Lambda:4+

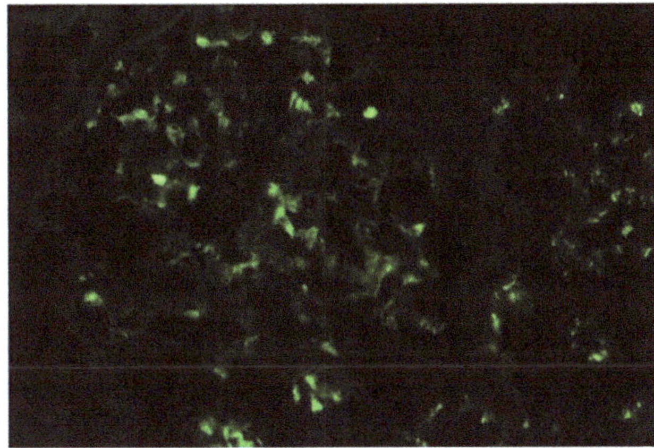

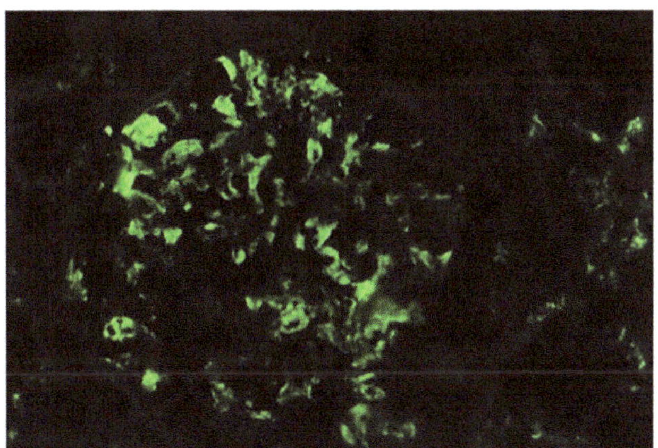

Figure 2:37.6: Immunofluorescence:Glomerulus: Lambda light chain restriction: showing significant mesangial smudgy deposits as comapred to Kappa light chain, which has insignificant deposits.

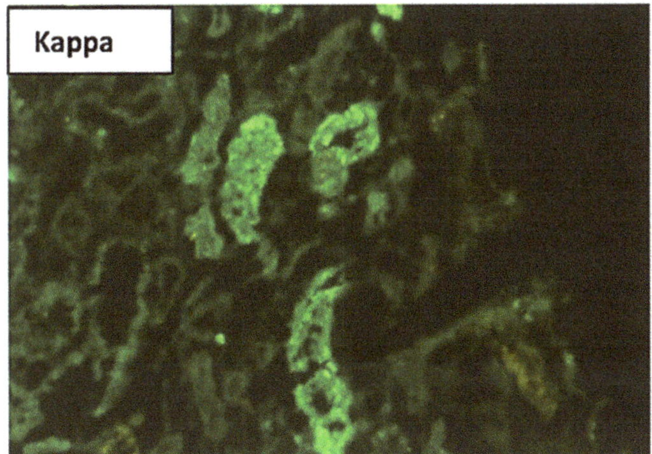

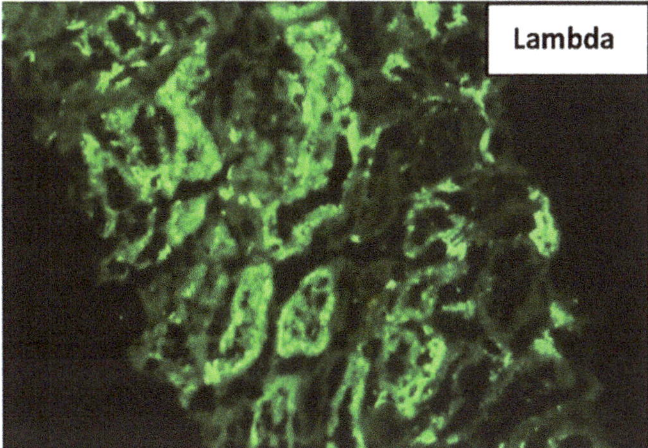

Figure 2:37.7: Immunofluorescence:Lambda light chain restriction in cytoplasm of tubular epithelial cells.

Interpretation:

Primary diagnosis: Amyloid light chain (AL) amyloidosis-Lambda light-chain restricted.

Additional findings: Lambda light chain restriction in the cytoplasm of the tubular epithelial cells causing Proximal Tubulopathy.

Ancillary studies: Congo red stain is positive in glomeruli and vessels.

Additional investigations: Serum Immunofixation electrophoresis (quantitative): Monoclonal M band was seen, Free light chain assay showed Lambda light chains elevated. Beta 2 Microglobulin levels: elevated, Bone marrow biopsy: showed 20% of plasma cells.

CASE 38

History: 36 years old male, non-diabetic, non-hypertensive, nonsmoker and non-alcoholic. He had past h/o fall from tree 3 years back requiring open reduction and internal fixation of the fractured tibia and fibula. He has a chronic draining sinus in the skin in the same leg. He has been treated with antibiotics on multiple occasions for the same with some relief and then recurrence. He now is having progressive increase in pedal edema for last 2 months. He is normotensive BP: 100/70 mm of Hg.

Investigations: Serum creatinine: 3.8 mg/dl. Urine analysis: Protein:3+, RBCs: 4 to 7/HPF. 24 hour urine protein: 6 gm. USG: Bilateral enlarged kidneys.

Clinical diagnosis: Nephrotic range proteinurea with microscopic hematuria without hypertension with renal dysfunction.

Differential diagnoses: Membranous nephropathy / AA Amyloidosis.

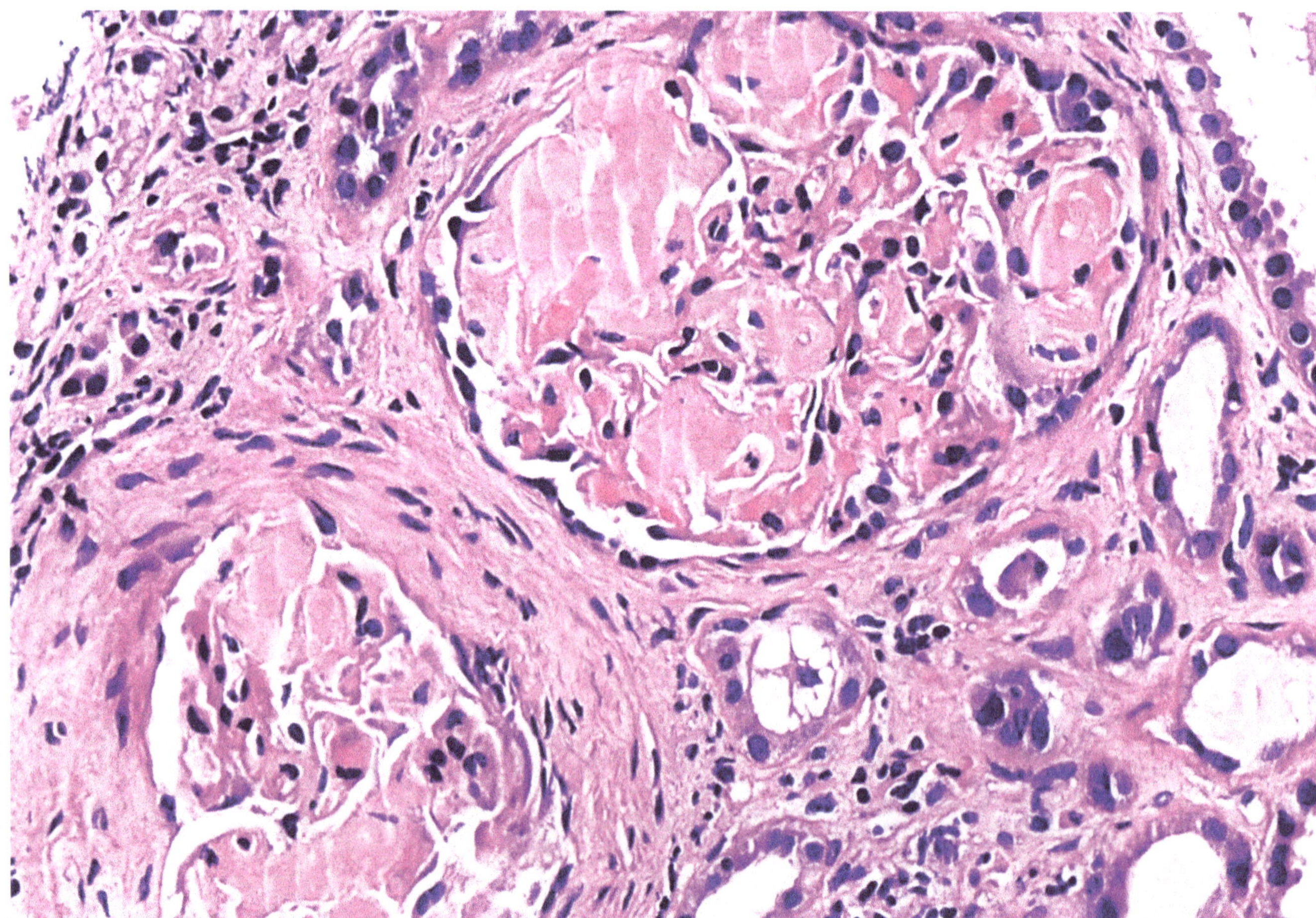

Figure 2:38.1: H&E Stain: 10x: Glomeruli: Pale, waxy eosinophilic deposits in mesangium focally exceeding the diameter of adjacent capillary lumina forming acellular nodules.

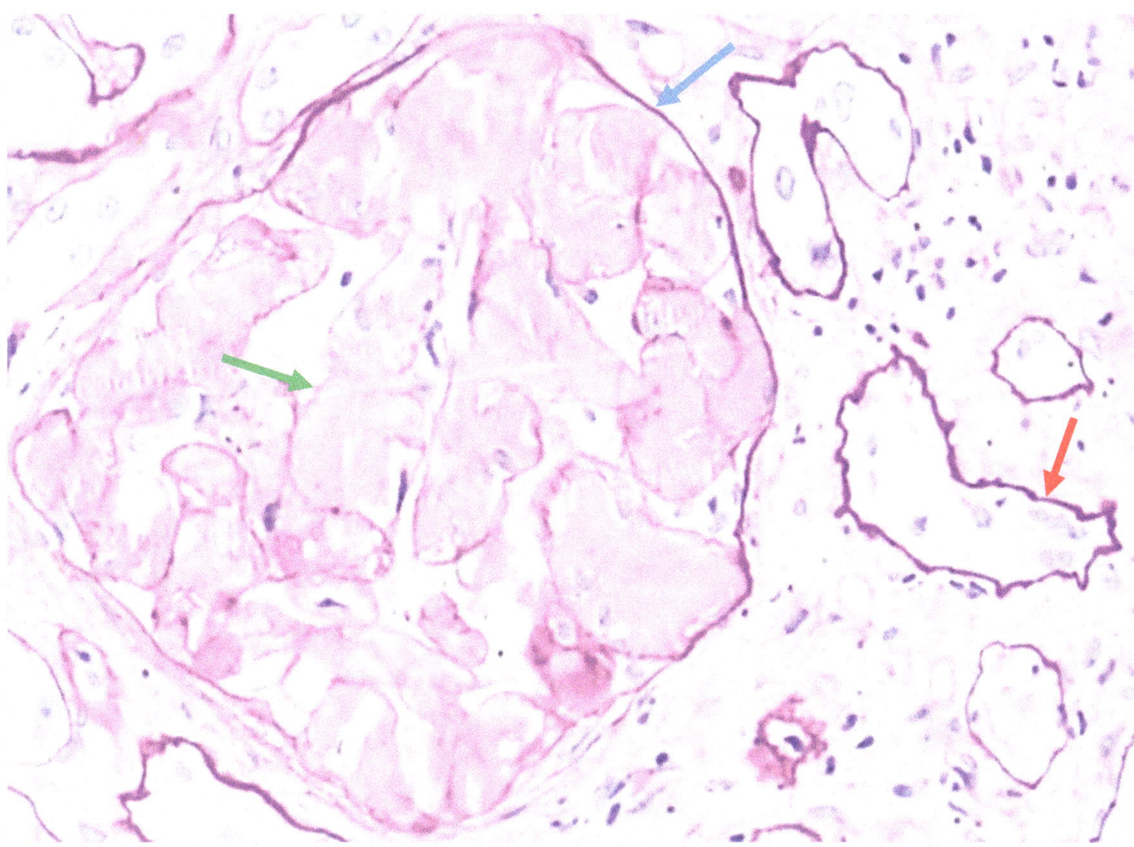

Figure 2:38.2: PAS Stain: 20x: Glomerulus: PAS-negative material in mesangium, look at GBM (green arrow) & TBM (red arrow) and Bowman capsule (blue arrow) are PAS positive.

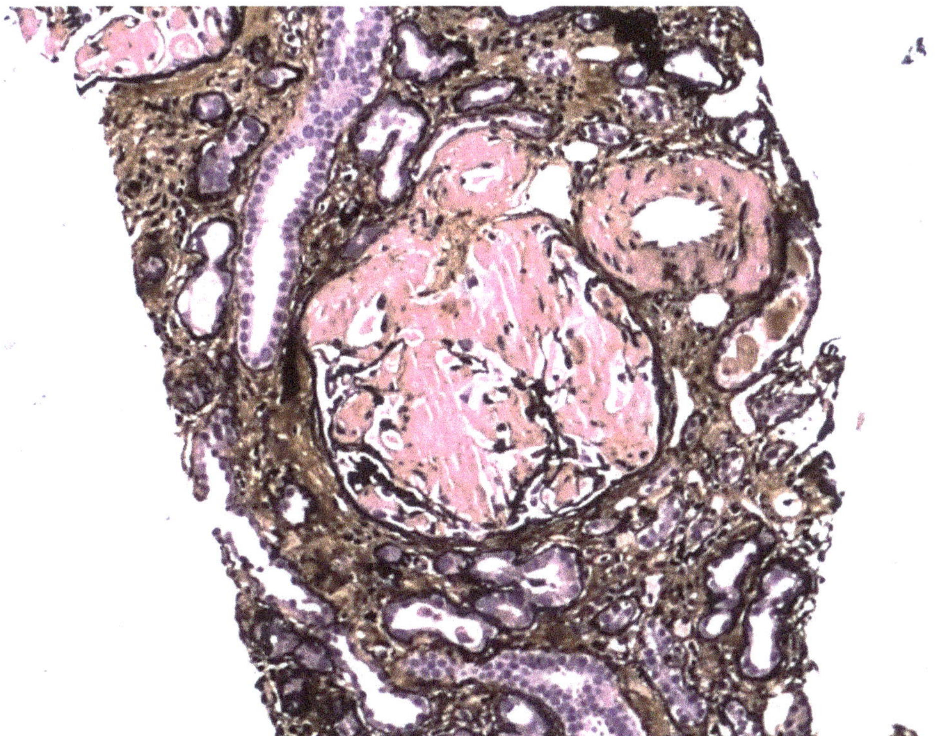

Figure 2:38.3: PASM Stain: 20x: Glomeruli: Pale Silver-negative material in mesangium and around the artery.

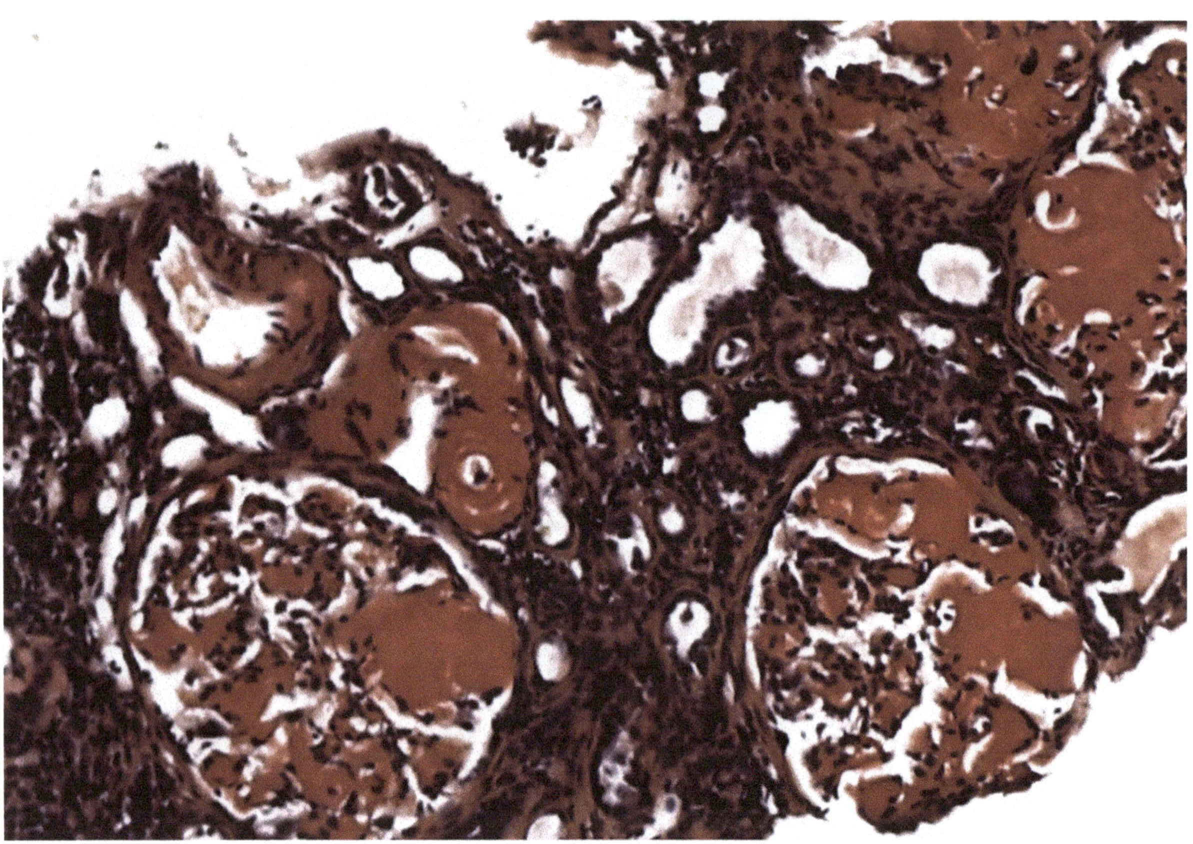

Figure 2:38.4: Congo Red Stain: 20x: Glomeruli: Congophilic deposits in mesangium and arterioles.

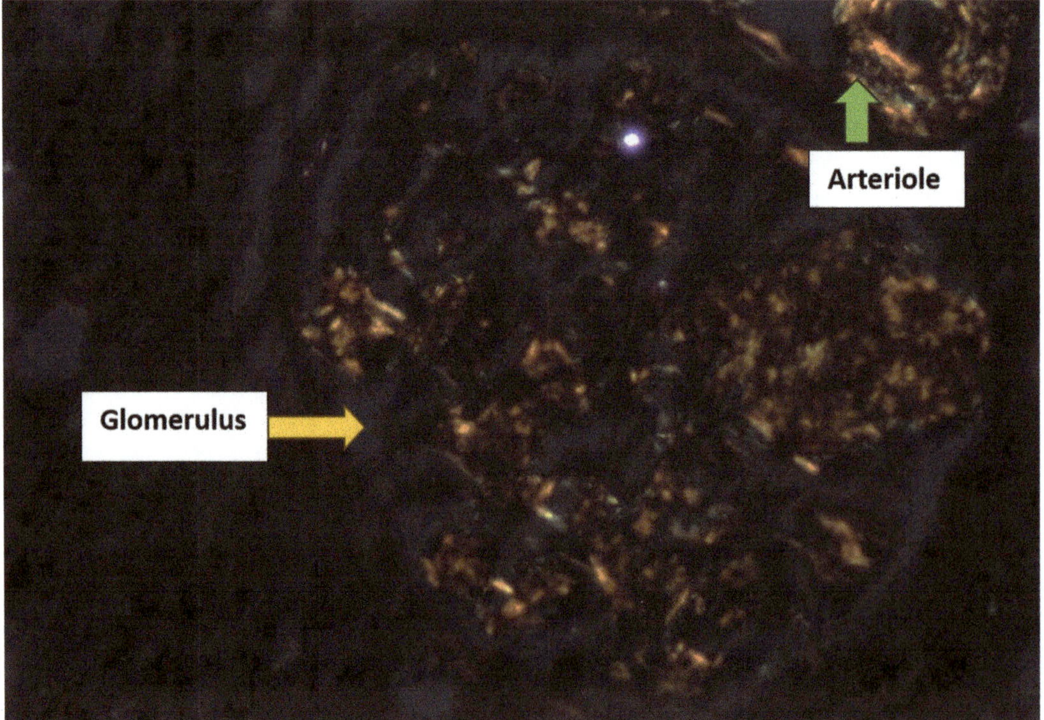

Figure 2:38.5: Congo Red Stain under polarization :20x: Apple-green -reddish birefringence confirming Amyloid.

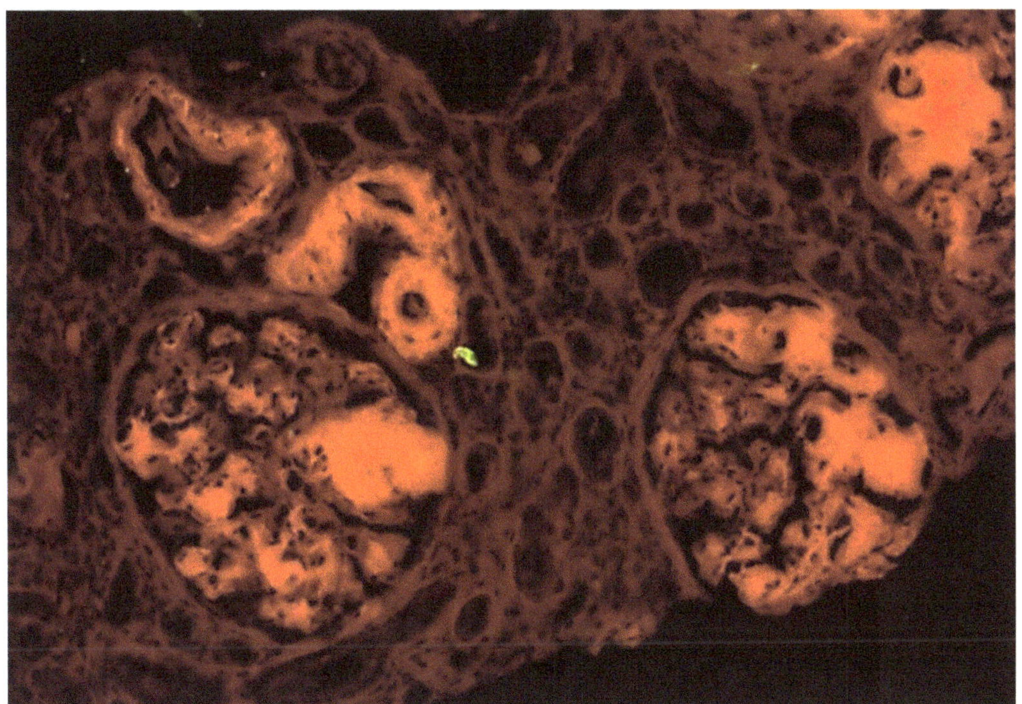

Figure 2:38.6: Congo Red Stain: 10x: Under Immunofluorescence microscope Glomeruli and arterioles: bright red deposits of Amyloid.

Immunofluorescence:

IF: 20x:No Light Chain Restriction

Kappa: negative

Lambda :negative

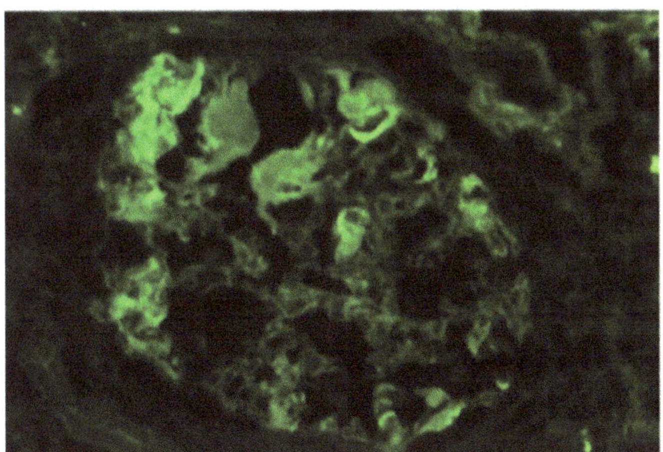

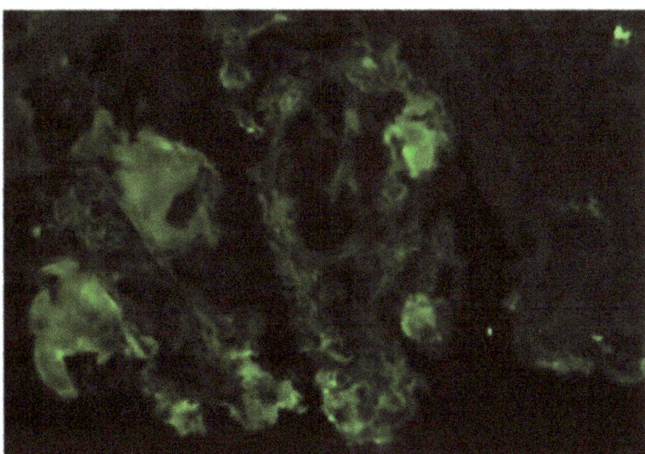

Figure 2:38.7: Immunofluorescence: No light chain restriction is seen.

Immunohistochemistry :AA Amyloid

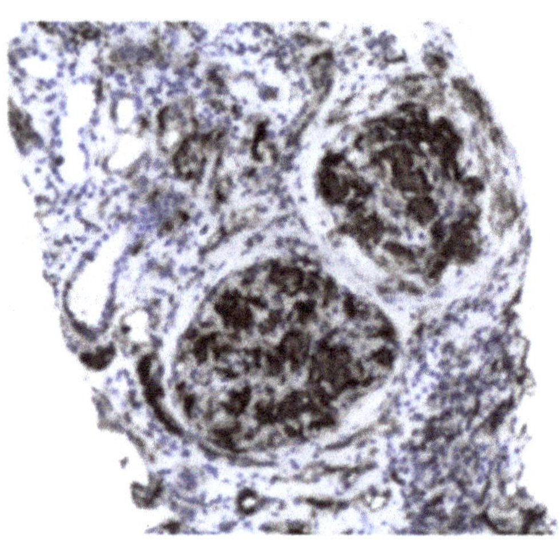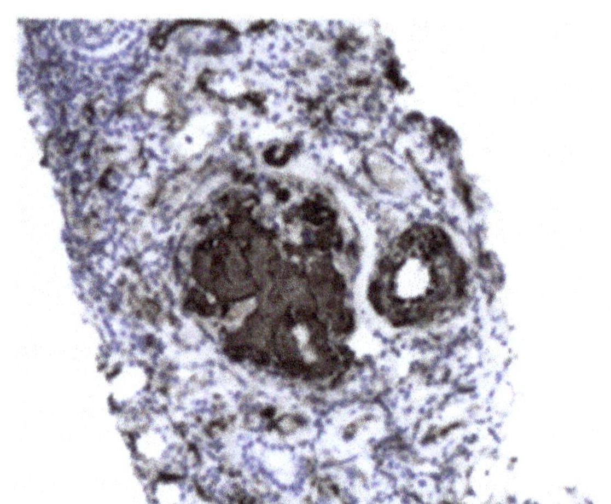

Figure 2:38.8: IHC: AA Amyloid:10x: positive in glomeruli and vessel.

Interpretation: Deposit glomerulopathy with no immunoglobulin light chain restriction and IHC AA-Amyloid positivity.

Final Diagnosis: AA Amyloidosis, secondary to Chronic osteomyelitis.

Pathology Pearls

Table 2:38.1: Differentiation between Amyloidosis, Fibrillary glomerulonephritis & Immunotactoid glomerulopathy.

Sr. No.	Features	Amyloidosis	Fibrillary GN	Immunotactoid glomerulopathy
1.	**Congo red stain**	+	Usually negative	-
2.	**Immunofluorescence**	Light chain restriction if AL amyloid	Polyclonal with IgG &C3c	Usually monoclonal
3.	**IHC-DNA JB9**	-	+	-
4.	**Electron microscopy**	Randomly arranged non branching fibrils 8 to 15 nm	Randomly arranged non branching fibrils 14 to 22 nm	Parallel arrays of Microtubules with large central lumen >30nm

Electron Microscopy:

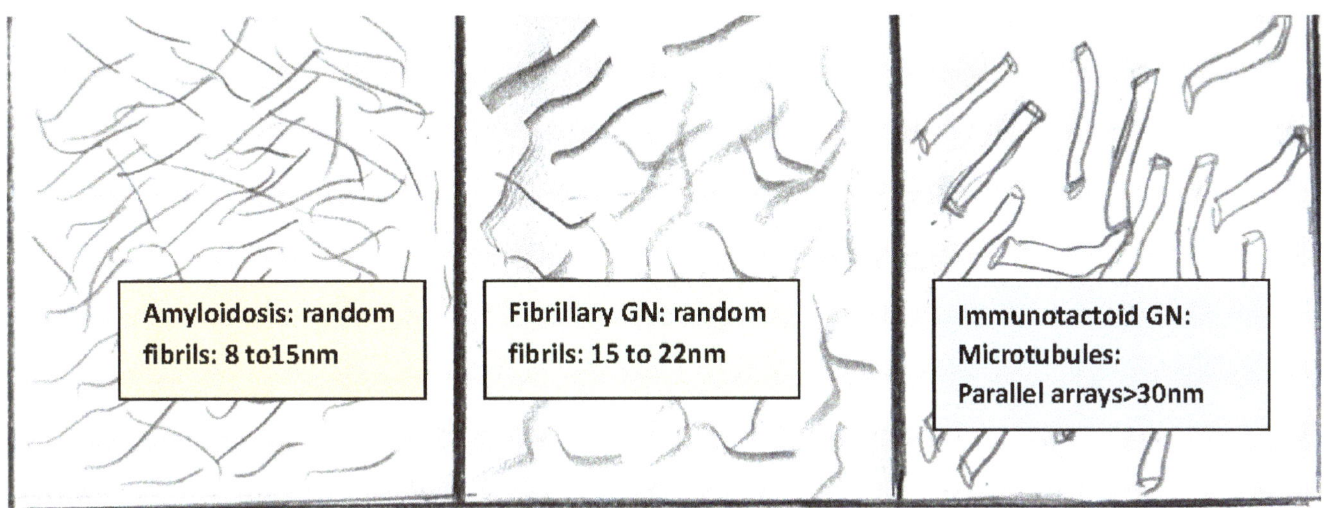

Figure 2:38.9: Diagrammatic representation of electron microscopic appearance of fibrils.

History: 46 years old female, non-diabetic, non-hypertensive, nonsmoker, no other addictions. She presented with progressive facial puffiness and pedal edema for last one month. No fever. She had noticed mild reddish tinge of urine on and off. She has no other urinary complaints. No history of indigenous medicine use or NSAIDs or any heavy metal exposure. She has no systemic symptoms of collagen vascular disease. She has no weight loss or B symptoms. BP is 140/90 mm of Hg.

Investigations: Serum Creatinine: 1.5 mg/dl, Urine analysis: protein: 3+, RBCs: plenty/HPF, Pus cells: 4-5/HPF, Serum albumin: 3.4gm/dl, total cholesterol: 250mg/dl, LDL: 185mg/dl, HDL: 28mg/dl, Trigycerides: 300mg/dl.

Clinical diagnosis: Nephrotic syndrome with hypertension and renal dysfunction without systemic features of collagen vascular disease

Differential diagnoses: Membranous nephropathy/MCD /FSGS/IgA Nephropathy.

Light microscopy:

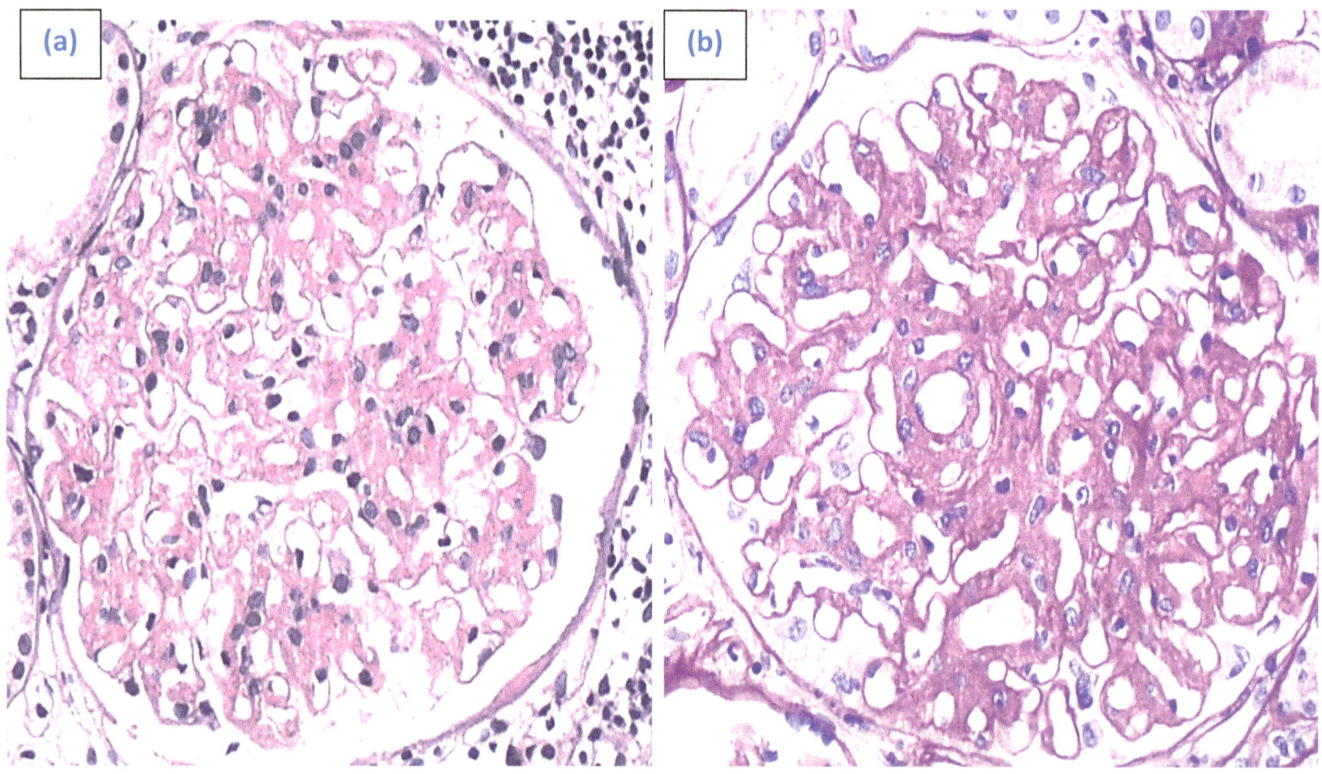

Figure 2:39.1: Glomerulus 20x: **(a)** H&E stain **(b)** PAS-stain: Mesangial widening with eosinophilic and pale PAS-positive material in the mesangium.

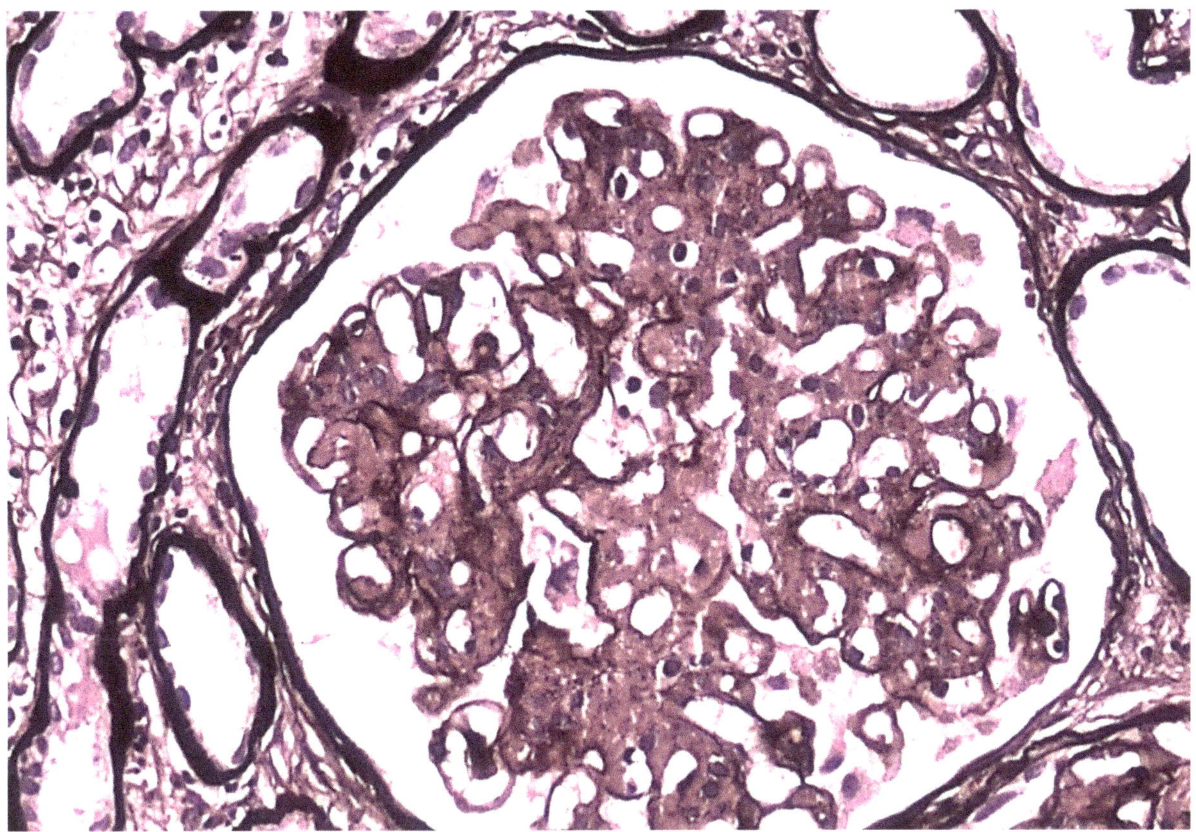

Figure 2:39.2: PASM Stain: 20x: Glomeruli: The material in the mesangium is Silver negative.

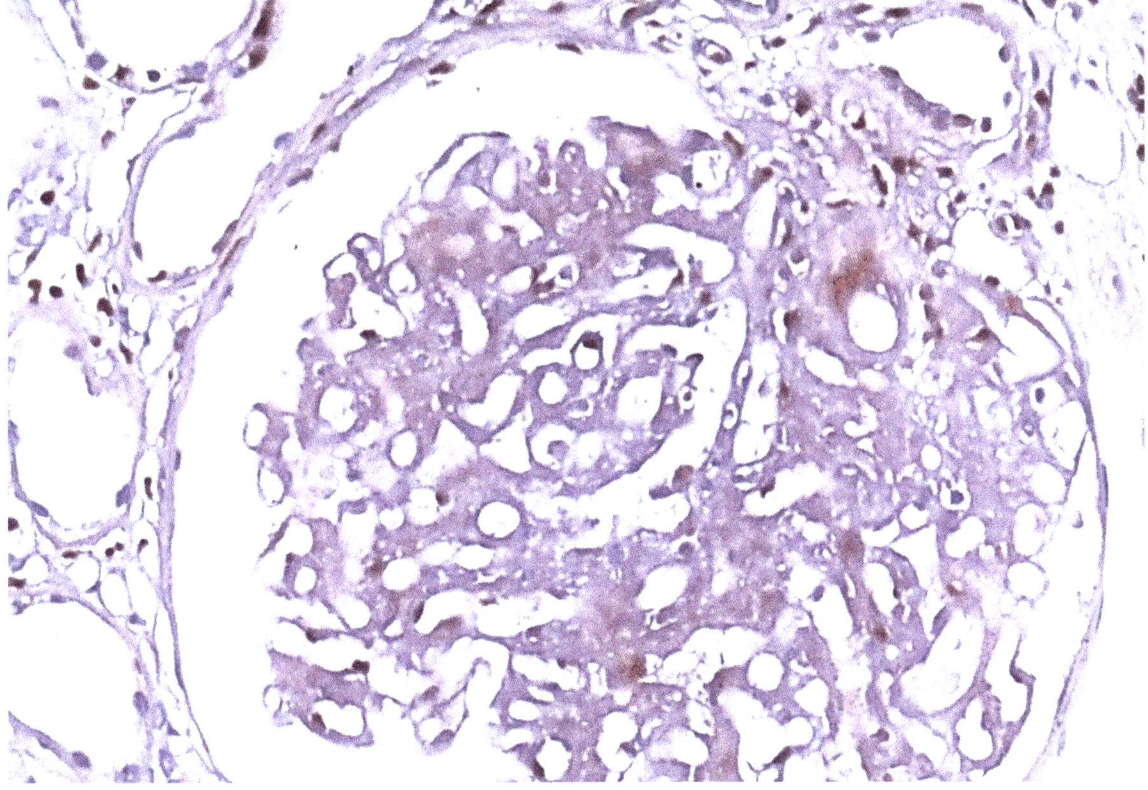

Figure 2:39.3: Masson Trichrome Stain: 20x: Glomerulus: The material appears bluish red in the mesangium.

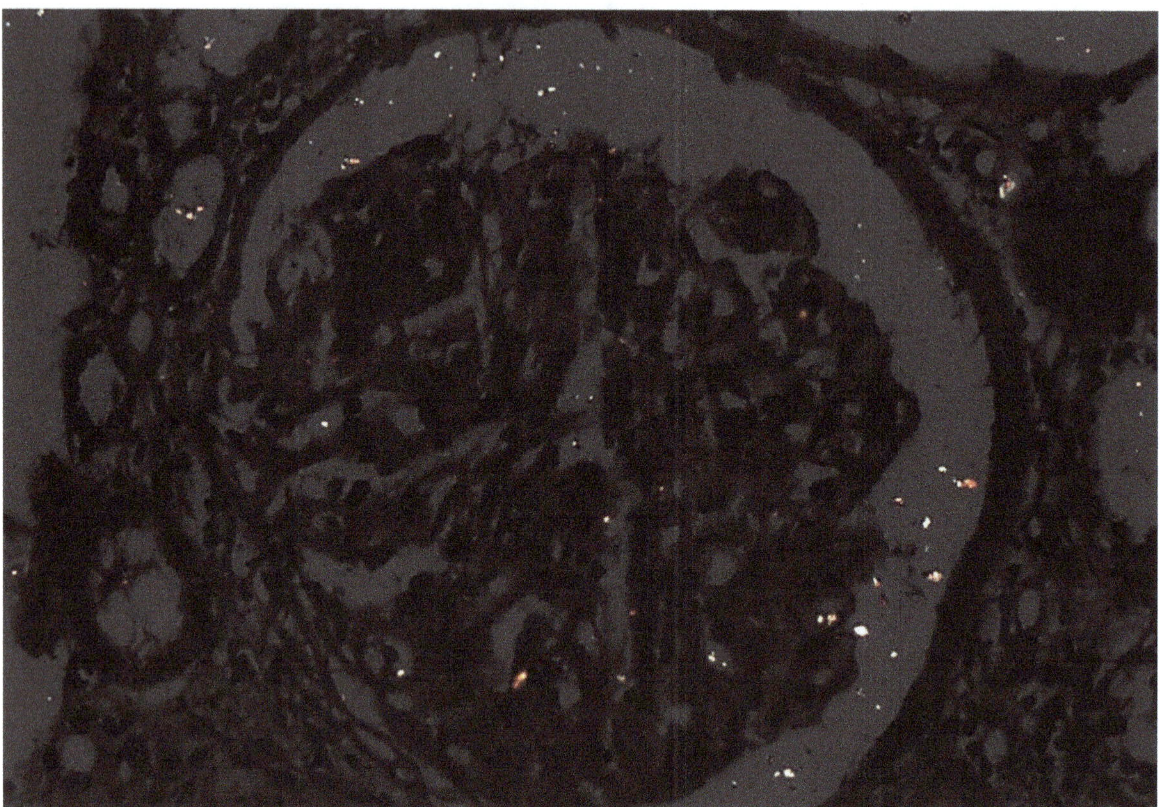

Figure 2:39.4: Congo red stain:20x: Glomeruli: under polarizer: no birefringence: negative for Amyloid.

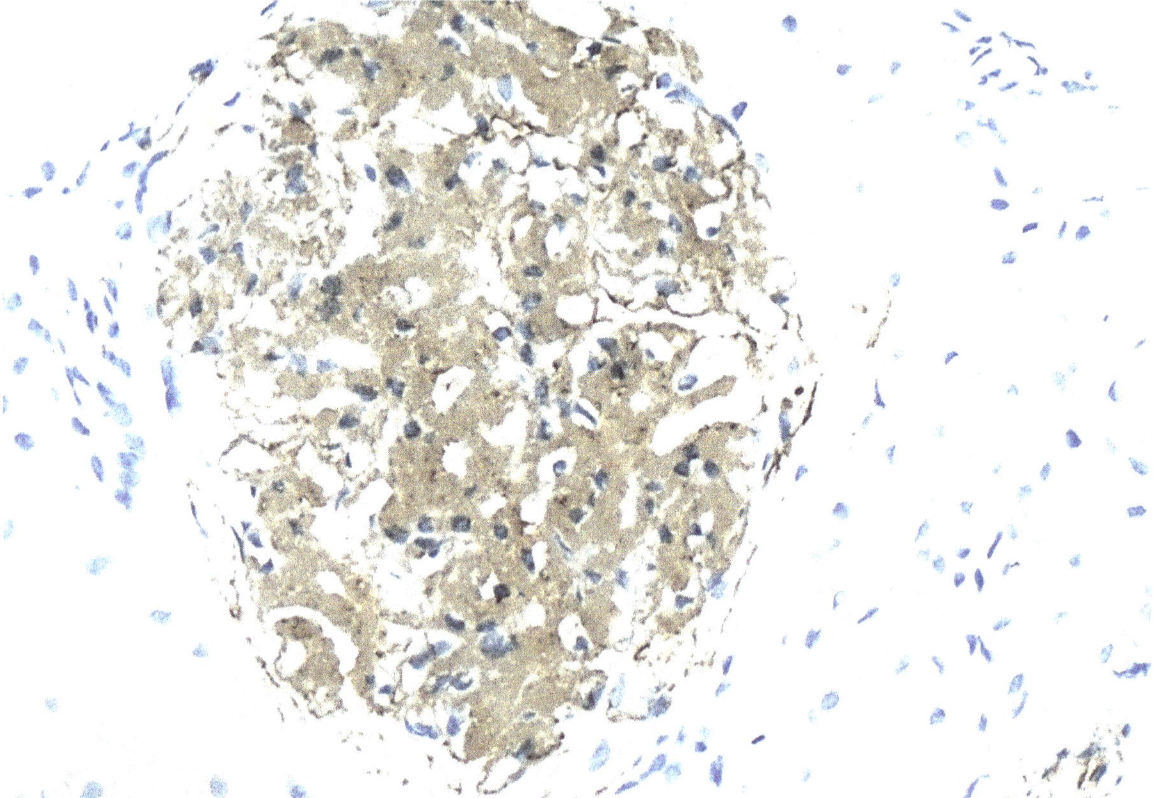

Figure 2:39.5: Immunohistochemistry: DNAJB9 stain: Glomerular deposits are positive with flbrillary glomerulonephritis.

Immunofluorescence:

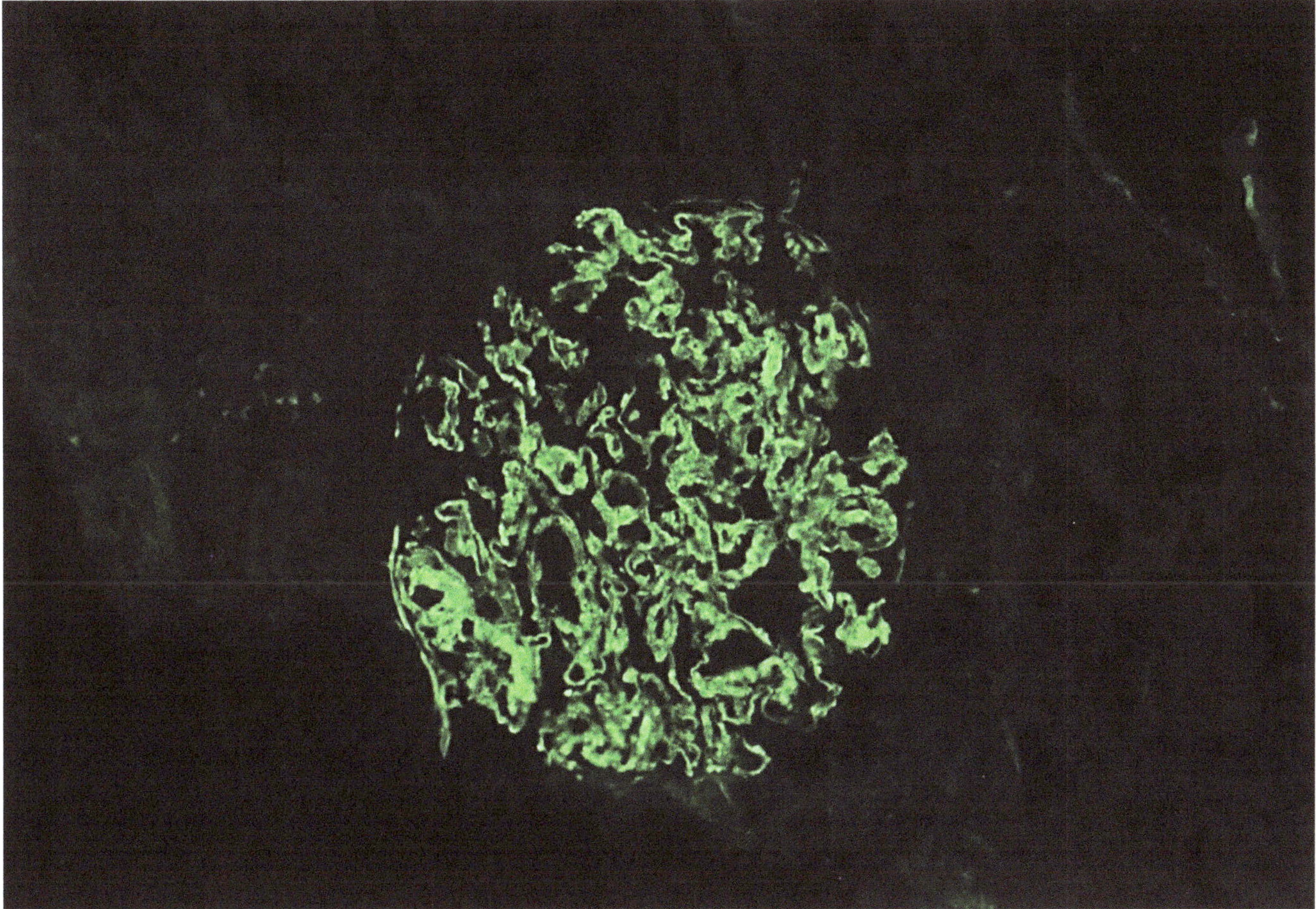

Figure 2:39.6: Direct Immunofluorescence: IgG:20x: Glomerulus: Capillary wall and some mesangial smudgy deposits.

Interpretation: Deposit glomerulopathy (possibility of Fibrillary GN /Immunotactoid GP).

Additional investigations:

Electron microscopy: Accumulation of randomly oriented, non -branching fibrillary structures measuring from 16-21nm in mesangial and focal subendothelial regions consistent with Fibrillary Glomerulopathy.

IHC FOR DNA JB9: Positive staining in the mesangium.

C3 and C4: Normal, ANA Profile: Negative, Serum immunofixation electrophoresis: No monoclonal gammopathy, HIV: Neg, HCV: Neg, HBsAg Neg, Papanicolaou smear: negative for intraepithelial lesion or malignancy, Mammogram: Normal, Stool Occult blood: Negative, Chest X-ray: Normal. Peripheral smear: no atypical cells.

Final Diagnosis: Fibrillary Glomerulonephritis.

CASE 40

History: 31 years old male, non-diabetic and non-hypertensive, nonsmoker and non-alcoholic. He presented with headache and blurring of vision in emergency department. He was found to have BP:220/120 mm of Hg. Fundus examination revealed bilateral papilloedema. He has no urinary complaints. No history of any drug use. No history suggestive of any active infection or infection in recent past. No h/o diarrhea. No history of palpitations, syncopal episodes or fainting episodes. No history of skin tightening at fingertips or face, no h/o Raynaud's phenomenon, no arthritis or skin rash. No family history of kidney disease. Both parents are hypertensive.

Investigations: HB: 9 g/dl, TLC: 5,500/cu mm, Platelet: 1.0 Lakh/cu mm, Peripheral smear: occasional schistocytes. LDH 500 IU/L: elevated. Creatinine: 7 mg/dl. Urine analysis: urine protein: +, RBCs:5b to 6/HPF, no e/o muddy brown casts, Potassium: 3.5 mEq /L, USG: Normal size kidneys, Doppler: No Renal artery stenosis. Plasma metanephrine and Normetanephrine levels: both normal, Plasma aldosterone and Renin levels: both normal.

Clinical Diagnosis: Malignant Hypertension with AKI & thrombocytopenia probably associated with TMA.

Light microscopy:

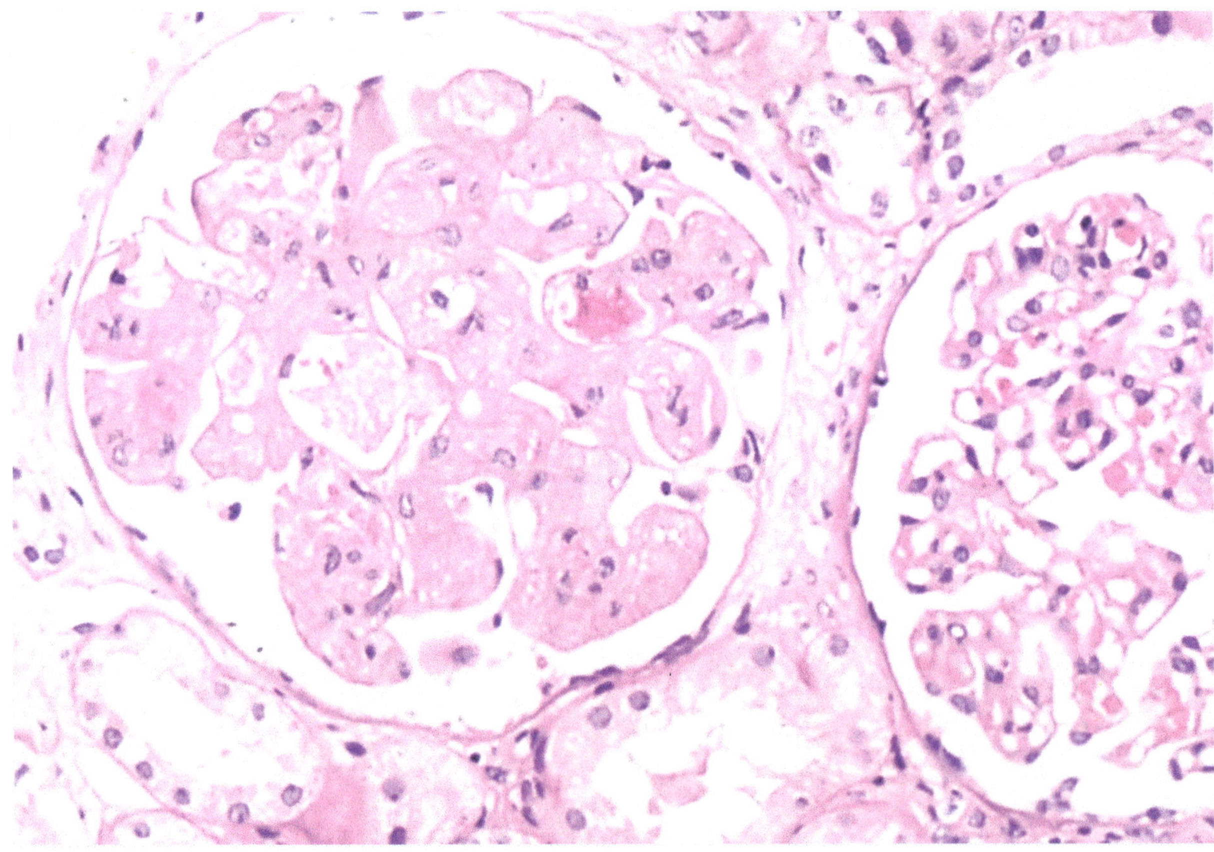

Figure 2:40.1: H&E Stain:20x: Glomeruli: Mesangiolysis-fibrillary appearance of mesangium (left sided glomerulus); Normal glomerulus (to the right).

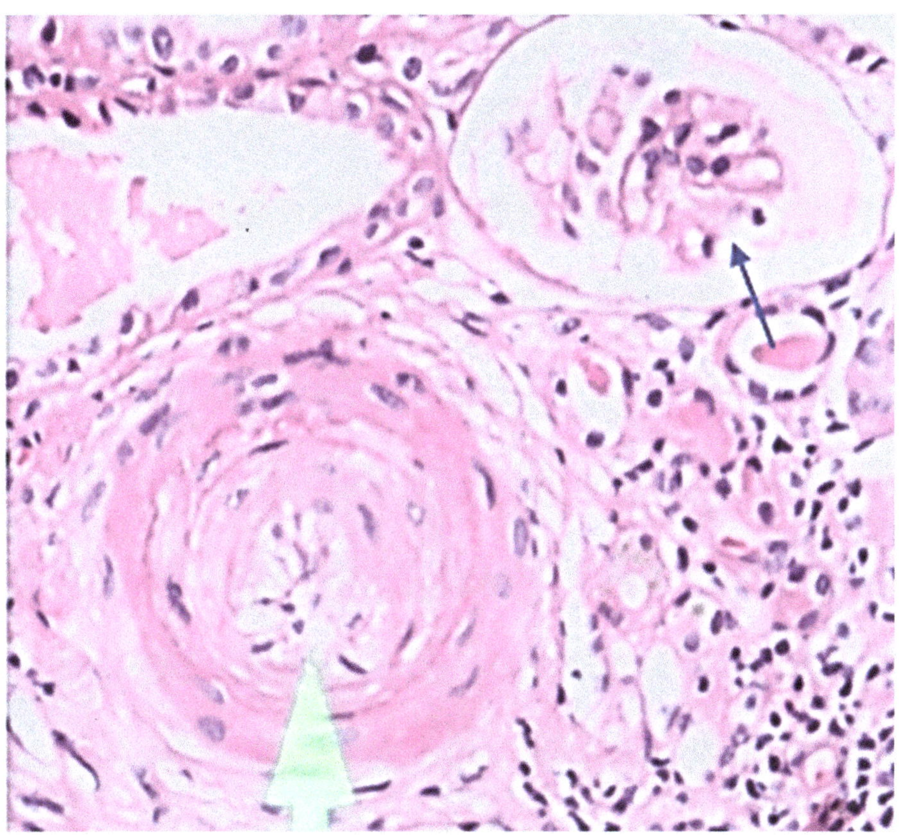

Figure 2:40.2: H&E Stain: 20x: Arteriole (green arrow): Myointimal hyperplasia (onion skinning) and ischemic glomerulus (blue arrow).

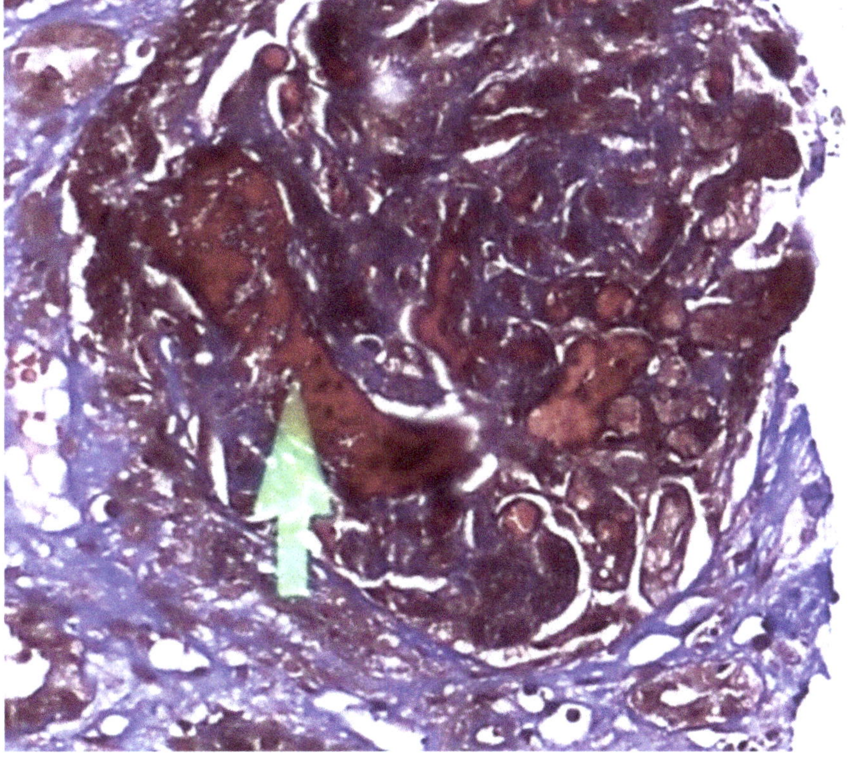

Figure 2:40.3: Masson Trichrome: 40x: Other Glomerulus: Fibrin thrombi: Fibrin is fuchsinophilic and fibrillar in appearance.

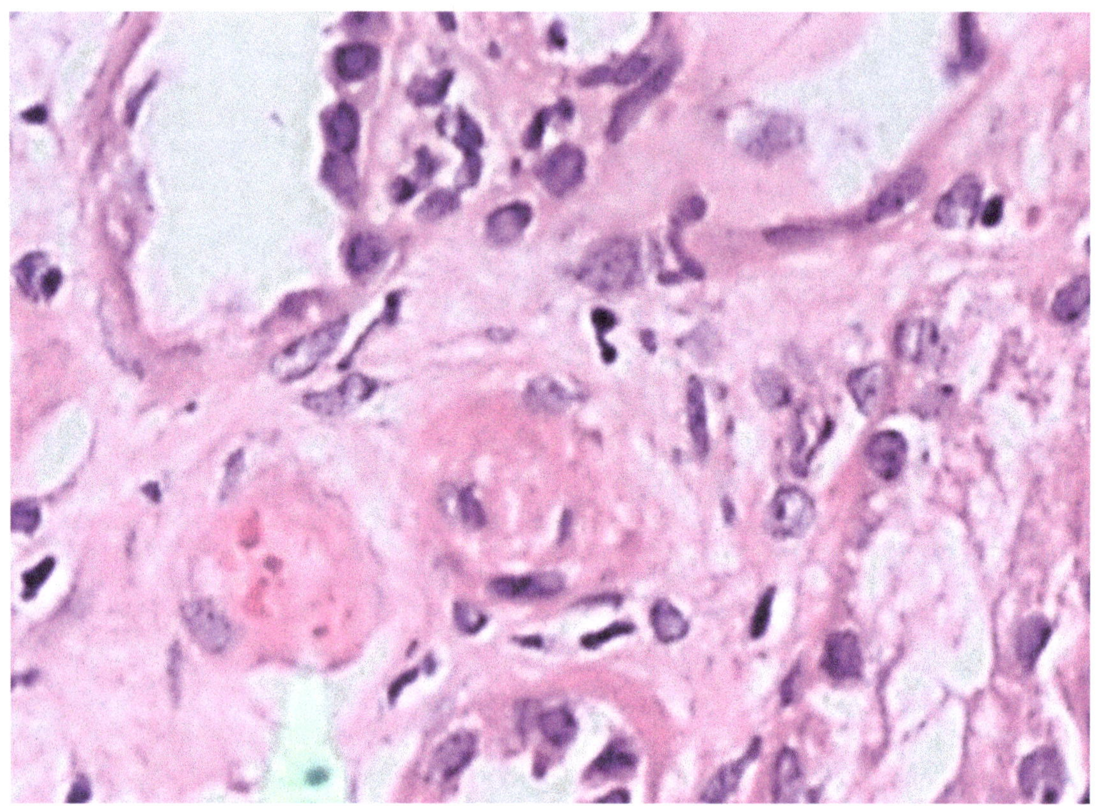

Figure 2:40.4: H& E Stain: Fibrin thrombi in arterioles with fragmented RBCs.

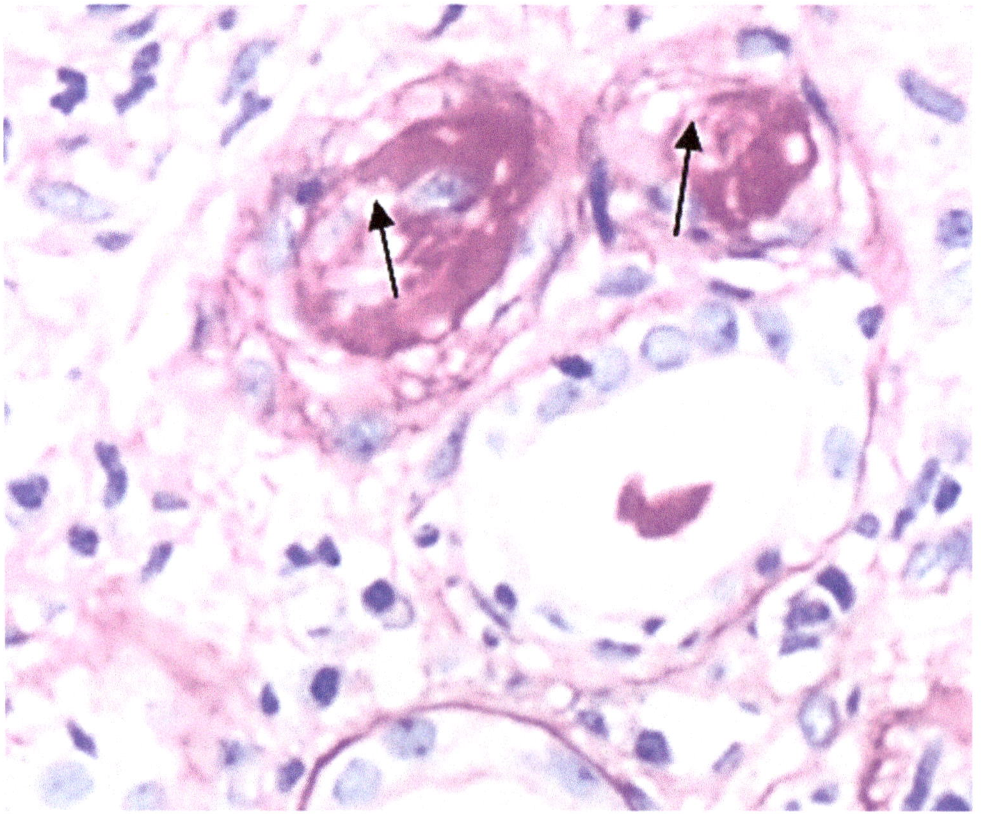

Figure 2:40.5: PAS Stain:20x: arteriole: strong PAS-positive fibrin thrombi.

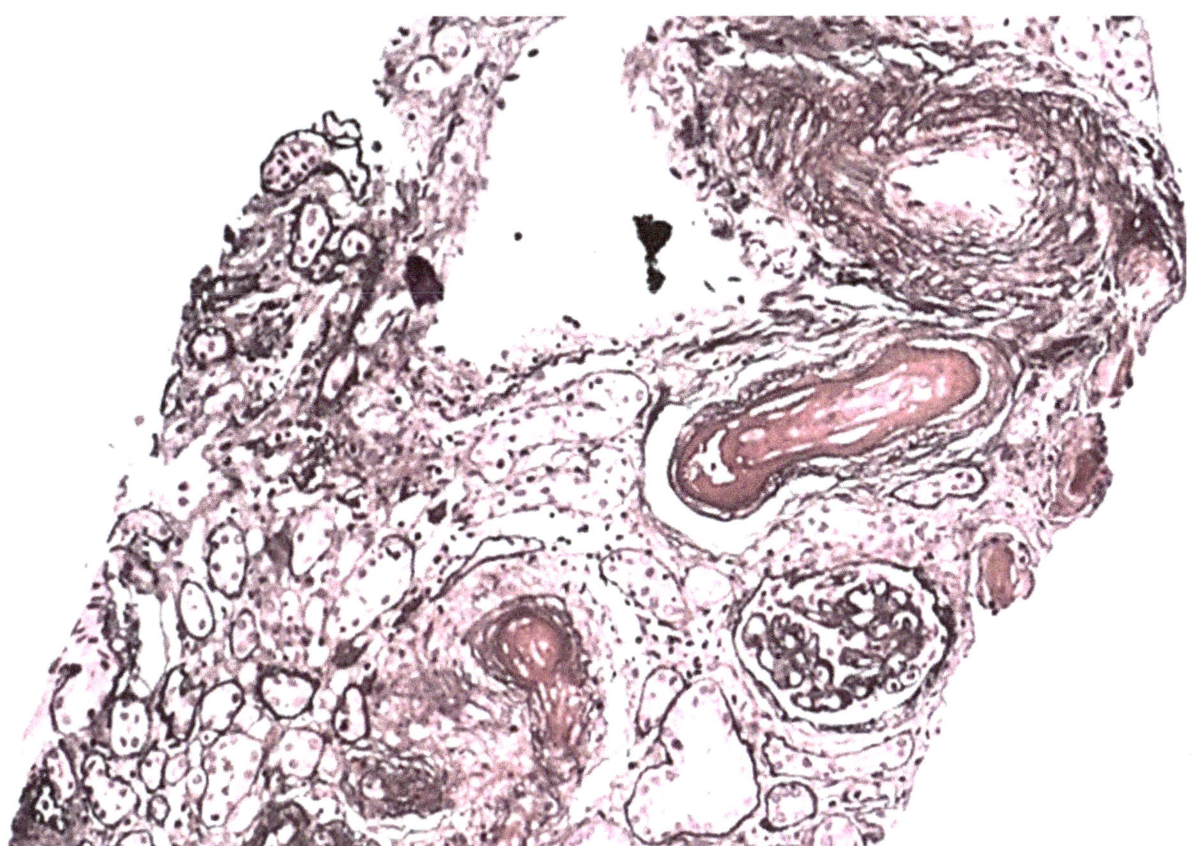

Figure 2:40.6: PASM Stain: 10x: arterioles: Silver negative fibrin thrombi.

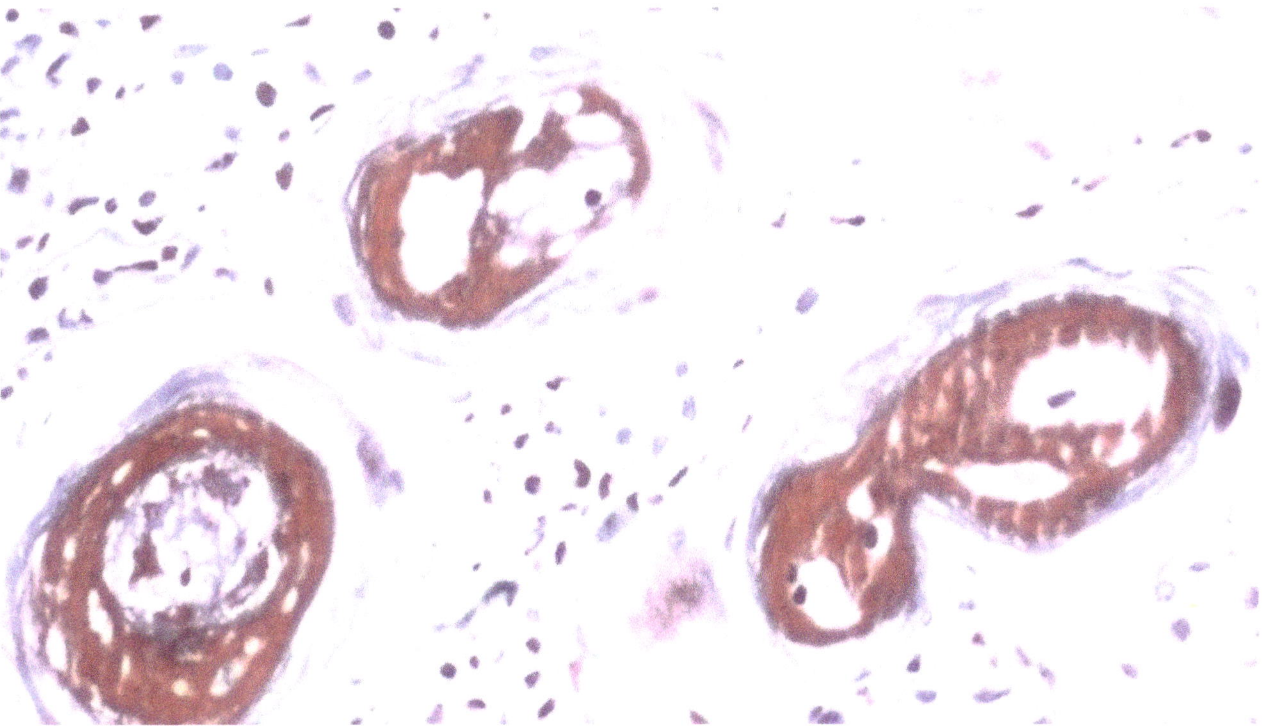

Figure 2:40.7: MT Stain:20x: arterioles: partial to near total luminal occlusion by fuchsinophilic (reddish) fibrin thrombi.

Interpretation: TMA due to Malignant Hypertension, to rule out Compliment mediated TMA(CM-TMA).

Additional evaluation in this case of TMA:

Test	Result	Comments
ADAMTS Activity	58%	Activity <10% – s/o TTP, rarely seen in sepsis and systemic cancer as well. Activity 11% - 60%: Can be seen less often with TTP, often with sepsis/Cancer. Activity 55-60%: Can be seen in other TMAs >60%: NO TTP.
ANA Profile	Negative	SLE/APS and Scleroderma can be associated with TMA
Serum Complement factor H (CFH) Autoantibody	Elevated > 1:1000 titre	Treat till titre < 1:1000, May need immunosuppressive meds if titres persistently high. Less chance of relapse.
Genetic testing for 5 Complement genes: CFH, CFI, CFB, MCP, C3	Not detected.	1. If a pathogenic sequence variant is detected in one of the genes, CM-TMA Confirmed. Continue Anti complement therapy till stable renal function. 50% relapse risk after stopping treatment. A relapsed case or one with a family history of TMA needs indefinite therapy. 2. Sequence variant of uncertain significance in one of the genes: CM-TMA Probable: <50% risk of relapse on stopping therapy. A relapsed case or one with a family history of TMA needs indefinite therapy. 3. No sequence variant detected: CM -TMA – Unlikely. Consider stopping therapy after stable renal function unless it's a relapse or there is a family history of TMA.
Stool culture	Negative for *E. coli* O157: H7 or O104:H4.	Special agar is required for E.Coli. It may not detect Shigella species. Bacterial shedding may have already stopped at presentation, so other tests should be done to detect Shigella toxin.
Stool Shiga toxin protein assay	Negative	It is done in patients with a history of diarrhoea.
Stool for Shiga toxin genes (STX1 and STX2)- DNA PCR	Negative	Can be done on stool or plate colonies. It is rapid and more reliable. Used by Public Health Labs. For early detection to control epidemics.

Final Diagnosis: Complement mediated Thrombotic microangiopathy due to complement factor H autoantibody.

Pathology Pearls

*An increased number of neutrophils in the glomerular capillaries can be seen in some cases; this feature may be prominent in patients with classic HUS.

** Collapsing GN with TMA: Collapsing glomerulopathy is common in the setting of thrombotic microangiopathy of the native kidney.

***French score to rule out TTP: Platelet count <30,000/microL and serum creatinine <2.25 mg/dL predicts a 94 % chance of having ADAMTS13 activity <10 percent, suggesting TTP.

Reference

*Inward CD. Howie AJ, Fitzpatrick MM, etal. Renal histopathology in fatal cases of diarrhea-associated haemolytic uraemic syndrome. British Association for Paediatric Nephrology. Paediatr Nephrol 1997;11(5):556-559.

** David Buob, et.al, Kidney International (2016)90,1321-1331.

*** Thrombotic thrombocytopenic purpura: Toward targeted therapy and precision medicine. Coppo P, Cuker A, George JN Res Pract Thromb Haemost. 2019;3(1):26.

CASE 41

History: 28-years old female, with no past h/o diabetes or hypertension or any other medical or surgical illness, primigravida, with normal ANC checkup till 28 weeks of gestation, presented with headache, abdominal right quadrant pain, nausea and blurring of vision. She was having bilateral pedal edema for last 4 weeks. She was found to have elevated BP: 170/100 mm of Hg. There is no history of fever, arthritis, skin rash and oral ulcers. She has shortness of breath on minimal exertion. Decreased air entry at bases and mild fine bilateral basal crepitations on auscultation. She was manged with diuretics, antihypertensives and Magnesium sulphate. Next day she had worsening shortness of breath and decreased urine output with rising creatinine levels, so an elective caesarean section was done. Low birth weight baby was born. Post delivery there was no improvement in urine output, and she was started on dialysis. There was no recovery of renal function at the end of 1 week despite improvement in BP and general condition.

Investigations: Hemoglobin (Hb): 8.5 g/dl, TLC: 5,000/cu mm, Platelet count:98,000/cu mm. Peripheral smear showed schistocytes. Prothrombin time: 15 seconds, INR: 1.2, APTT: 32 seconds, serum creatinine: 6 mg/dl. Urine Protein: 4+. Serum Uric acid: 9 mg/dl. UPCR: 5 g/g. LDH: 650IU/L, total Bilirubin: 2.5mg/dl, Indirect bilirubin: 1.8 mg/dl, SGOT: 250 U/L, SGPT: 200 U/L, blood sugar: 170 mg/dl. USG: No hydroureteronephrosis, no renal artery or vein thrombosis.

Clinical diagnosis: Post partum AKI-AKIN Stage -III Pre-eclampsia/ HELLP syndrome.

Light microscopy:

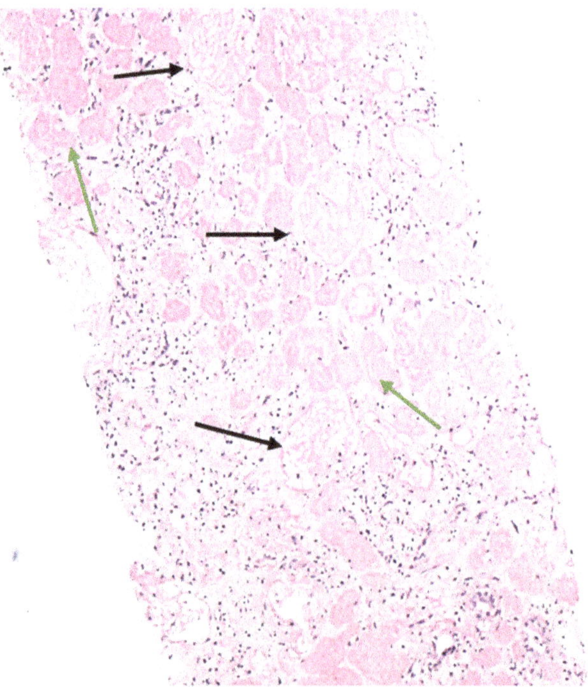

Figure 2:41.1: H&E Stain: 4x: Diffuse Cortical necrosis with ghost outlines of glomeruli (**black** arrows) and tubules. Tubules containing necrotic debris (**green** arrows) with loss of cellular details.

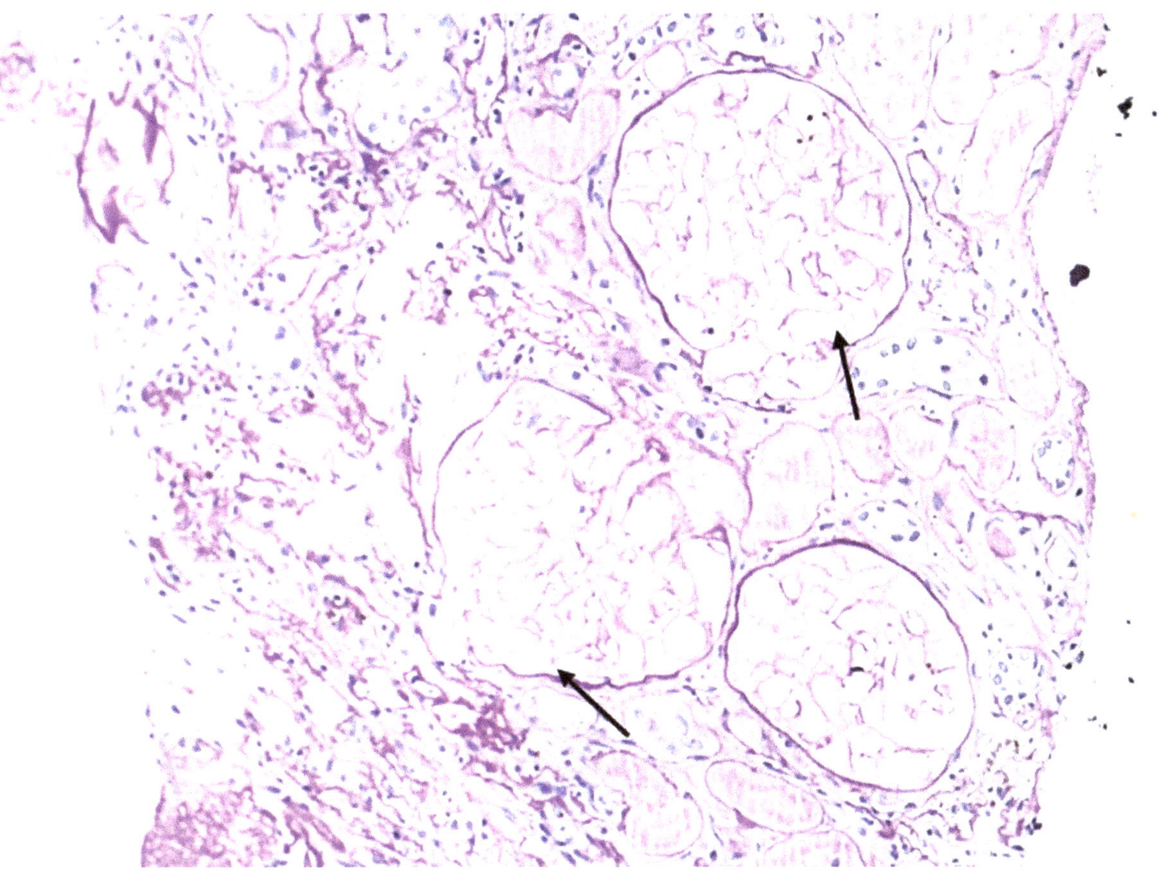

Figure 2:41.2: PAS Stain: 20x: Diffuse Cortical necrosis with ghost outlines of glomeruli.

Interpretation: Diffuse Cortical Necrosis.

Additional investigations: ANA Profile: negative, C3 & C4 levels: normal.

Final diagnosis: Severe Preeclampsia with HELLP Syndrome leading to AKI due to acute diffuse renal cortical necrosis.

Table 2:41.3: Differentiating some mimicking etiologies.

Parameters	HELLP	HUS/TTP	Acute fatty liver of pregnancy
LDH	≥600	>1000	variable
SGOT & SGPT	≥ 2 times upper normal limit	<100 IU/L	Elevated
Hypoglycemia	Less	Less	50% -100%
DIC	Less	Rare	+(20%)
VW factor multimers	-	80% -90%	-
ADAMTS 13	-	<5% in TTP	-

History: 50 years old male, non-diabetic and non-hypertensive, chronic smoker, non-alcoholic, a farmer by occupation, was admitted with a history of Russel viper snake bite. He was managed with Anti snake venom, antibiotics, and hydration. He started having decreased urine output from day 2 and became anuric, needing dialysis support. His bleeding diathesis improved over next one week, but he continued to be dialysis dependent at the end of 2 weeks. BP 150/90 mm of Hg.

Investigations: Serum creatinine:10.5mg/dl, Urine analysis (oliguric): Protein: 2+, CUE: RBCs: 1 to 2/HPF, WBCs: 4 to 6/HPF, USG findings: Right kidney: 9.4cm, Left kidney: 9.1cm, raised echogenicity.

Clinical diagnosis: AKI due to vasculotoxic snake bite, AKI-AKIN Stage -III.

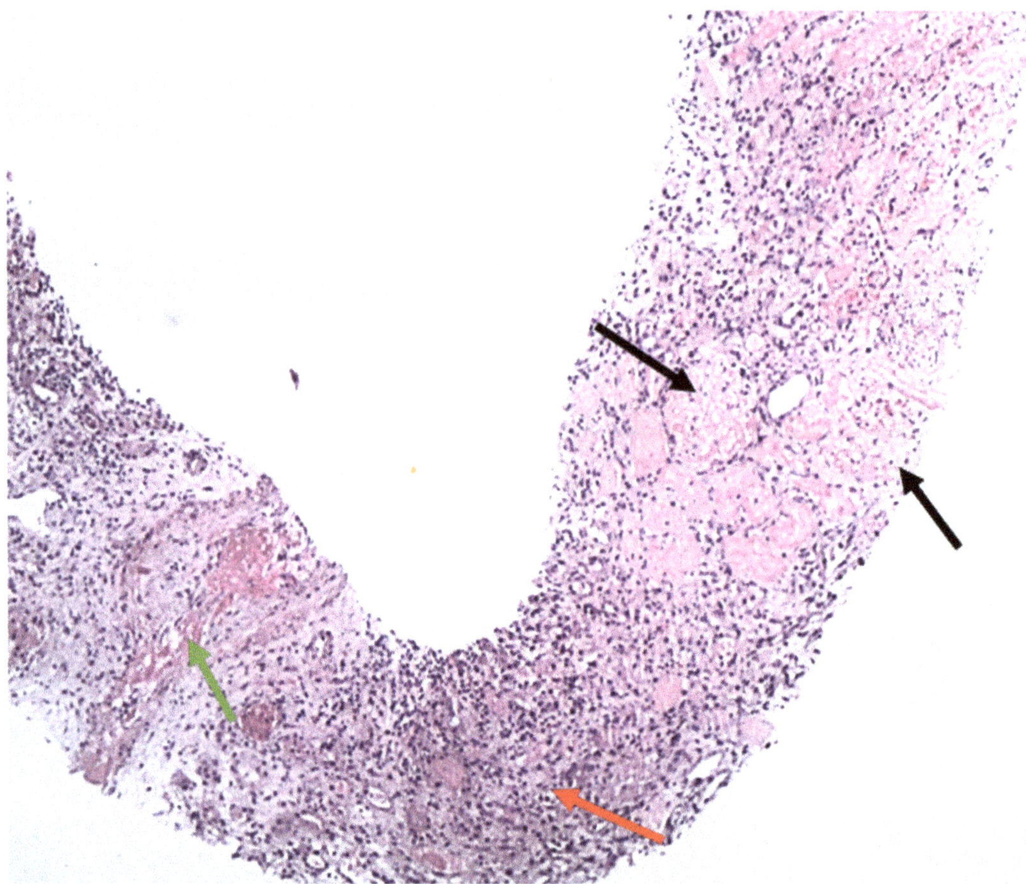

Figure 2:42.1: H&E Stain: 10x: Diffuse cortical necrosis showing ghost outlines of glomeruli, tubules with loss of cellular details (**black** arrows) & the large artery at the corticomedullary junction showing necrosis of muscle layer (**green** arrow) with luminal occlusion by fibrin deposition. 10% viable portion near the medulla show mild interstitial inflammation (**red** arrow).

Interpretation: Diffuse renal Cortical Necrosis post vasculotoxic snake bite.

CASE 43

History: 28 years old female, primigravida, had uneventful pregnancy followed by normal vaginal delivery, Post partum developed severe hemorrhage needing multiple blood transfusions and uterine packing. She developed pulmonary edema needing diuretic infusion and oxygen support. There was a progressive decline in urine output over the next 24 hours and a suboptimal response to diuretics. She was initiated on dialysis. No history of seizures or hypertension. No history of any joint pains or skin rash in the past. No history of jaundice. BP 110/70mm of Hg. Urine output increased to 500 ml per day but still dialysis dependent at end of 2 weeks, hence a renal biopsy was done.

Investigations: Serum Creatinine:6mg/dl, patient is anuric, viral markers: non-reactive, USG findings: B/L:11cm kidneys, prothrombin time 16 seconds, INR 1.3. APTT: 33 seconds. Total Bilirubin: 1.3 mg/dl, SGOT: 45U/L, SGPT: 50U/L, 2D ECHO: Severe global hypokinesia of Left ventricle with Ejection Fraction: 30%.

Clinical diagnosis: 1. AKI-AKIN Stage III 2. Post partum hemorrhage 3. post partum cardiomyopathy.

Light microscopy:

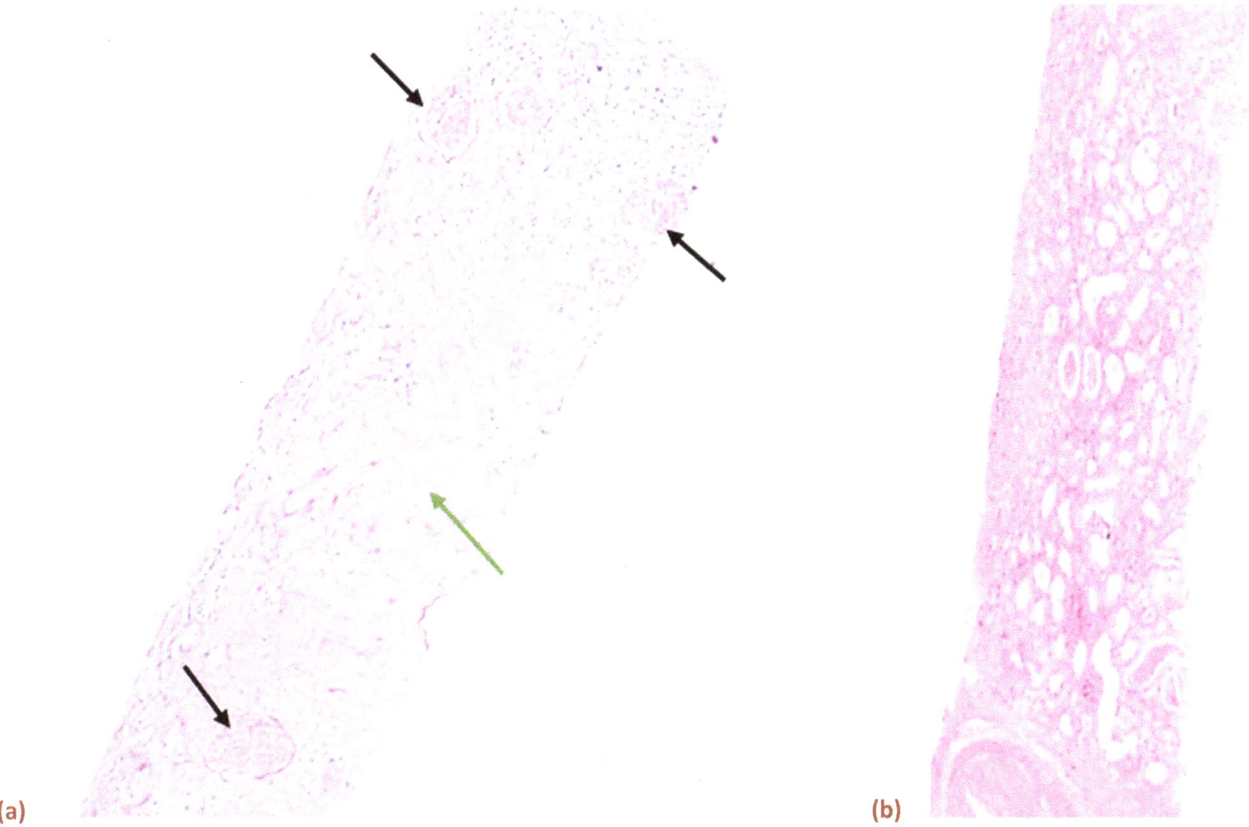

(a)   (b)

Figure 2:43.1: (a) PAS Stain: 4x: Necrotic area with ghost outlines of glomeruli (**black** arrows) & tubules (**green** arrow)
(b) H&E Stain: 4x: viable cortical area of the biopsy.

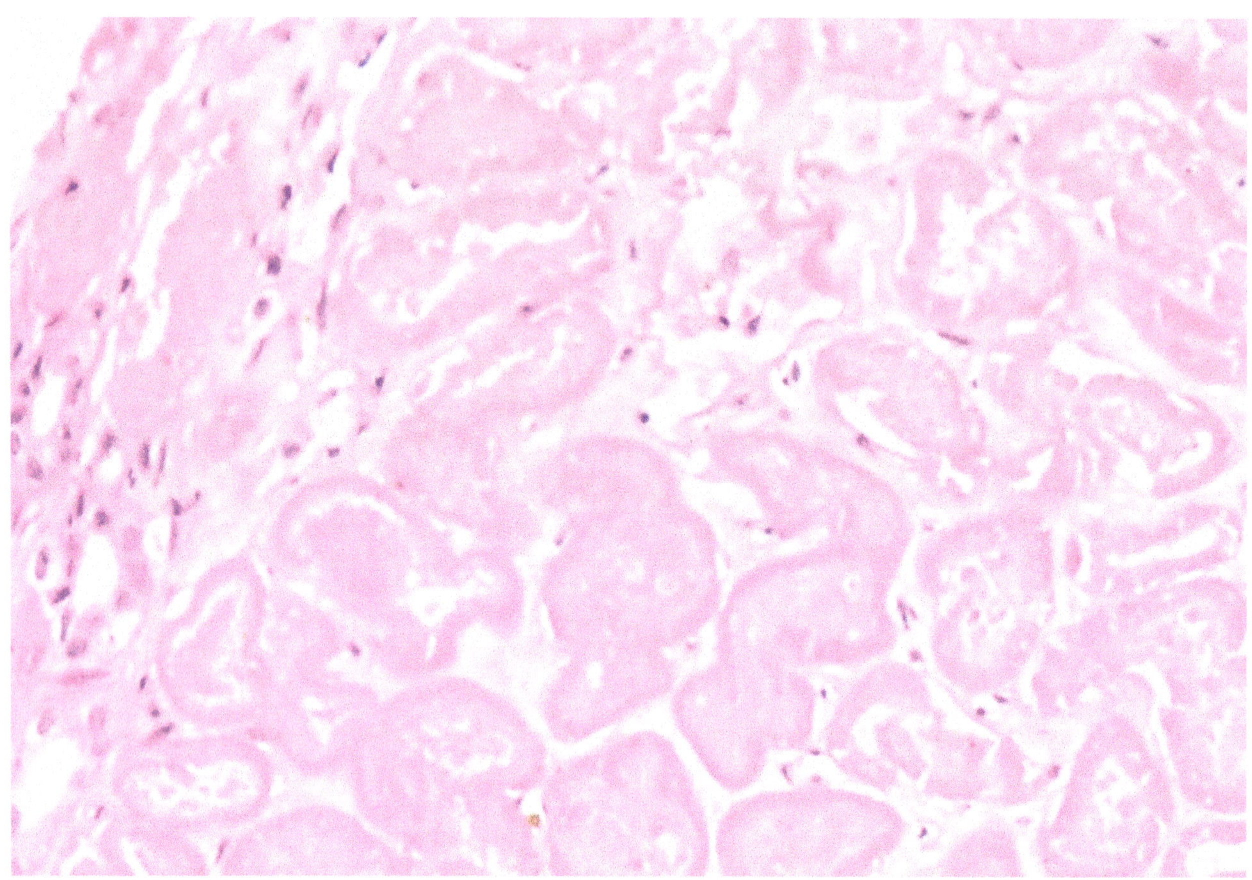

Figure 2:43.2: H&E Stain: 40x: Ghost outlines of tubules, loss of cellular details.

Interpretation: Post partum haemorrhage induced AKI with Patchy Cortical Necrosis.

CASE 44

History: 27 years old male, non-diabetic, hypertensive, Presented with facial puffiness, abdominal distension, pedal edema, hypertensive, BP 130/90 mm of Hg.

Investigations: Serum creatinine:0.7 mg/dl, UPCR:3g/g, Urine analysis: Protein: 3+, RBCs: 8-10/ HPF, Pus cells:2 to 3/HPF, serum albumin:2g/dl, serum cholesterol:250mg/dl, serum TG:270mg/dl, HDL:35mg/dl, LDL:150mg/dl, VLDL: 50 mg/dl, HIV: Non-reactive, HBSAg: Non-reactive, HCV: Non-reactive.

Clinical diagnosis: Steroid Resistant Nephrotic syndrome with microscopic hematuria with hypertension without renal dysfunction.

Differential diagnoses: FSGS.

Light microscopy:

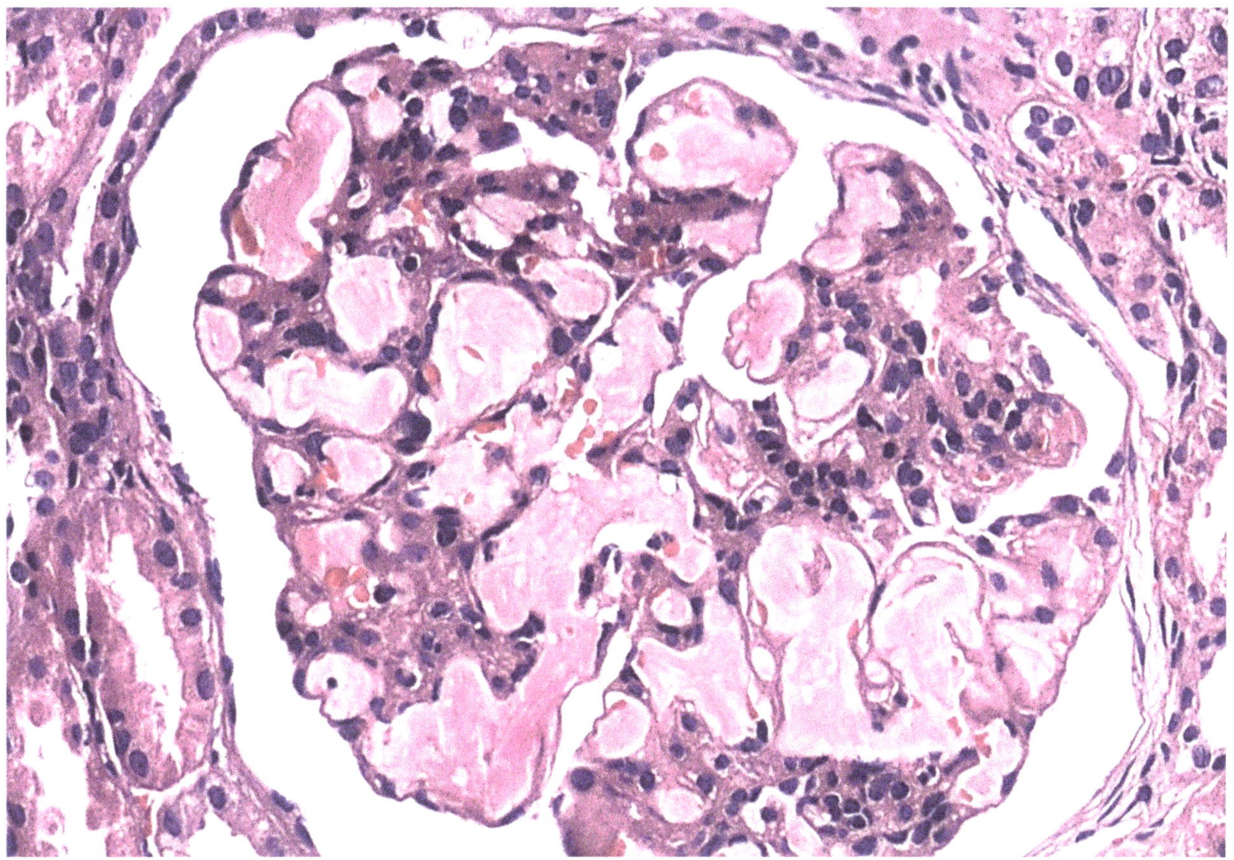

Figure 2:44.1: H&E Stain:20x: Glomerulus is enlarged and shows dilated glomerular capillaries containing pale acellular having a vague laminated appearance of lipoprotein thrombi.

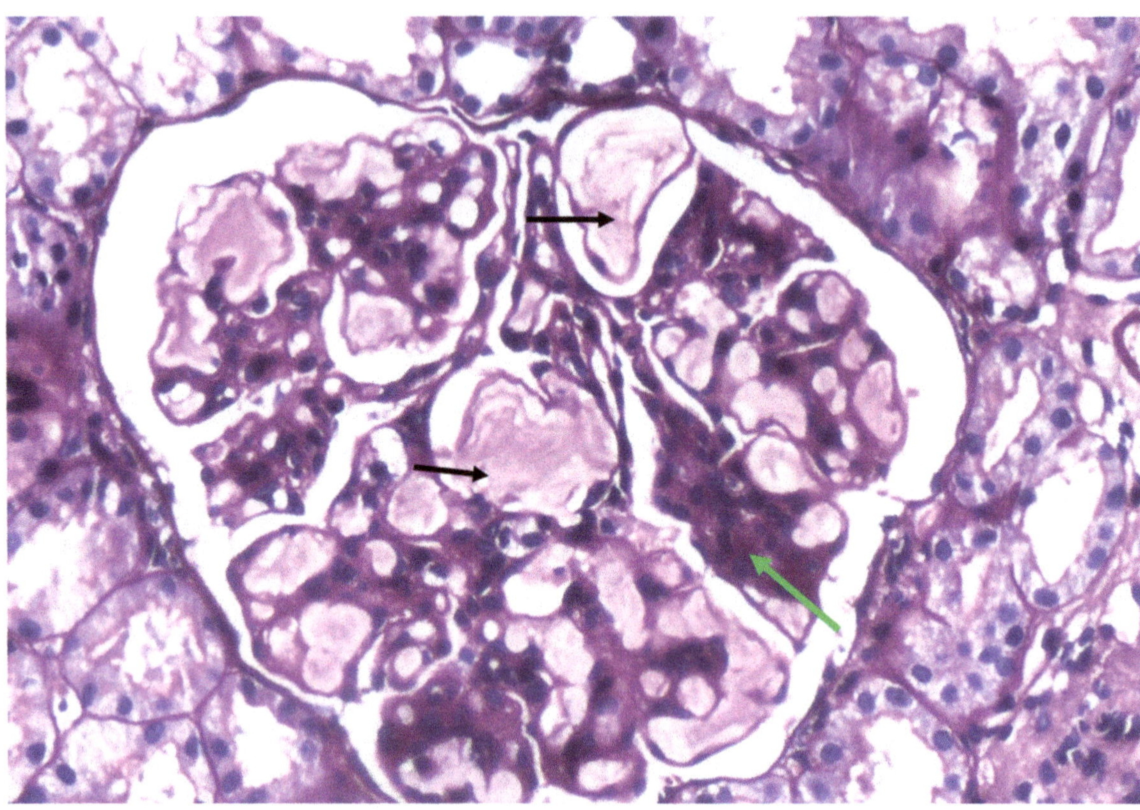

Figure 2:44.2: PAS Stain:20x: Glomerulus showing weak PAS positive lipoprotein thrombi (**black** arrows). There is mild mesangial hypercellularity (**green** arrow).

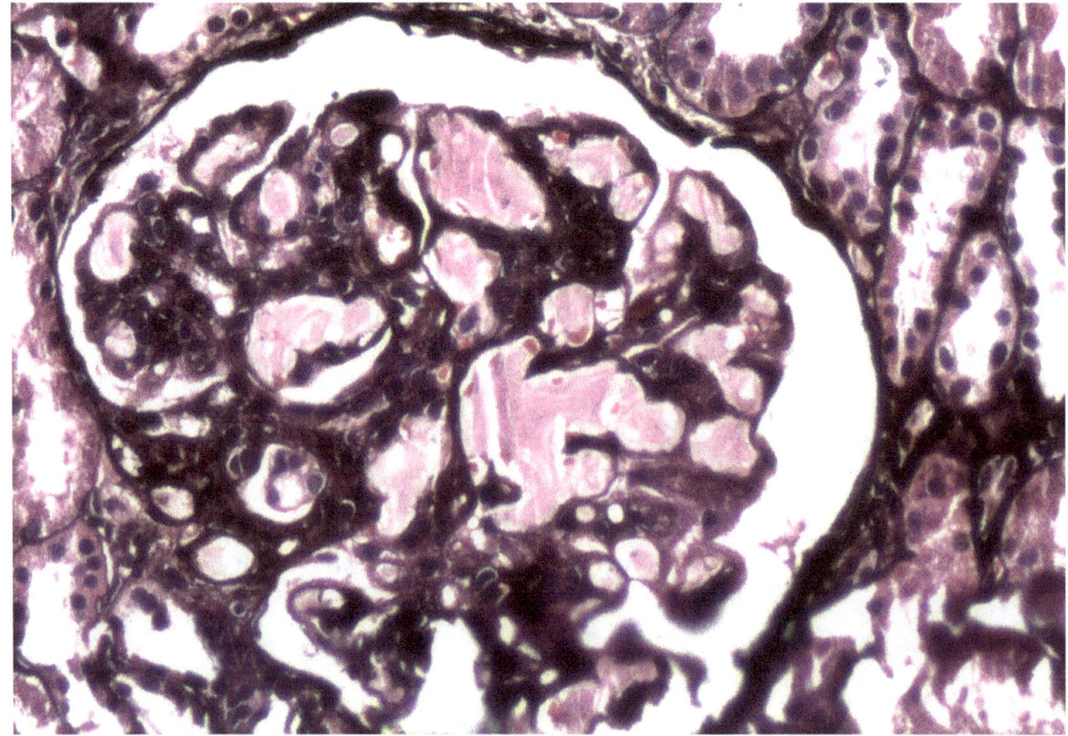

Figure 2:44.3: PASM Stain:20x: Glomerulus showing Silver-negative lipoprotein thrombi. The basement membranes appear mildly thickened.

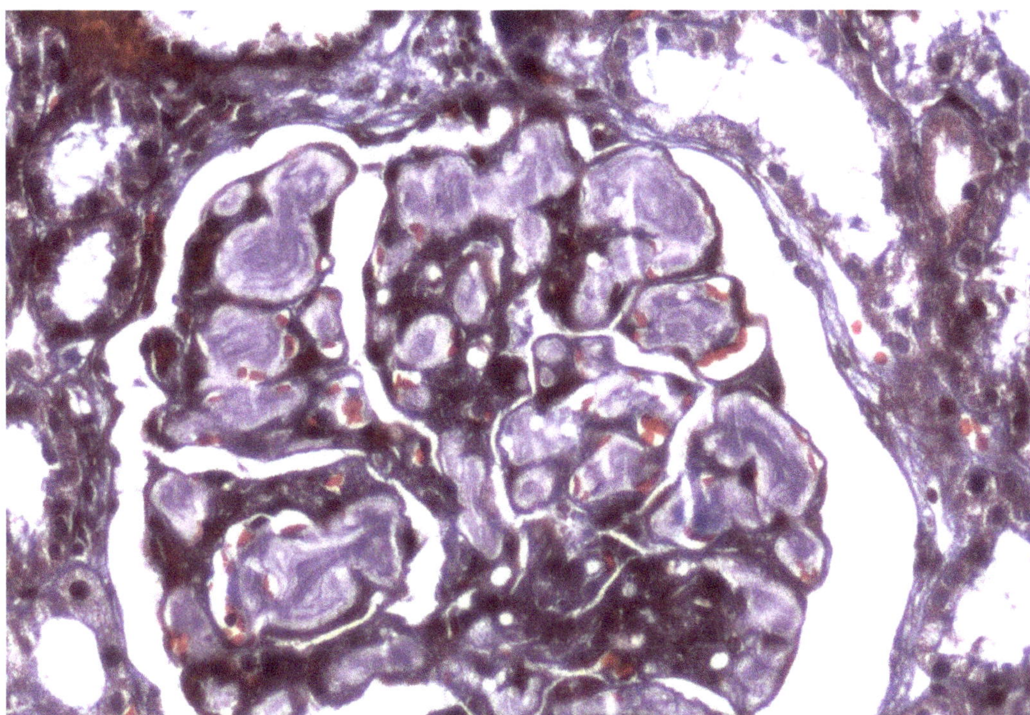

Figure 2:44.4: MT Stain:20x: Glomerulus showing pale blue lipoprotein thrombi. Note: Fibrin thrombi would have been fuchsinophilic (reddish).

Additional stains:

1. Congo red stain: These thrombi are not congophilic.

2. Oil red O stain: frozen section: positive for Lipid showing reddish capillary thrombi.

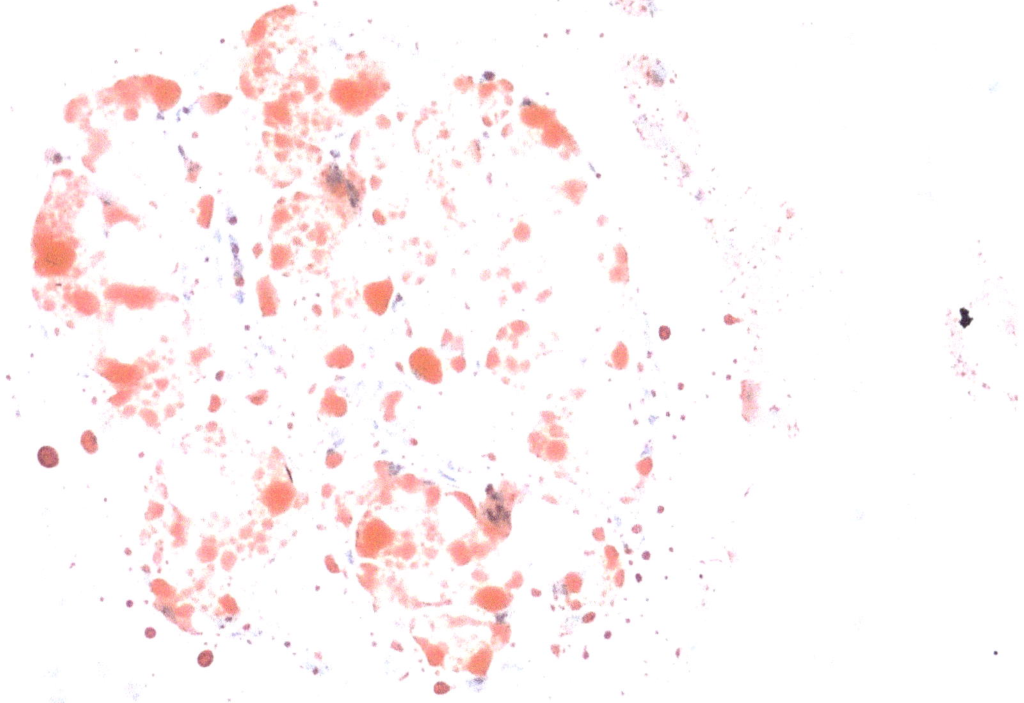

Figure 2:44.5: Oil red O stain on frozen section 20x: Positive for Lipid showing reddish capillary thrombi.

Immunofluorescence:

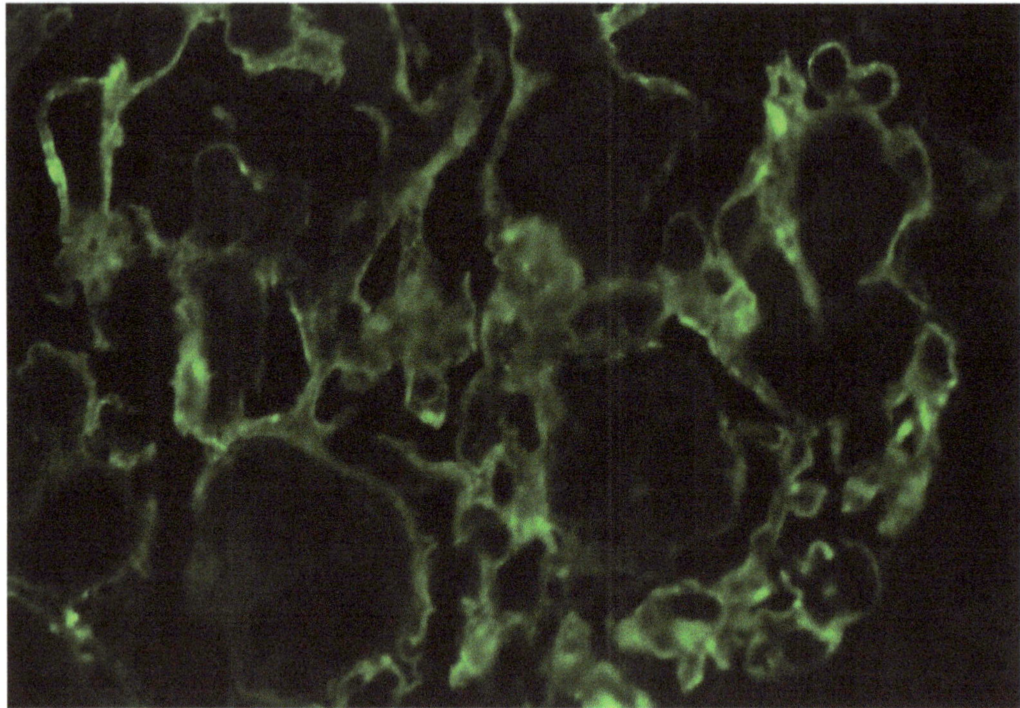

Figure 2:44.6: IF:20x: Negative for Immunoglobulins and complements.

Interpretation: Suggestive of Lipoprotein glomerulopathy.

Additional investigations:

Whole Exom Sequencing: Apolipoprotein E gene mutation is seen.

Electron microscopy: Dilated glomerular capillaries showing granules and vacuoles, forming concentric lamellate, giving finger-print appearance.

Final diagnosis: Lipoprotein Glomerulopathy.

DEFINITIONS

Acute tubular injury:

Denudation and flattening of the lining epithelium along with loss of the brush border. Necrosis is not seen.

Acute tubular necrosis:

Ischemia/toxin mediated coagulative necrosis of tubular epithelium.

Tubulitis:

Inflammatory cells infiltrating the basolateral aspect of tubular epithelium.

Tubular casts:

Tubules act like Molds in which different coagulated proteins and elements form casts in tubular lumens. E.g. Red cells casts, WBC casts, PAS-positive hyaline casts, pigmented casts.

Tubular atrophy:

Wasting of tubules due to ischemia, obstruction or severe cellular injury.

PATTERNS

Patterns of Tubular Atrophy (3 types):

1. **Thyroidization pattern:** It is more common in chronic pyelonephritis and chronic kidney disease (CKD) (Figure 3.1).
2. **Classic pattern:** There is wrinkling and thickening of the basement membranes and also loss of the brush border (Figure 3.2).
3. **Endocrinization pattern:** Small tubules with narrow or no tubular lumina, showing cuboidal epithelial cells with little or no basement membrane thickening, resembling endocrine gland histology e.g. parathyroid gland. This pattern is commonly seen in renal artery stenosis (Figure: 5:5.2)

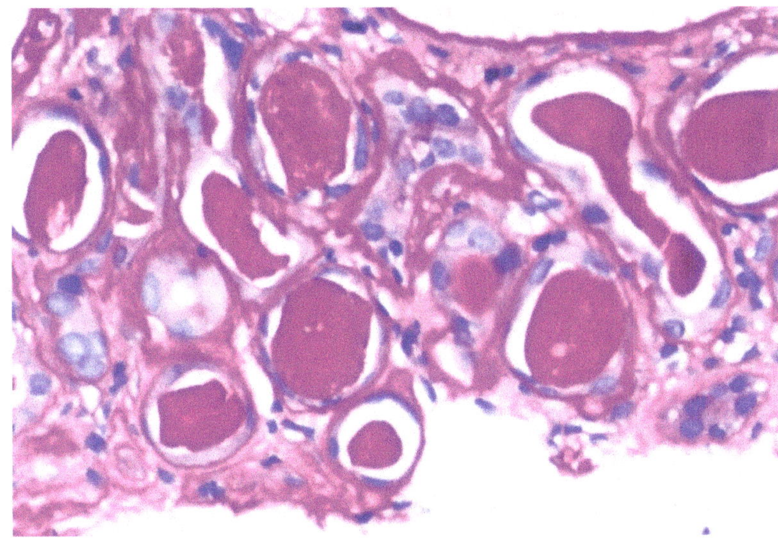

Figure: 3.1: PAS Stain 40x: Thyroidization pattern of tubular atrophy, the tubules show a flattened lining epithelium and contain PAS-positive casts(colloid-like) mimicking thyroid gland parenchyma.

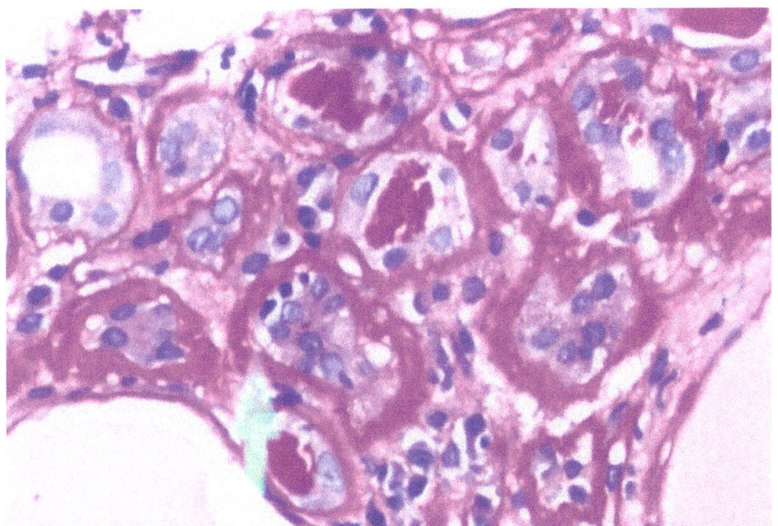

Figure: 3.2: PAS Stain 40x: Classic pattern of atrophy with thickening and wrinkling of tubular basement membranes

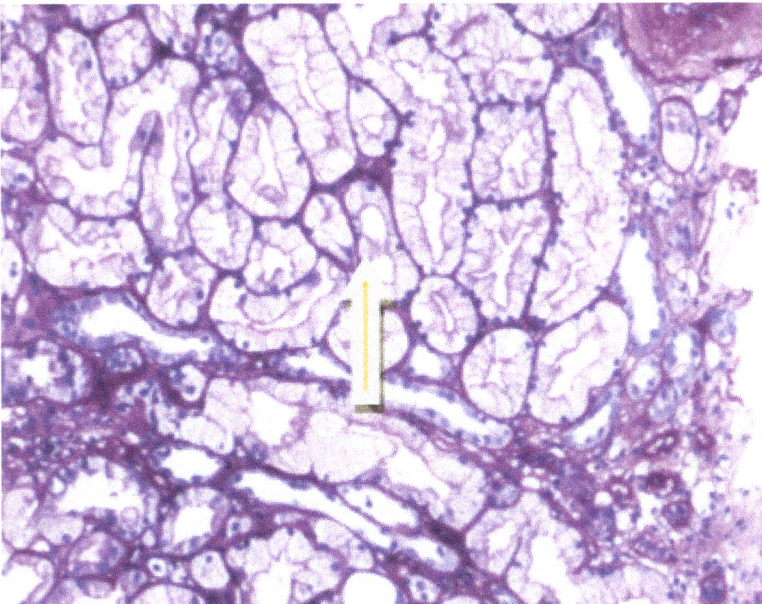

***Hydropic change/osmotic nephrosis:**

Figure: 3.3: PAS Stain 20x: Isometric tubular vacuolizations of proximal tubular epithelial cells

Reference

Hydropic change: Hydropic change may be seen in patients who have received hypertonic solutions such as sucrose solutions, mannitol, high molecular weight dextrans, radiopaque contrast material, hydroxyethyl starch, or intravenous immunoglobulin.: Heptinstall's Pathology of Kidney, Seventh edition, Chapter 03: Primer on the Pathologic Classification and Diagnosis Of Kidney Disease: Vacuolar change:page-105.

*Hyaline degeneration of tubules seen in nephrotic range proteinuria:

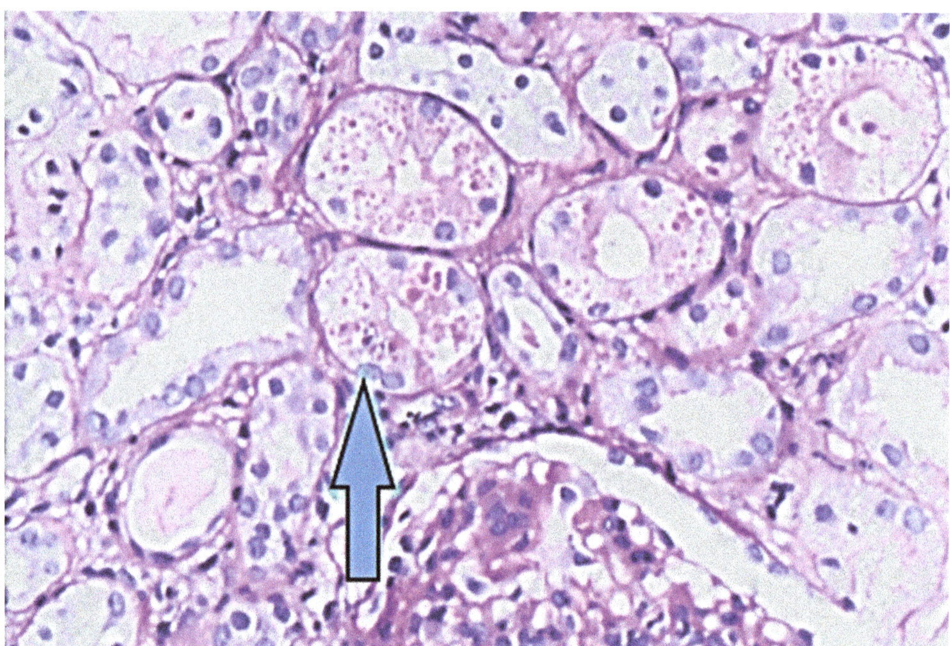

Figure: 3.4: PAS Stain: 20x: PAS-positive Lipid resorption droplets in proximal tubules, which are eosinophilic on H&E, fuchsinophilic on MT Stain.

CASE 1

History: A 26-year-old male, non-alcoholic, was treated for acute pancreatitis a month back; he continues to get on and off abdominal pain, nausea, vomiting, and poor oral intake. He has now developed pedal edema for the last four days. BP is 110/80 mm of Hg.

Investigations: Serum creatinine: 2.24mg/dl, CUE: protein: 2+, pus cells: 15 to 16/HPF, RBCs: 03 to 04/HPF, 24 hour urine protein: 2478mg, USG: Right kidney: 10.7cm, Left kidney: 10.8 cm, increased echogenicity, serum cholesterol: 220 mg/dl, Triglycerides: 474mg/dl, Liver function test: normal, serum albumin: 4.2g/dl, C3, C4: normal, ANA profile: negative.

Clinical diagnosis: Subnephrotic proteinuria with renal dysfunction, suspected AKI/ Glomerulonephritis.

Differential diagnoses: 1. ATN/AIN 2. Autoimmune Pancreatitis with glomerulonephritis 3. IgG4-related tubulointerstitial nephritis.

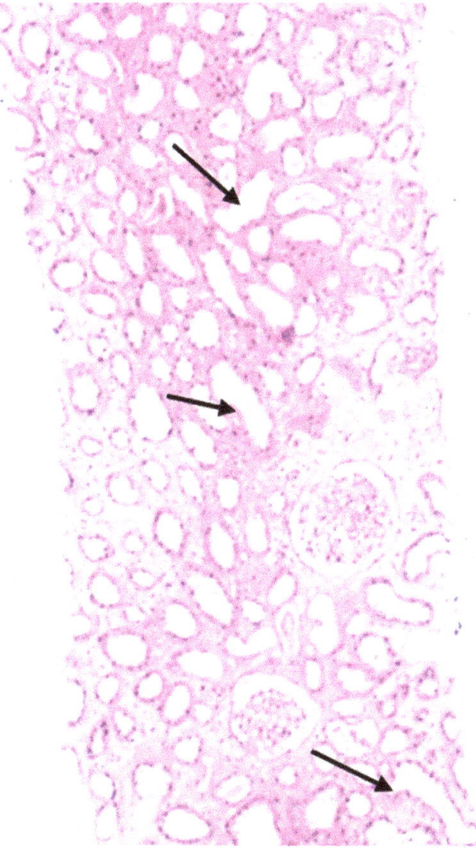

Figure 3:1.1: H&E stain: 10x: Tubular injury: loss of the brush border of tubules.

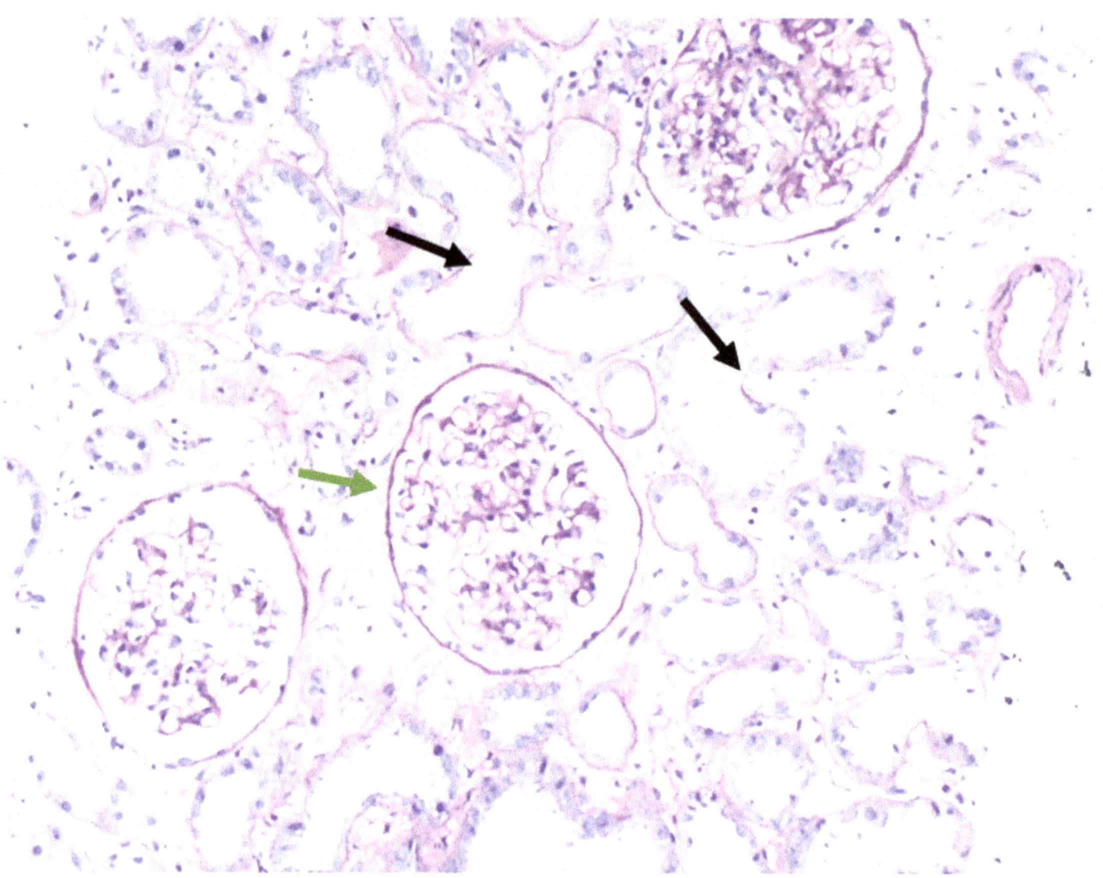

Figure 3:1.2: PAS Stain: 20x: Flattening and denudation of the lining epithelium along with loss of the brush border (**black** arrows). The glomeruli appear normal (**green** arrow).

Interpretation: Moderate Acute Tubular Injury

Final Diagnosis: AKI due to ischemic ATN (Prerenal)

CASE 2

History: 3 months and 14 days old female, full term normal vaginal delivery, low birth weight= 2 Kg, cried normally at birth, born of non-consanguineous marriage, presented with failure to thrive. There is no family history of any metabolic or renal disease.

Investigations: Hb: 7.5 gm/dl, Total leucocyte count: 5,000/cu mm, Platelet count: 2.5 Lakh/cu mm. Serum creatinine: 5mg/dl, Spot Urine protein to creatinine ratio: 1.2 g/g, Urine analysis: Protein: 2+, RBCs: 8 to 10/HPF, WBCs: 4 to 6/HPF, Crystals: Oxalate ++, USG findings: Right kidney: 4.6cm, Left kidney: 4.8cm, CMD-lost, normal sized echogenic kidneys.

Clinical Diagnosis: Failure to thrive with AKI-AKIN Stage 3 with Sub Nephrotic range proteinuria with microscopic hematuria and oxalate crystalluria.

Differential diagnoses: AKI due to Ischemic ATN/ CKD due to – Genetic disorders like Cystinosis/ Oxalosis/ARPKD/CAKUT.

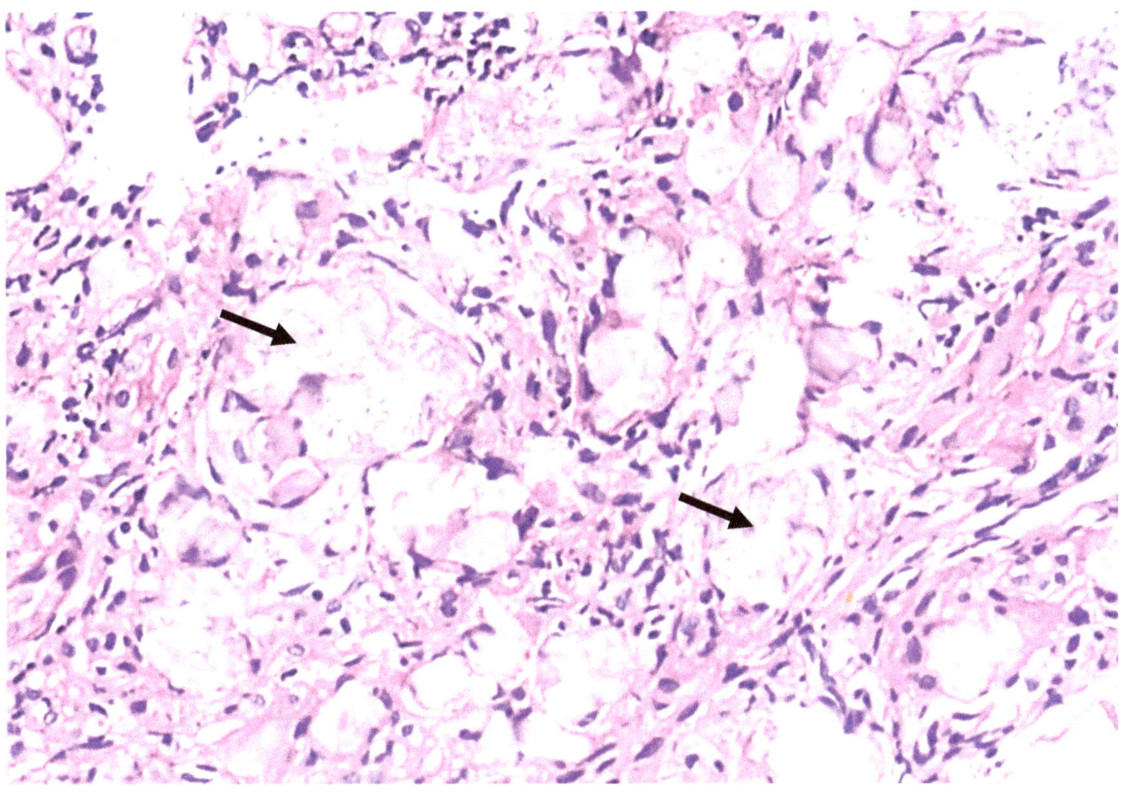

Figure 3:2.1: H&E Stain 20x: Tubules with Oxalate crystals (**black** arrows).

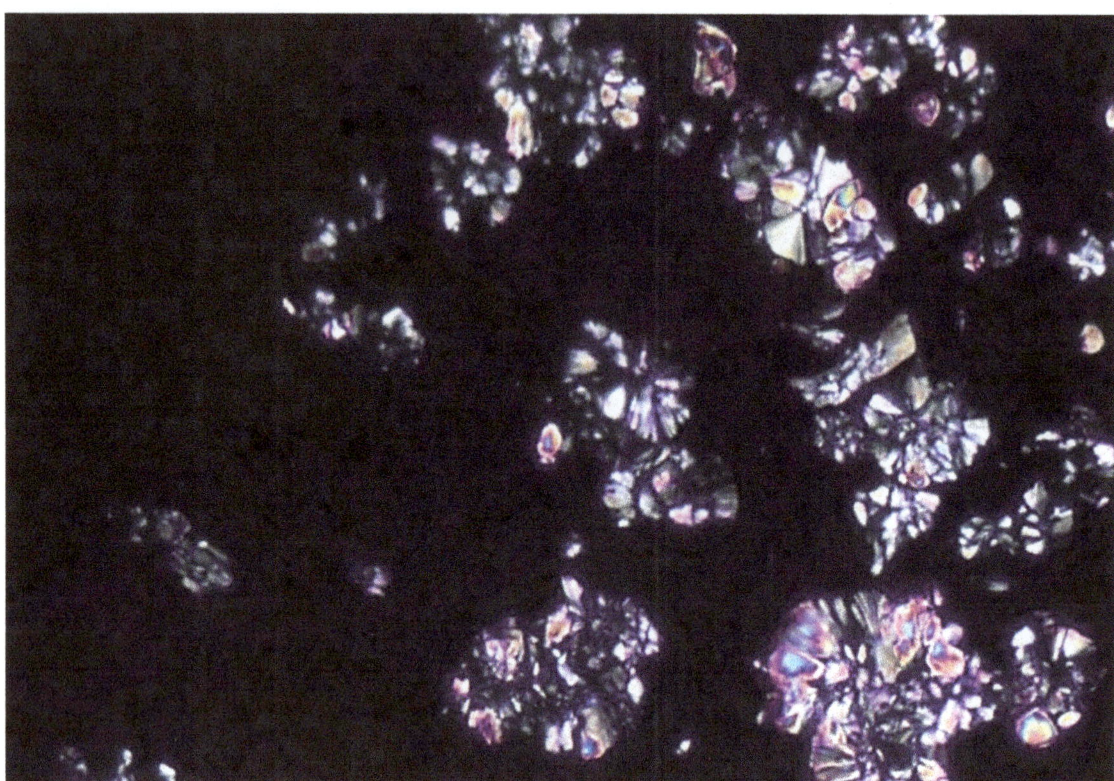

Figure 3:2.2: H&E Stain 20x: Tubules: Oxalate crystals under polarizer.

These crystals are clear with refractile quality shaped as plates, fine spicules and exhibit bright birefringence under polarization, suggestive of Calcium oxalate crystals

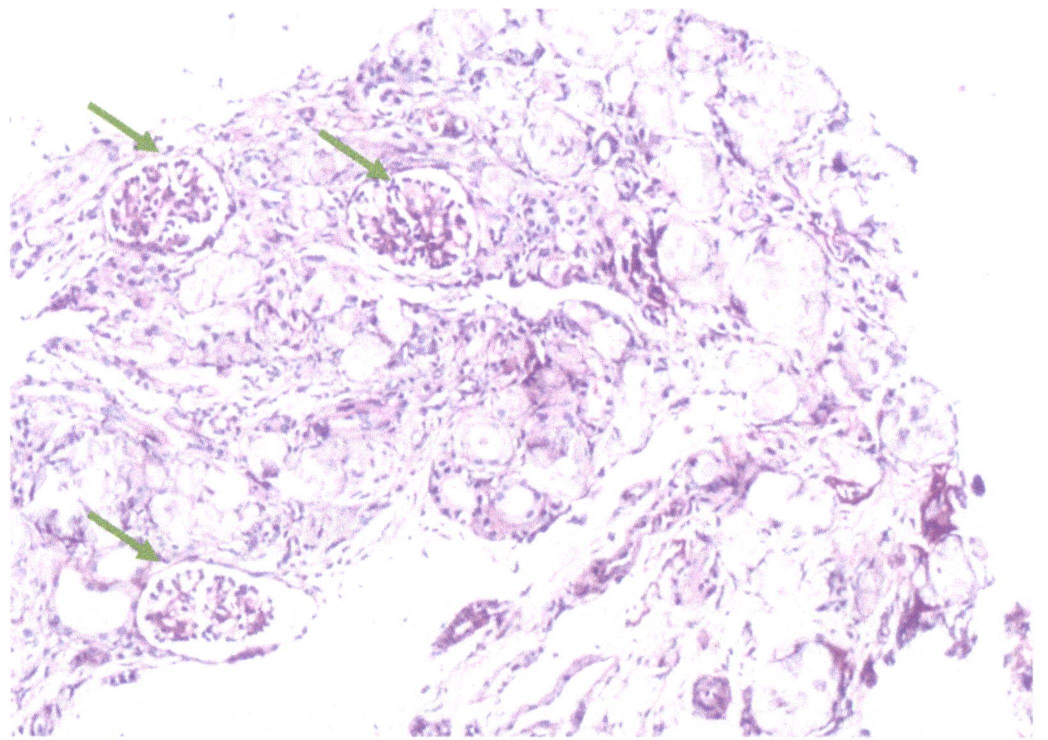

Figure 3:2.3: PAS Stain 10x: Many Infantile type of glomeruli (green arrows).

Immunofluorescence: IF study shows no significant immune deposits.

Interpretation: Oxalate Nephropathy

Additional investigations:

1. **Genetic testing:** Whole exome sequencing: mutation of the gene AGXT: Alanine Glyoxylate Transferase

Final diagnosis: Primary hyperoxaluria type 1.

CASE 3

History: 57-year-old male, a chronic alcoholic, non-smoker, non-diabetic, and non-hypertensive, presented with a history of generalized weakness for the last few months. For gastritis, he has been using Proton pump inhibitors daily for the last few years. He has chronic diarrhea, 2-3 bowel movements in medium to large volume daily, without any crampy abdominal pain or fever, not accompanied by vomiting or blood in the stool. He has lost 3 Kilograms of weight in the last 3 months. He is lethargic and looks pale with pedal edema. No jaundice. On evaluation, he was found to have normal Liver function except for hypoalbuminemia. He is anemic and has renal dysfunction with hypokalemia and hypomagnesemia.

Investigations: Serum creatinine:3.1mg/dl, urea:130mg/dl, serum potassium: 3mEq/L, Serum Magnesium 1.2 mEq/L, Serum albumin: 2.5 g/dl, serum Bilirubin: 0.8 mg/dl, SGOT:55U/L, SGPT: 35U/L, Serum Vitamin B12 level: 150pg/ml. Urine analysis: Protein 1+, RBCs: 1 to 2/HPF, Pus cells: 1 to 2/HPF.

The patient had persistent renal dysfunction with Serum Creatinine 2.5mg/dl at the end of one month; hence, a renal biopsy was done.

Clinical Diagnosis: Prerenal AKI, now AKD/Acute Kidney disease (Renal dysfunction of 1-3 months duration) with nutritional deficiencies related to chronic alcoholism and prolonged PPI use, causing chronic diarrhea and associated electrolyte abnormalities.

Differential diagnoses: ATN/AIN/CKD

Light microscopy:

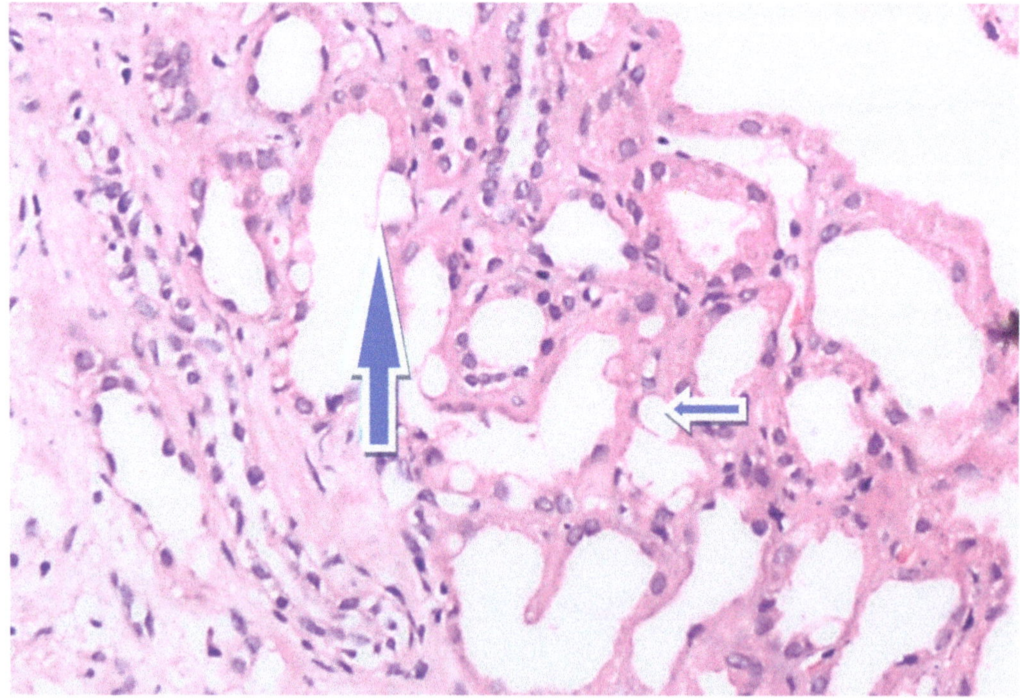

Figure 3:3.1: H&E Stain 20x: Hypokalemic Nephropathy: These tubular epithelial cell cytoplasmic vacuolizations are coarse, clear, and irregular in size.

Immunofluorescence: IF study shows no significant immune deposits.

Interpretation: Hypokalemic Nephropathy.

Additional reading

Hypokalemic nephropathy generally requires one month to develop and is reversible with potassium repletion. Prolonged hypokalemia can cause severe changes like interstitial nephritis and fibrosis, tubular atrophy, and cyst formation, especially in the renal medulla. Once these chronic changes develop, correcting potassium may not reverse the pathology but reduce the speed of progression of CKD. Low dietary potassium and low urinary potassium excretion are associated with the progression of chronic kidney disease. A Urinary Potassium of < 25 meq/day or Spot Urinary Potassium to creatinine ratio < 22 meq/g suggests extrarenal causes for hypokalemia.

CASE 4

History: 35-years old female, farmer by occupation, had fever with chills, dysuria, Vomiting, and bilateral loin pain. She is non-diabetic and non-hypertensive. She was treated at a local hospital with IV Antibiotics, IV Fluids, and IV analgesics – NSAIDs. She was later found to have worsening renal function. She was referred to a higher centre for further management. Patient had improvement in fever, but renal function continued to worsen. There is no h/o arthritis, skin rash, or oral ulcer. Dialysis was initiated, and a renal biopsy was done.

Investigations: Hb: 10 gm/dl, TLC: 13,000/cu mm, Platelet count: 5 lakhs/cu mm, serum creatinine: 10 mg/dl, CRP: 50 mg/dl, Urine analysis: Protein: 2+, Pus cells: 40 to 50/HPF, RBCs: 10 to 12/HPF, Pus cell casts: 2 to 3/HPF, Urine culture: Sterile.

Clinical Diagnosis: Acute Pyelonephritis versus Acute interstitial nephritis related to antibiotics / NSAIDs.

Light microscopy:

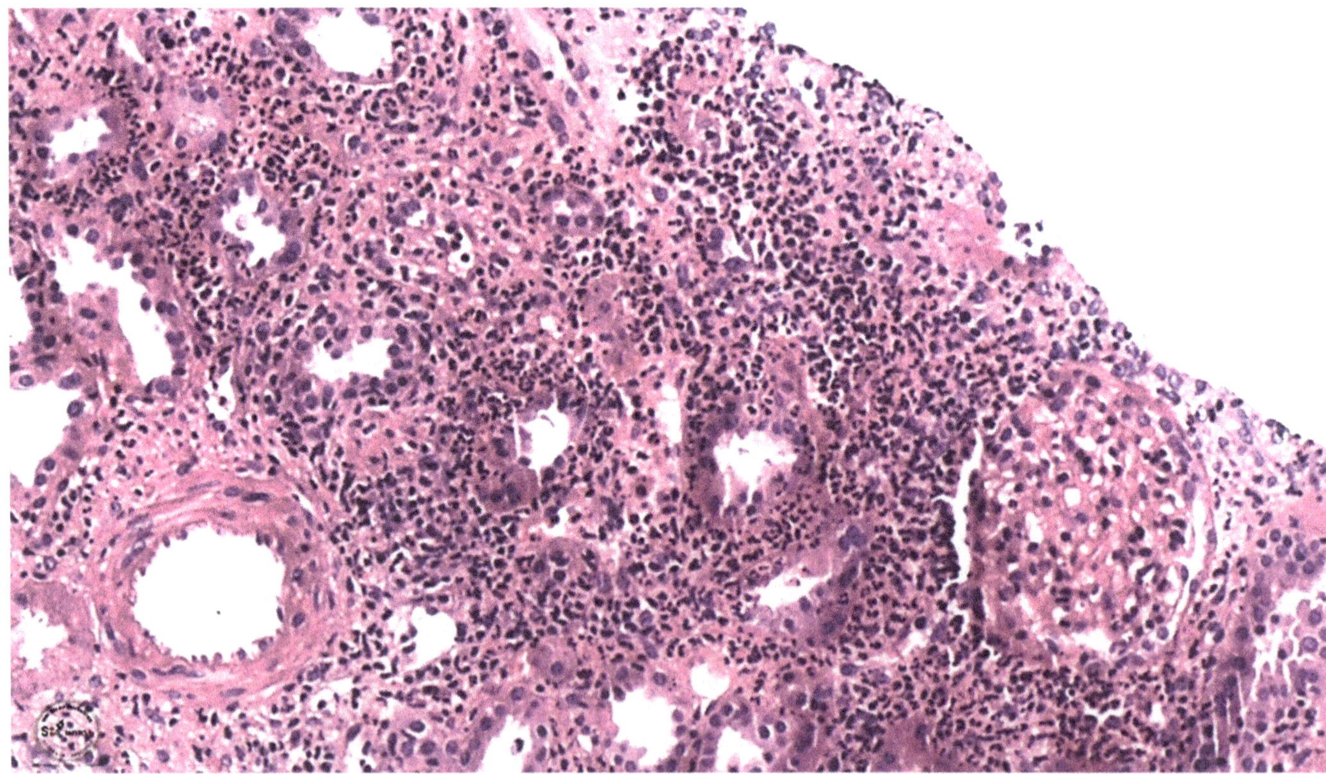

Figure: 3:4.1: H&E Stain 10x: Diffuse neutrophilic interstitial inflammation. The glomerulus and artery are normal.

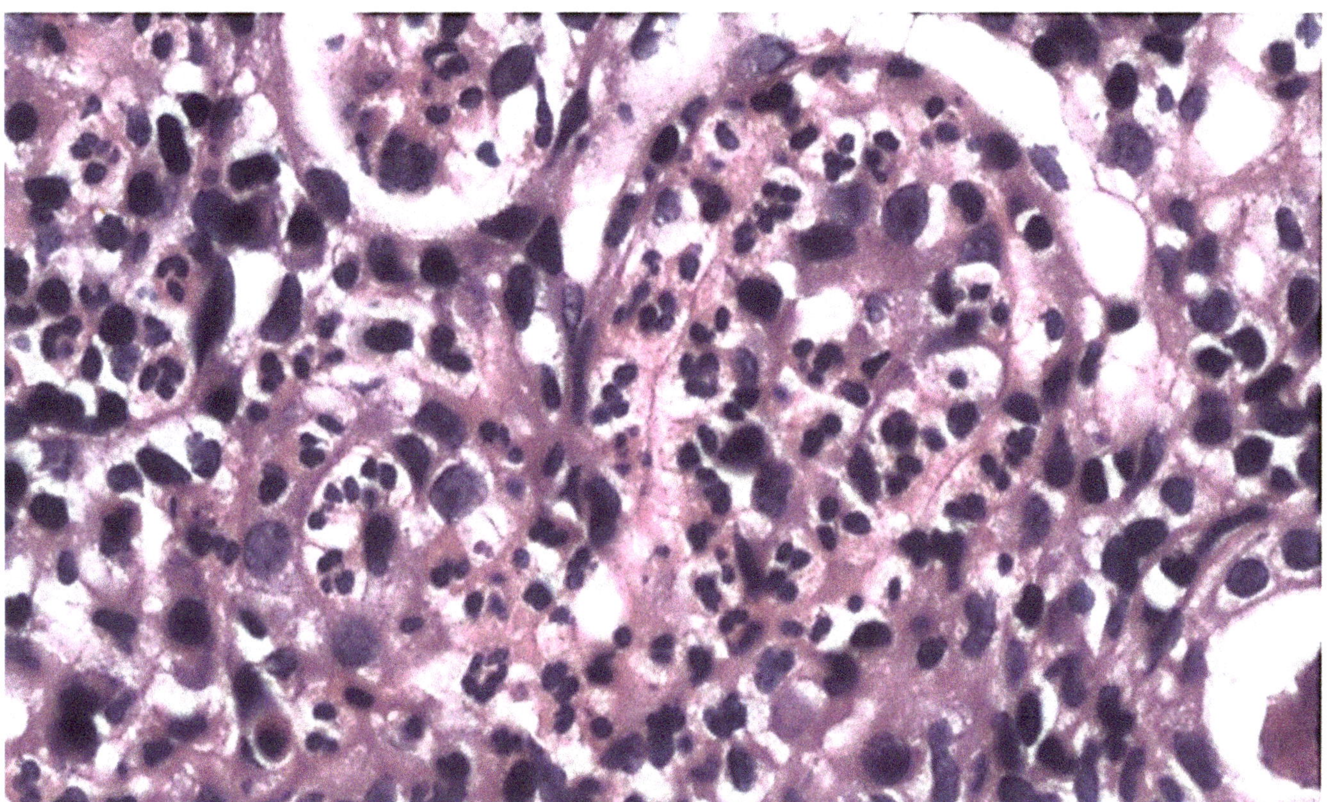

Figure 3:4.2: H&E Stain: 40x: Tubules: Neutrophilic tubulitis and neutrophils in tubules.

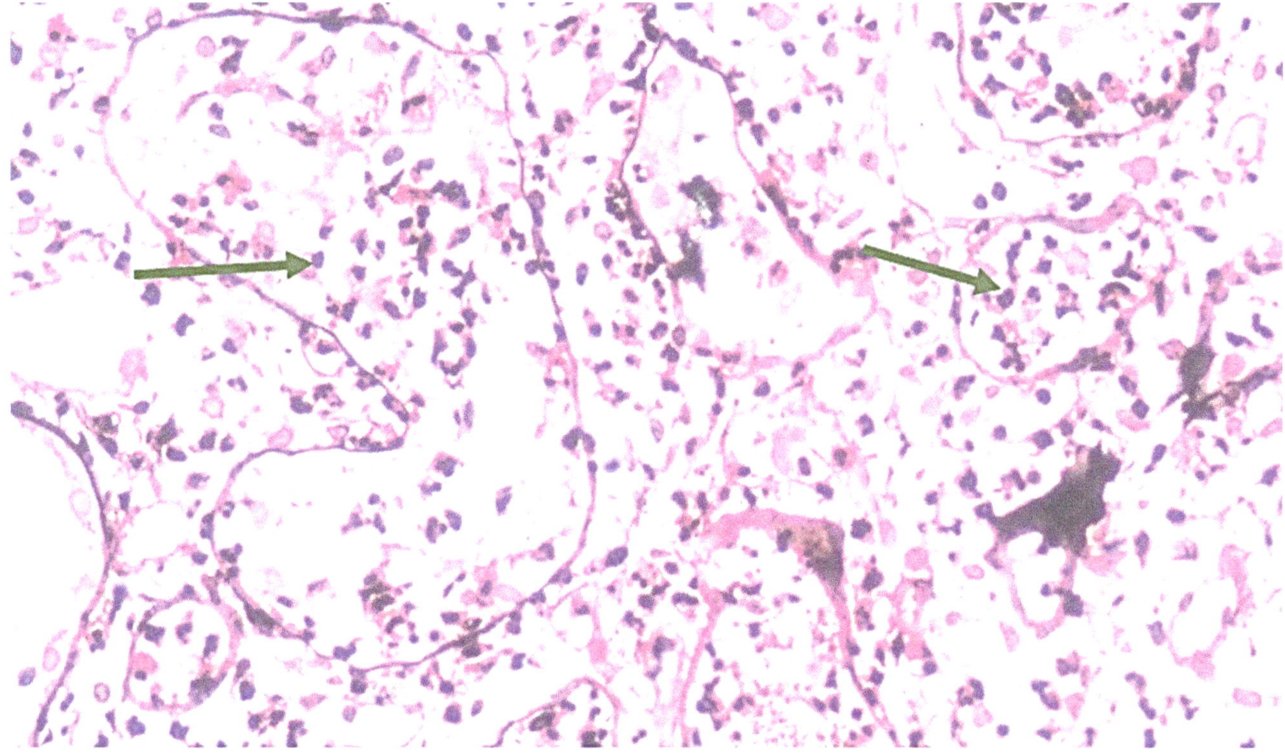

Figure: 3:4.3: PASM Stain: 20 x: Tubules: neutrophilic casts.

Immunofluorescence: IF study shows no significant immune deposits.

Interpretation: Acute pyelonephritis

Pathology Pearls

*In acute pyelonephritis, neutrophils appear first in peritubular capillaries. This is followed by capillary wall rupture, with leakage of fluid and cells into the interstitium.

Reference
*Microvascular injury and Repair in acute human bacterial pyelonephritis, Ivanyi B, Thoenes W. et.al, Virchows Arch A Pathol Anat Histopathol 1987;411:257.

History: A 46-year-old female, non-diabetic and non-hypertensive, had a fall and vertebral wedge fracture with slip disc and compressive myelopathy for which she needed surgical decompression and vertebroplasty. She was started on Calcium supplements, Vitamin D supplements and IV Zoledronate yearly once.4months later, she came with easy fatiguability, backache and shortness of breath on minimal exertion. She was pale on inspection, without any crepitations or adventitious sounds in the lungs. BP 100/60 mm of Hg.

Investigations: Hb: 6.5 g/dl, TLC: 4,600/cu mm, Platelet count: 1.2 lakhs/cu mm. serum creatinine: 4.1 mg/dl, serum Calcium: 11 mg/dl, Vitamin D level: 35ng/ml, Urine analysis: Protein: 2+, RBCs:8 -10/HPF, Pus cells: 4-5/HPF. USG: Normal size kidneys, Parathyroid hormone (PTH): 55 pg/ml.

Clinical Diagnosis: AKI suspected CKD with severe anaemia/ Hypercalcemia – to rule out malignancy /paraproteinemia.

Light microscopy:

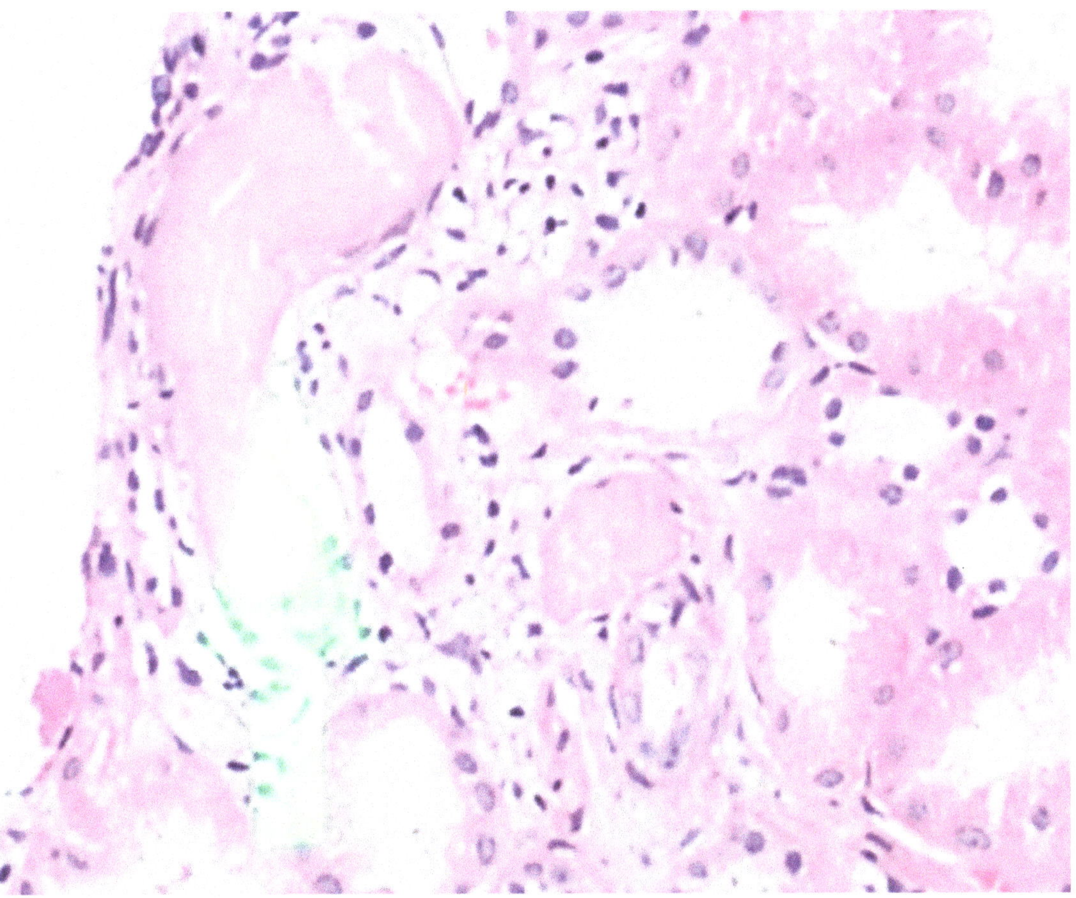

Figure: 3:5.1: H&E Stain 20x: Pale cast with fractured planes (green arrow).

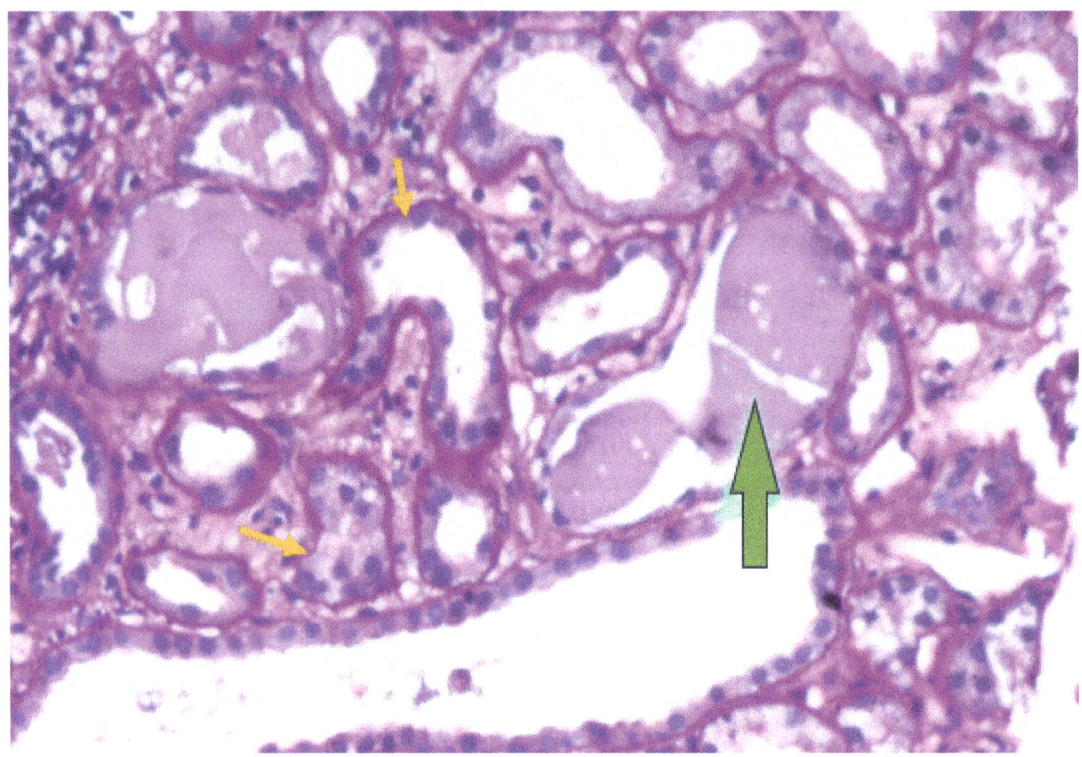

Figure: 3:5.2: PAS Stain 20x: Distal convoluted tubules (DCT): PAS negative casts with fractured planes (green arrow)Note the Tubular Basement Membranes (TBM) are PAS-positive(small yellow arrows).

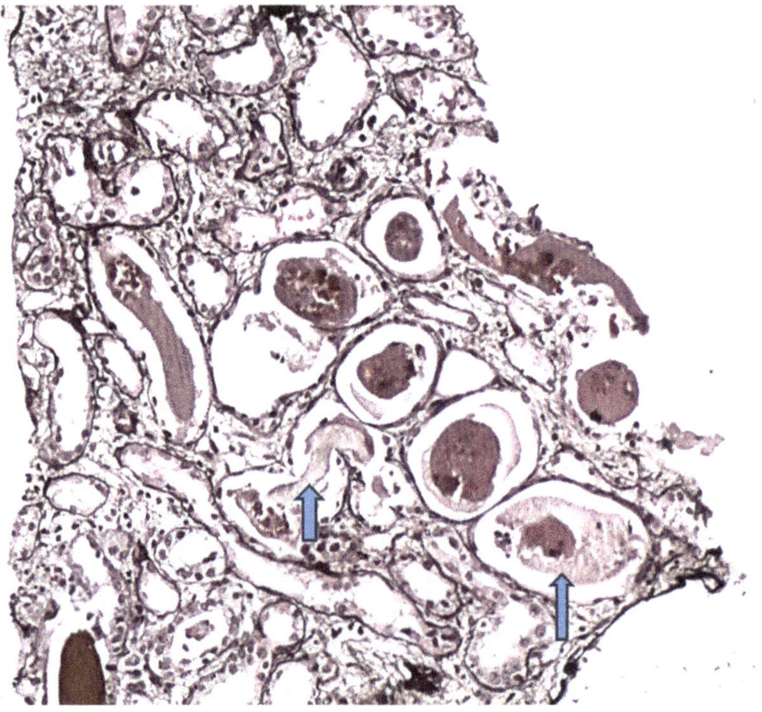

Figure: 3:5.3: PASM Stain:10x: DCT: Silver-negative tubular casts.

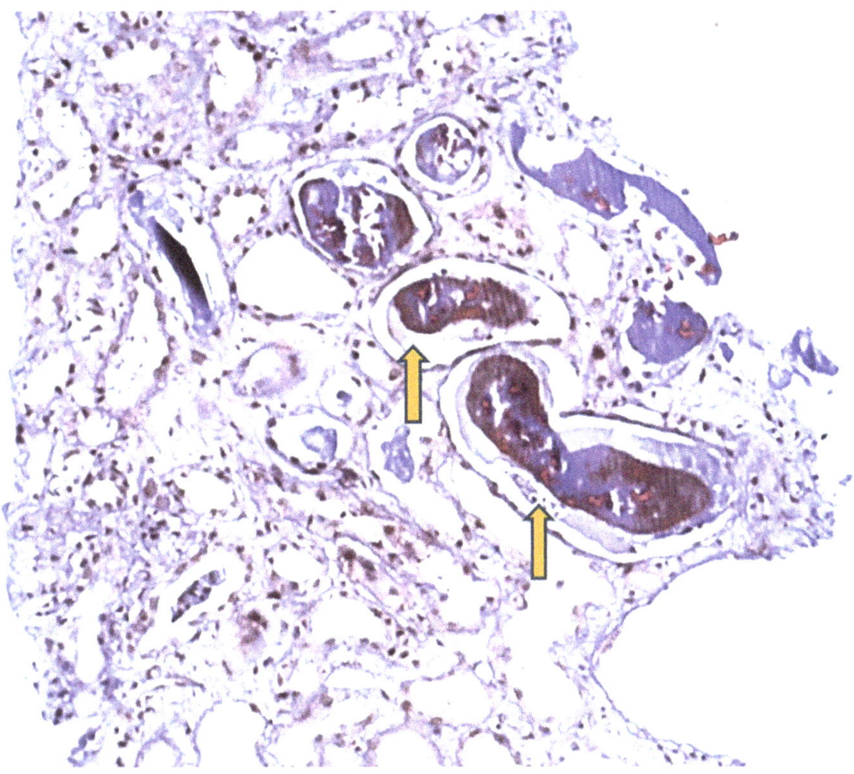

Figure: 3:5.4: Masson Trichrome Stain: 10x: DCT: Reddish-blue tubular casts.

Immunofluorescence: IF study shows no significant immune deposits in glomeruli and there is kappa light chain restriction in tubular casts.

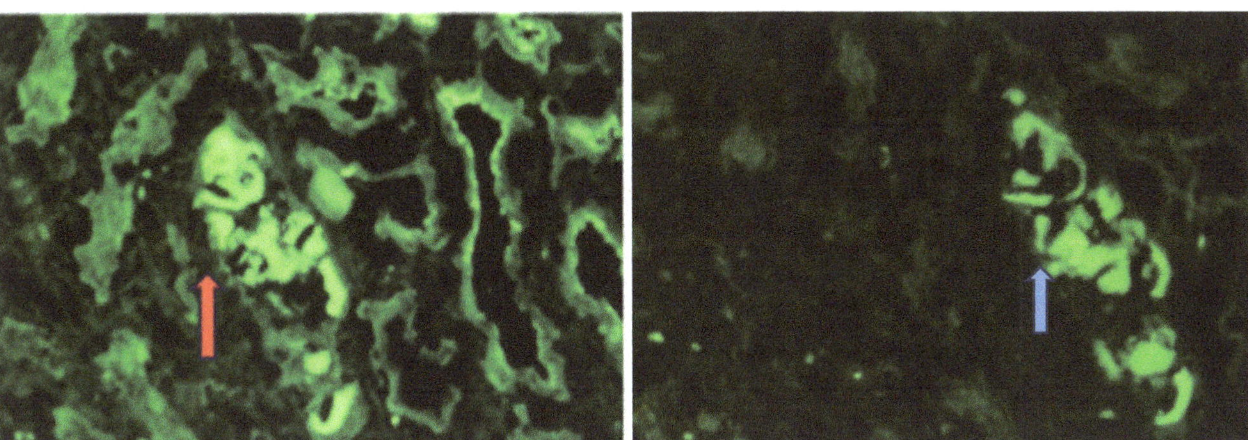

Figure: 3:5.5: Immunofluorescence 20 X: Kappa light chains being significantly positive (the difference of intensity should be ≥2 grades higher to call it restriction)in tubular casts with fractured planes as compared to Lambda light chains in tubular casts.

Interpretation:

Primary diagnosis: Light chain cast nephropathy (Kappa light chain restriction).

Pattern of injury: Acute tubular injury with approximately 30% of tubules involved by light-chain casts.

Additional findings: There is a mild tubulointerstitial change of chronicity (10%).

Serum immunofixation electrophoresis: IgG-Kappa M band, serum free light chain assay: Kappa light chains elevated, Beta-2 microglobulin: elevated, bone marrow biopsy: 25% of plasma cells.

CASE 6

History: A 25-year-old male with no baseline comorbid conditions was brought to the hospital with h/o multiple wasps bites all over exposed areas of his body. He had periorbital swelling, peri oral swelling, swelling all over his body, and shortness of breath. He has decreased urine output for the last 24 hours after the wasp stings. The last time he passed urine was 6 hours back, and it was cola coloured. BP 100/70. He was treated conservatively with IV Fluids, Analgesics and Antibiotics. He had persistent renal dysfunction at the end of 10 days, so renal biopsy was done.

Investigations: Hb: 11gm/dl, TLC: 15,000/cu mm, Platelet :1.9 lakhs/cu mm, serum creatinine: 3.6 mg/dl, Potassium: 6 mEq/L, Venous blood gas: Lactate 4 mEq/L, PaO2: 70mm Hg, PCO2: 35, mmHg Bicarbonates: 13 mEq/L.

Clinical Diagnosis: AKI post wasp bites – Could be wasp toxin mediated ATN, prerenal AKI, Myoglobinuria mediated AKI and rarely AIN.

Light microscopy:

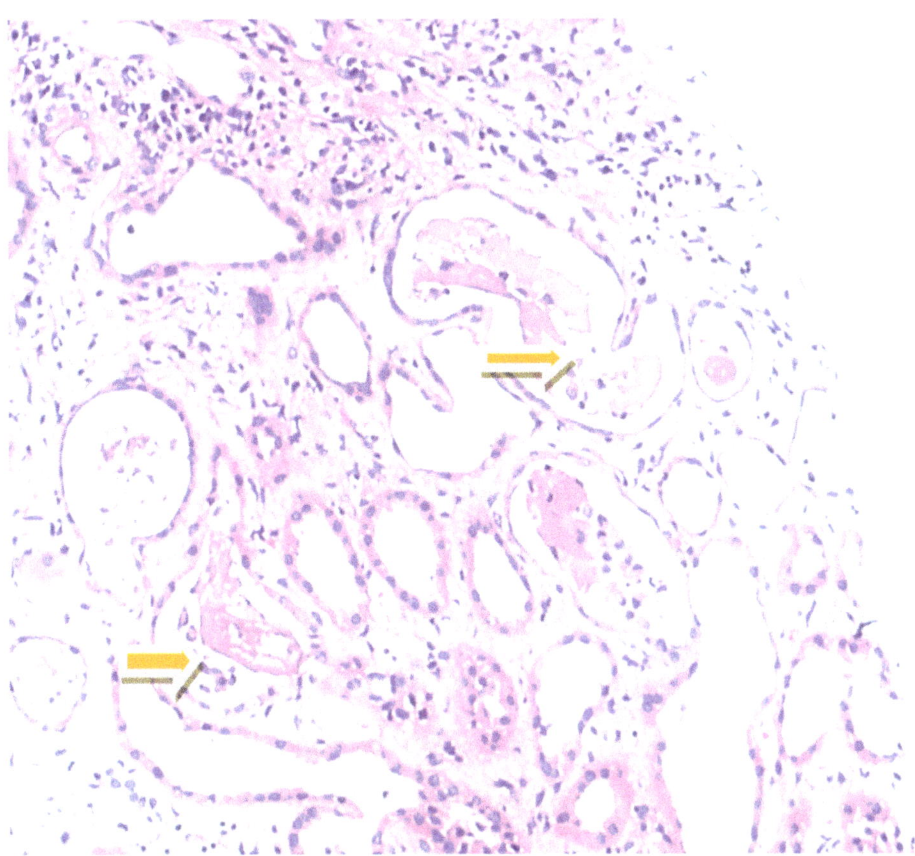

Figure: 3:6.1: H&E Stain 10x: Distal convoluted tubules (DCT): Pinkish granular casts: Myoglobin casts.

The morphology* of these casts ranged from light pink to dark red and slightly brown granular casts by haematoxylin and eosin stain.

Myoglobin casts

PASM Stain:40x:silver positive casts

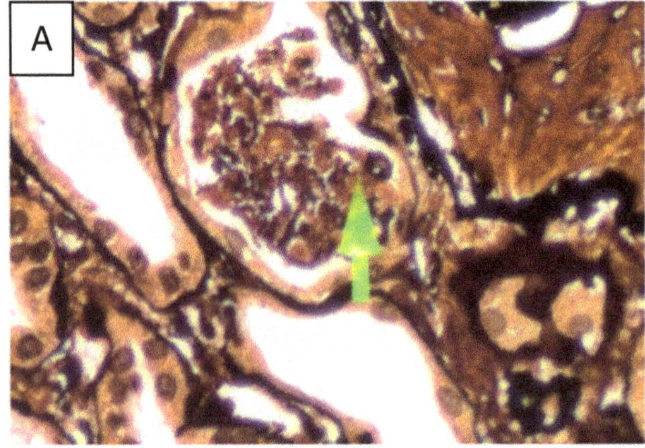

MT Stain-40x: fuchsinophilic casts

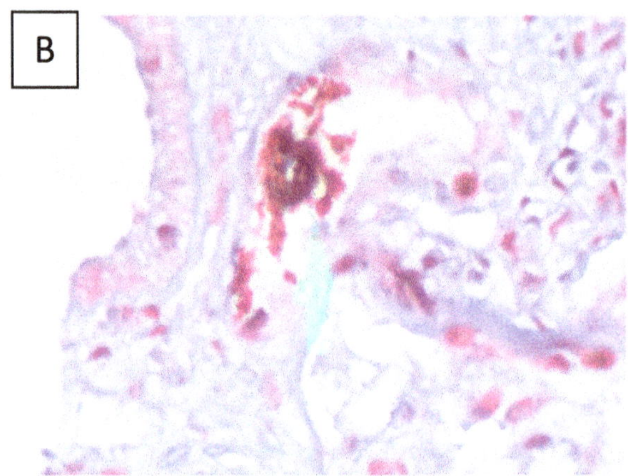

Figure: 3:6.2: PASM Stain: (A) 20x: Myoglobin casts partially argyrophilic and (B) Reddish with Masson trichrome.

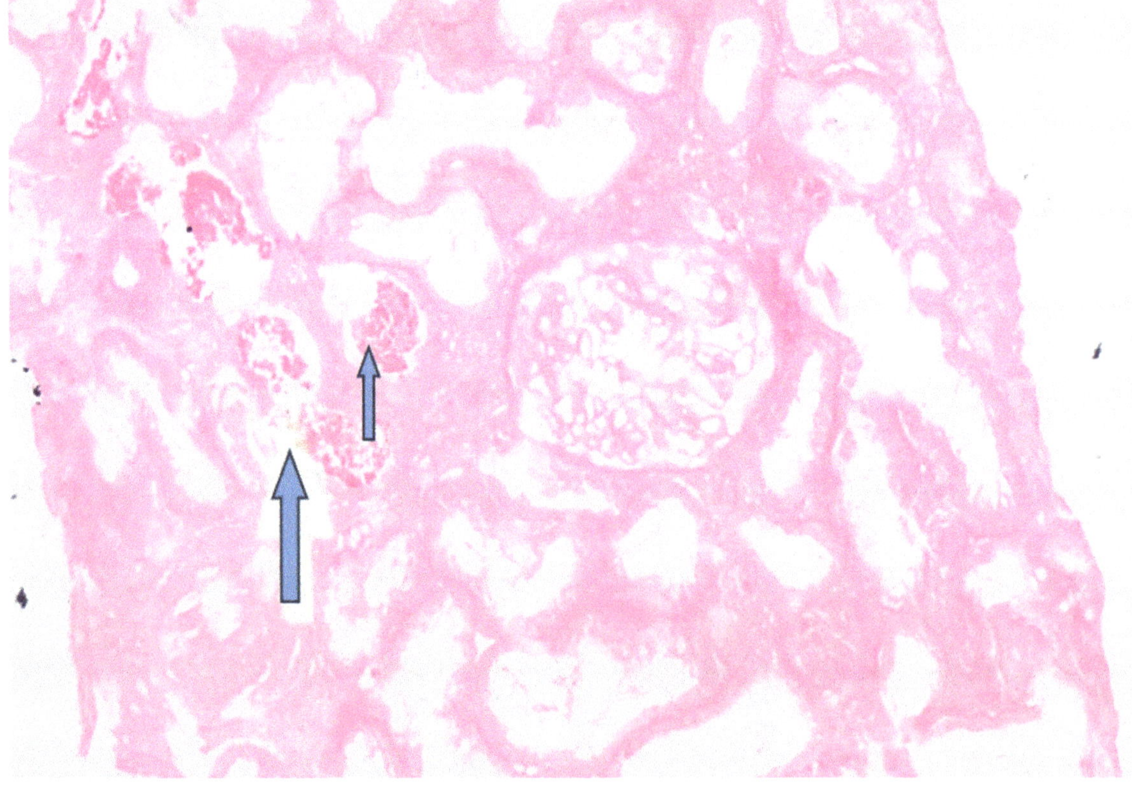

Figure: 3:6.3: Perl Stain 20x: Negative in the tubular casts.

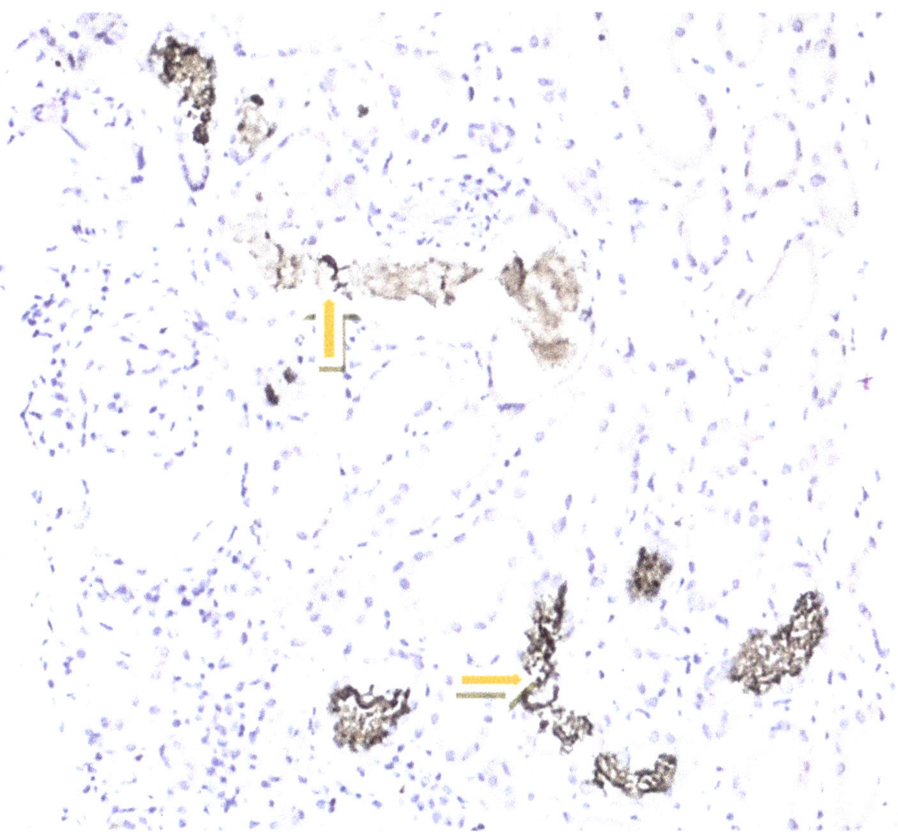

Figure: 3:6.4: Immunohistochemistry: Myoglobin stain 20x: Myoglobin cast nephropathy.

Interpretation: Myoglobin cast nephropathy.

***Reference**

Myoglobin casts in renal biopsies: immunohistochemistry and morphologic spectrum: Helen Liapis et. al, DOI: 10.1016/j.humpath.2016.02.026

CASE 7

History: 40 Years female presented with unexplained renal dysfunction picked on routine health check when performed for some generalised weakness and easy fatiguability. She is nonsmoker, non-alcoholic, non-diabetic and normotensive. She has no clinical features to suggest a secondary glomerulonephritis. Has not been using any indigenous medicines or pain killers. BP is 120/80 mm of Hg.

Investigations: Urine analysis: protein:2+, Glucose: 2+, RBCs: 8 to 10/HPF, Pus cells: 1 to 2/HPF, serum creatinine: 5 mg/dl, Sodium: 135mEq/L, Potassium: 3.4 mEq/L, Chloride: 111 mEq/L, serum albumin: 3.4g/dl, Globulin: 4.5g/dl, serum calcium: 9.8 mg/dl, Hb: 7 g/dl, HBA1c: 5.3%, viral screening is negative.

Clinical diagnosis: CKD-CIN/Proximal tubulopathy.

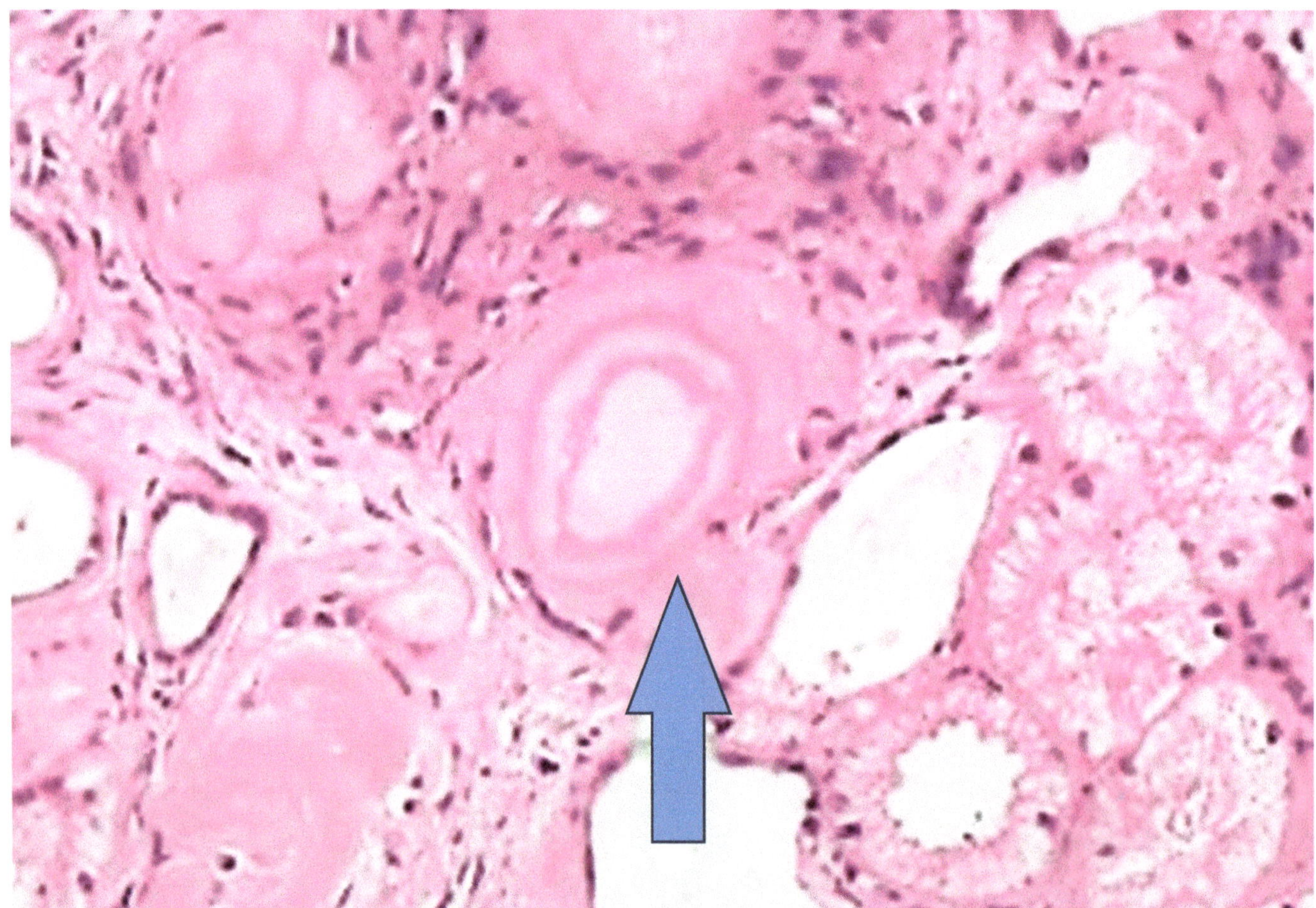

Figure: 3:7.1: Light microscopic appearance of distal tubular casts. Haematoxylin& Eosin(H&E) stain-(20x) tubular cast-central pale area and lamellated appearance.

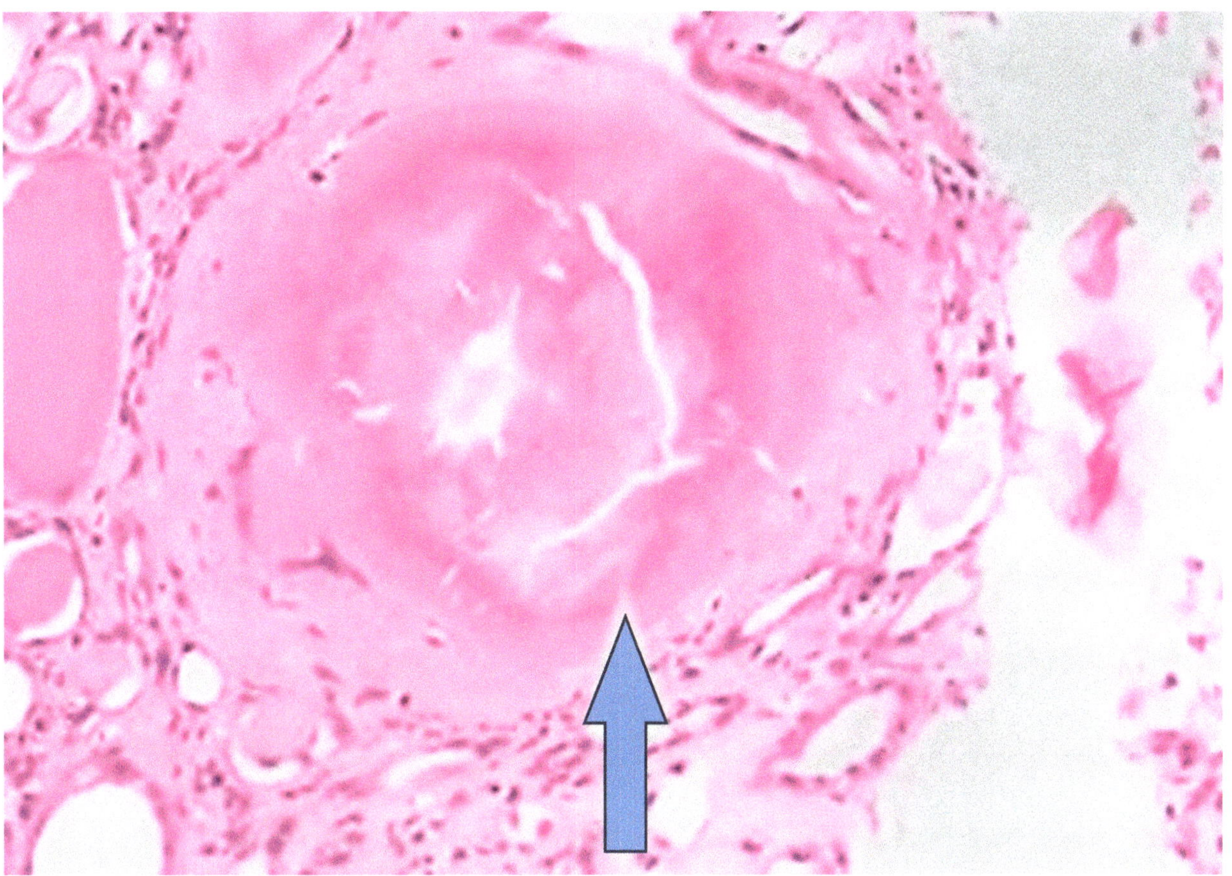

Figure: 3:7.2: H& E stain:(40x): Large cast with fractured planes.

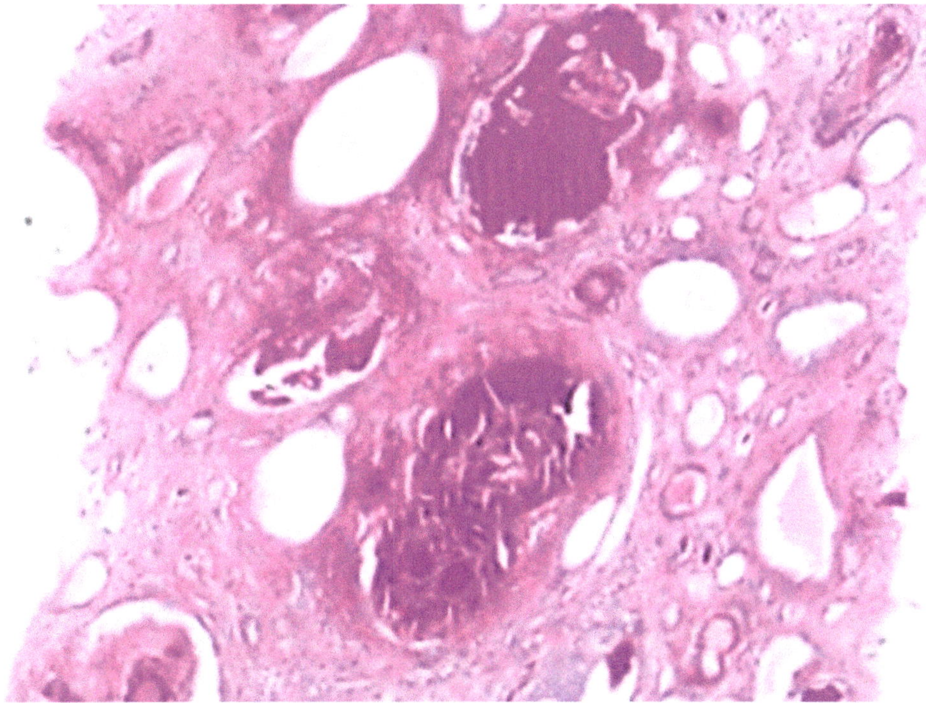

Figure: 3:7.3: Periodic acid Schiff (PAS) stain-(20x) alternate negative and positive appearance.

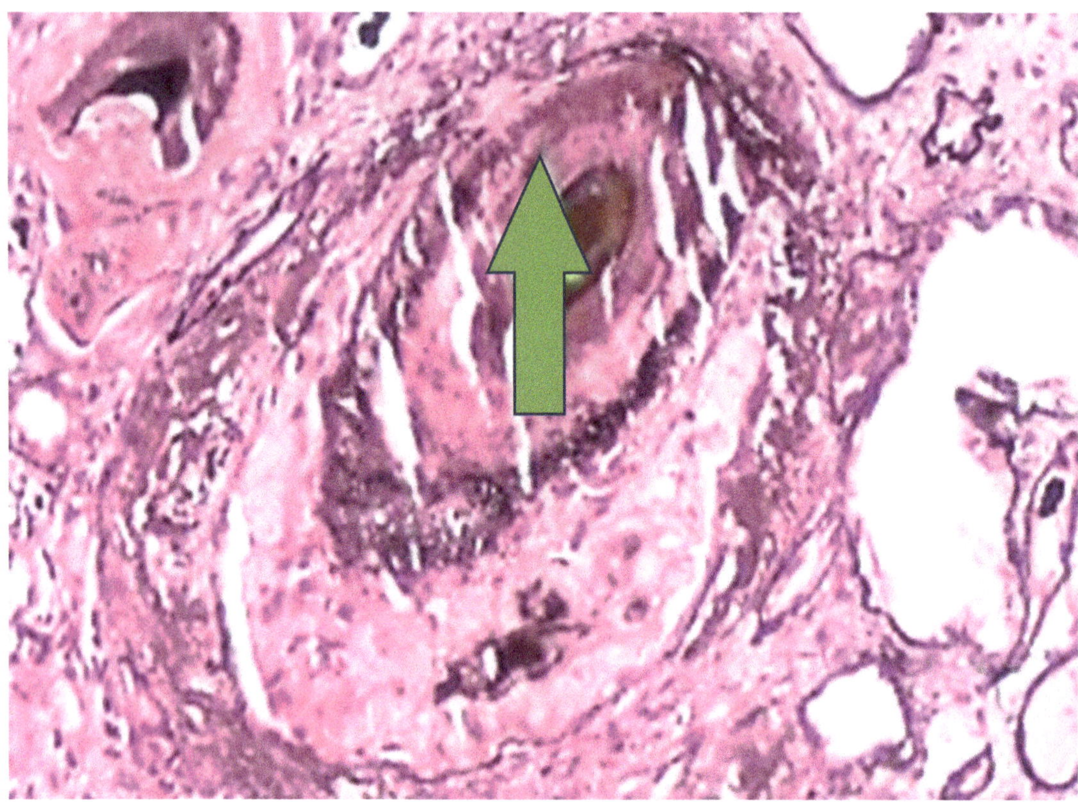

Figure: 3:7.4: PASM stain(20x) arrow showing spiculated silver positive periphery of the cast.

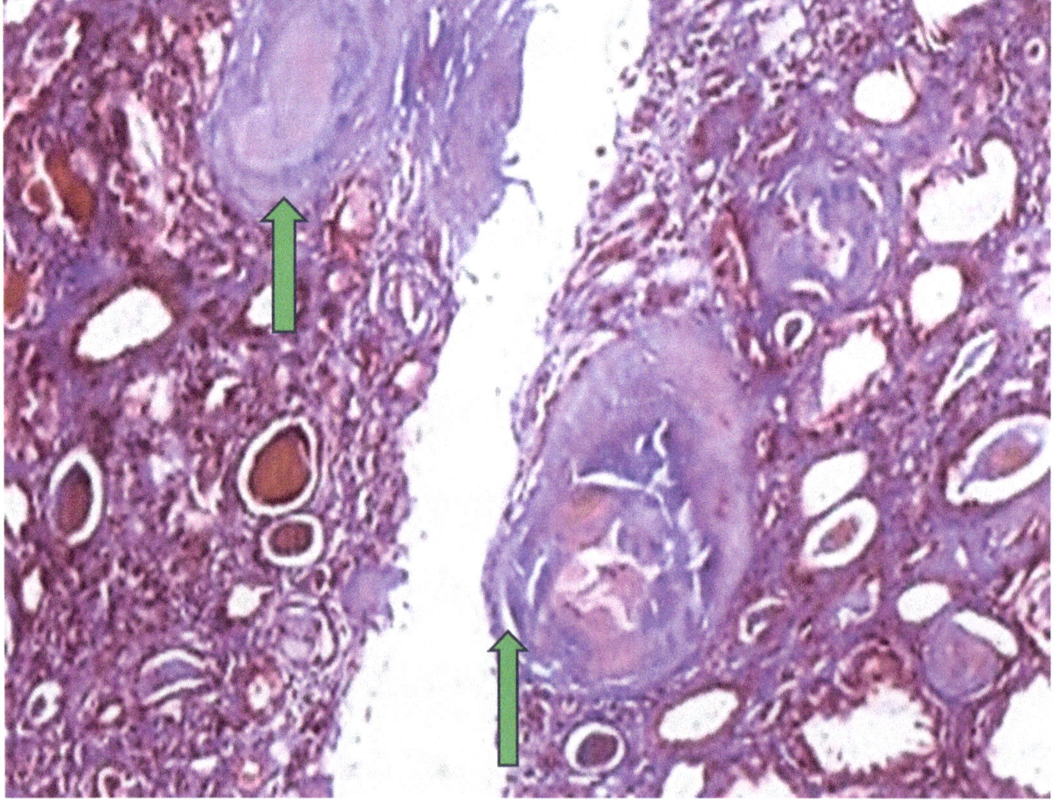

Figure: 3:7.5: Masson Trichrome (MT) stain: Bluish periphery of the cast.

AMYLOID CASTS:20x

CONGO RED STAIN-CONGOPHILIC CASTS

UNDER POLARIZER- REDDISH BIREFRINGENCE

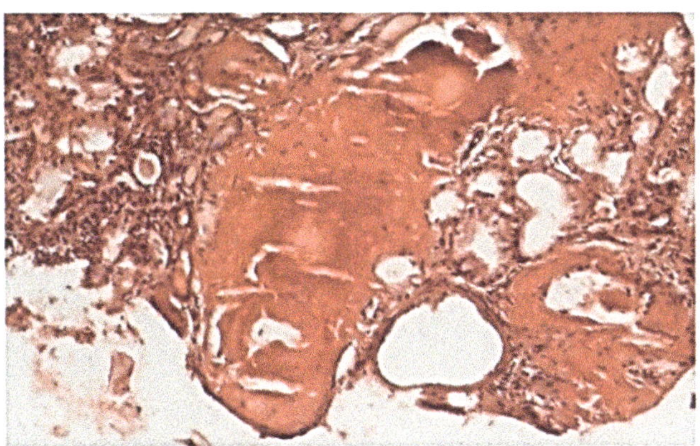

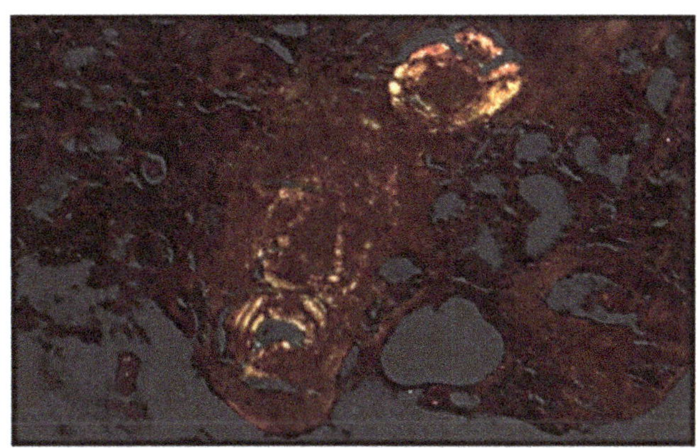

Figure: 3:7.6: Congo red stain: 20x: DCT: the tubular casts are congophilic and show reddish birefringence under polarizer

Immunofluorescence: If study shows kappa light chain restriction seen in many tubular casts and cytoplasm of Tubular epithelial cells (TEC). There is significant Kappa light chain staining along the GBM and Bowman capsule of glomeruli and along tubular basement membranes (TBM).

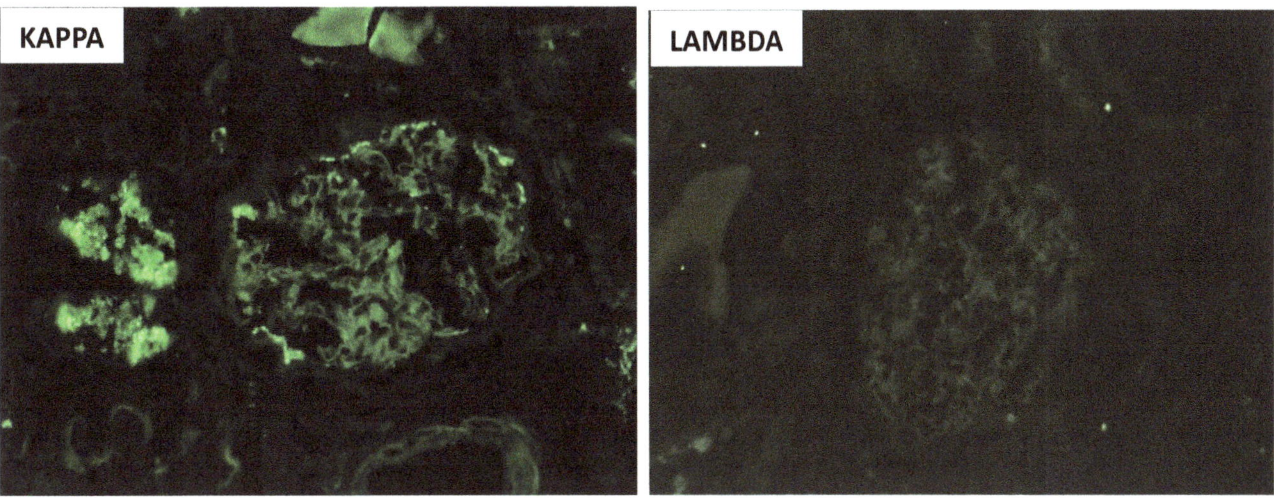

Figure 3:7.7: Immunofluorescence:20x: Kappa light chain stains positive along the GBM and TBM, but the Lambda light chain is negative.

TUBULAR CASTS-20x

KAPPA -RESTRICTED

LAMBDA-NO RESTRICTION

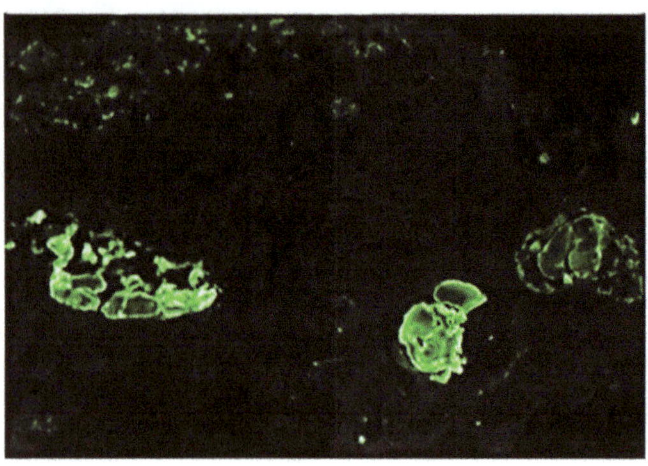
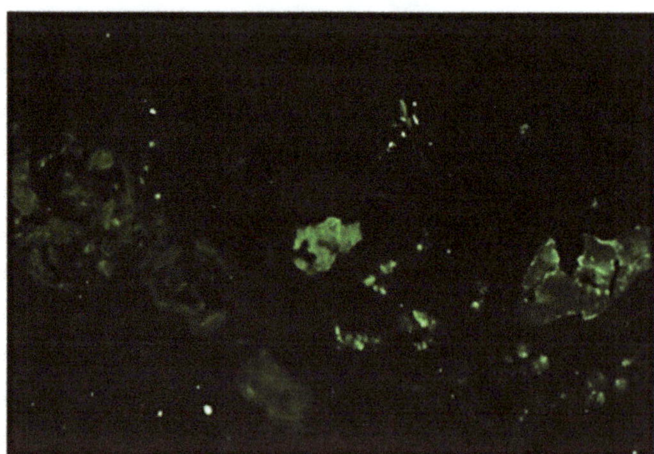

Figure 3:7.8: Immunofluorescence:20x: Kappa light chain shows strong positivity in tubular casts, whereas Lambda is negative in tubular casts.

KAPPA-TUBULES

LAMBDA-TUBULES

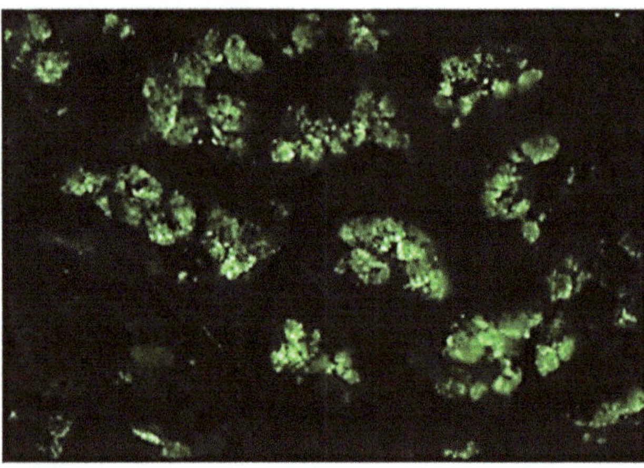
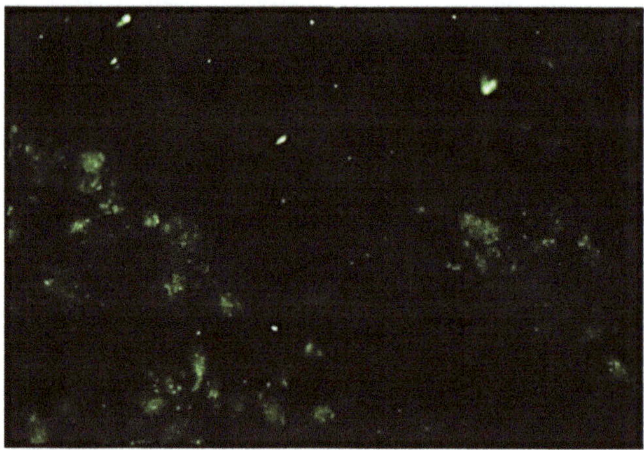

Figure 3:7.9: Immunofluorescence:20x: Kappa light chain shows strong positivity in the cytoplasm of tubular epithelial cells, whereas Lambda is negative.

Interpretation:

Primary diagnosis: Amyloid cast nephropathy, Kappa type

The pattern of injury: Acute tubular injury with approximately 30% of tubules involved by amyloidogenic light–chain casts

Additional findings: Mild tubulointerstitial change of chronicity (20%).

Ancillary studies: Congo red stain is positive in these 30% amyloidogenic tubular casts and negative in glomeruli, interstitium, and vessels.

Additional findings in this case:

A) There is also confluent staining for the Kappa light chain only along the glomerular capillary walls, Bowman capsule, tubular basement membrane, and along the vessel walls to some extent. This may be seen in the following two possibilities, which require an Electron microscope study to rule out and confirm:

1. The earliest evidence of a light chain deposition disease (LCDD), which often occurs concurrently with myeloma cast nephropathy, which on EM study shows fine granular, punctuate, powdery, electron-dense deposits (Randall-type deposits) distributed inside GBM, outside TBM and vascular basement membranes.

2. Light Chain Deposition by Immunofluroscence only: Artifactual IF staining if LM: no changes & IF: monotypic light chain staining and EM: no deposits.

   Monoclonal Immunoglobulin Deposition Disease: Differential diagnosis: page no.198, Colvin/ Chang, Diagnostic Pathology Kidney Diseases, Second Edition.

B) In view of Kappa light chain restriction in the cytoplasm of the tubular epithelial cells, Proximal Tubulopathy (Kappa light chain mediated) /Fanconi syndrome needs to be confirmed with Urine analysis (Albuminuria, Glucosuria, Phosphaturia, Bicarbonaturia) and ABG (Normal Anion Gap Hyperchloremic Metabolic acidosis).

Additional Investigations: Serum Immunofixation electrophoresis: IgG Kappa – M Band Present.

Final Diagnosis: Myeloma associated (Kappa light chain restricted) Amyloid cast nephropathy.

***Suggested reading:**

Unusual morphology of amyloid cast nephropathy in renal biopsy portending poor prognosis: Meyyappa Devan Rajagopal, et.al: BMJ Case Rep.2018 Dec 22;11(1): e225899. doi: 10.1136/bcr-2018-225899.

Case 8

History: 57 years old female, nondiabetic, and non-hypertensive, presented with frothy urine, loss of appetite, nausea, no pedal edema, no shortness of breath. No joint pains or skin rash. No h/o using NSAIDs or indigenous medicines. BP: 135/80 mm of Hg.

Investigations: Serum creatinine 1.9 mg/dl, Urine analysis: Protein 3+, RBC 4-5/HPF, pus cells: 2-3/HPF, 24 hours urine protein: 5332 mg/day. Serum Cholesterol 200 mg/dl, LDL:110 mg/dl, HDL: 40mg/dl, Triglycerides: 150mg/dl, C3 & C4: both normal, ANCA: Negative, ANA: Negative.

Clinical Diagnosis: Nephrotic range proteinuria with hypertension and renal dysfunction.

Differential diagnoses: Membranous nephropathy/IgA Nephropathy/FSGS.

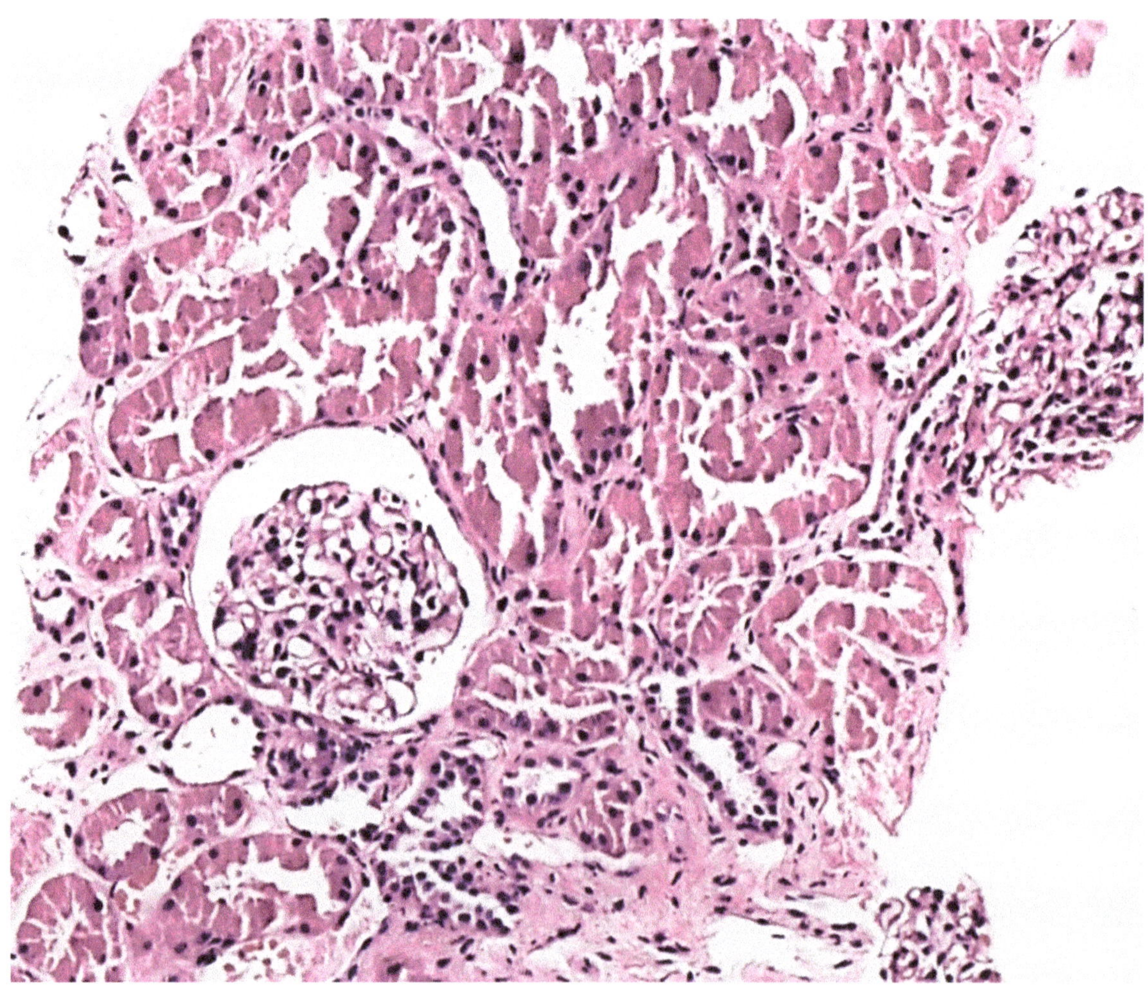

Figure 3:8.1: H&E Stain: 10x: Normal glomeruli and fragmentation and desquamation of tubular epithelial cells.

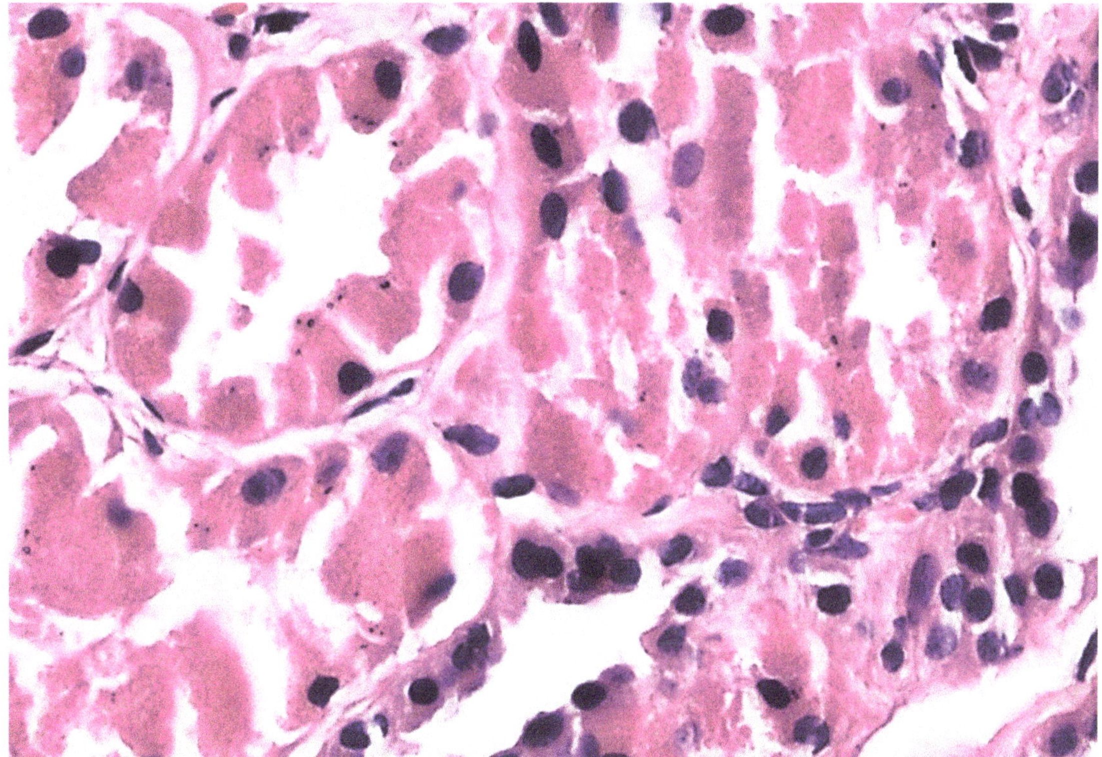

Figure: 3:8.2: H&E Stain: Tubules: 40x: Fragmentation of tubular epithelial cells.

IF

KAPPA CORE **LAMBDA CORE**

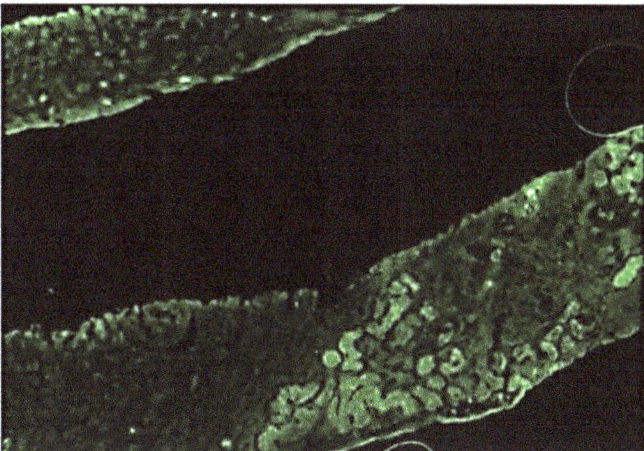

Figure: 3:8.3: Immunofluorescence: 4x: Lambda light chain shows strong positivity and Kappa is negative.

Immunofluorescence:10x

Kappa :negative in cytoplasm of tubular epithelial cells

Lambda :positive in cytoplasm of tubular epithelial cells

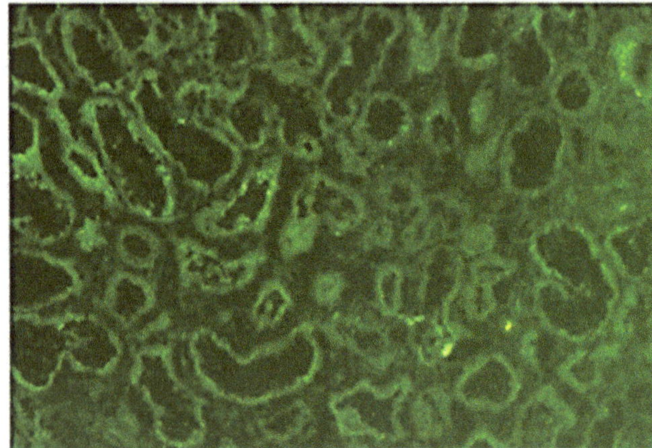 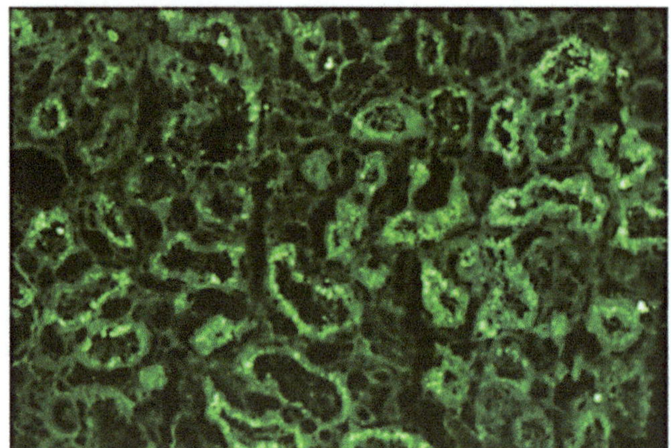

Figure: 3:8.4: IF: 20x: Kappa: TEC-tubular epithelial cells-TEC: negative, Lambda: TEC: 4+, Lambda light chain restriction.

Interpretation: Lambda Light chain Restricted Proximal tubulopathy.

Additional Investigations: Serum Immunofixation electrophoresis: IgG Lambda – M Band Present.

Final Diagnosis: Myeloma associated Lambda light chain proximal tubulopathy.

Suggested reading:

Proximal tubulopathy associated with crystalline inclusions: Kappa light chain related.
Proximal tubulopathy associated with non-crystalline inclusions: Lambda light chain related.
*Heptinstall's Pathology of the Kidney: seventh edition: chapter 22: Renal Diseases with Plasma Cell Dyscrasias: Page no. 960.

CHAPTER 4
Interstitial Diseases

DEFINITIONS

Interstitium: It is the space between the glomeruli, tubules and blood vessels.

Table 4.1

Sr. No.	Light Microscopy	Definition	Seen in
1.	Interstitial edema (light blue colour on MT Stain)	Expansion of interstitium by clear fluid	ATI, ATN, RVT, NS, AGN
2.	Interstitial fibrosis	Expansion of interstitium by collagen rich matrix and increased fibroblasts	CKD
3.	Interstitial leukocytes	Lymphocytes &/ Eosinophils	ATIN
		Neutrophils	Acute pyelonephritis
4.	Interstitial foam cells (Figure 2:2.1)	Macrophages with foamy cytoplasm and eccentrically placed nuclei	NS, Alport syndrome
5.	Interstitial neoplastic cells	Atypical cells with hyperchromatic, pleomorphic nuclei,+/-mitosis.	Malignancies: Haematological and solid organ: primary &/secondary

ATI: acute tubular injury, **ATN:** acute tubular necrosis, **RVT:** renal vein thrombosis, **NS:** nephrotic syndrome, **AGN:** acute glomerulonephritis, **CKD:** chronic kidney diseases, **ATIN:** acute tubulointerstitial nephritis.

CASE 1

History: 29 years old male, with h/o right great toe intense pain, swelling, redness and mild fever on and off for last 3 weeks. He has h/o similar gouty arthritis episode once in last one year. He was treated with Colchicine and Diclofenac in previous episode. He now has been started on Allopurinol for hyperuricemia, Colchicine and Paracetamol. He has now increased urinary frequency for last one week without dysuria. No edema in feet. No h/o any other Indigenous medicine use. He has renal dysfunction. BP: 110/70 mm of Hg.

Investigations: Urine analysis: Protein: +, Pus cells:8 to 10/HPF, Crystals: Uric acid crystals +. Serum creatinine:3.4mg/dl, Serum Uric acid: 12 mg/dl. USG abdomen: B/L Bulky kidneys, Urine culture: Sterile.

Clinical Diagnosis: AKI with sterile pyuria. Gouty arthritis.

Differential diagnoses: AIN due to? Drugs/Infection.? Urate Nephropathy.

Light microscopy:

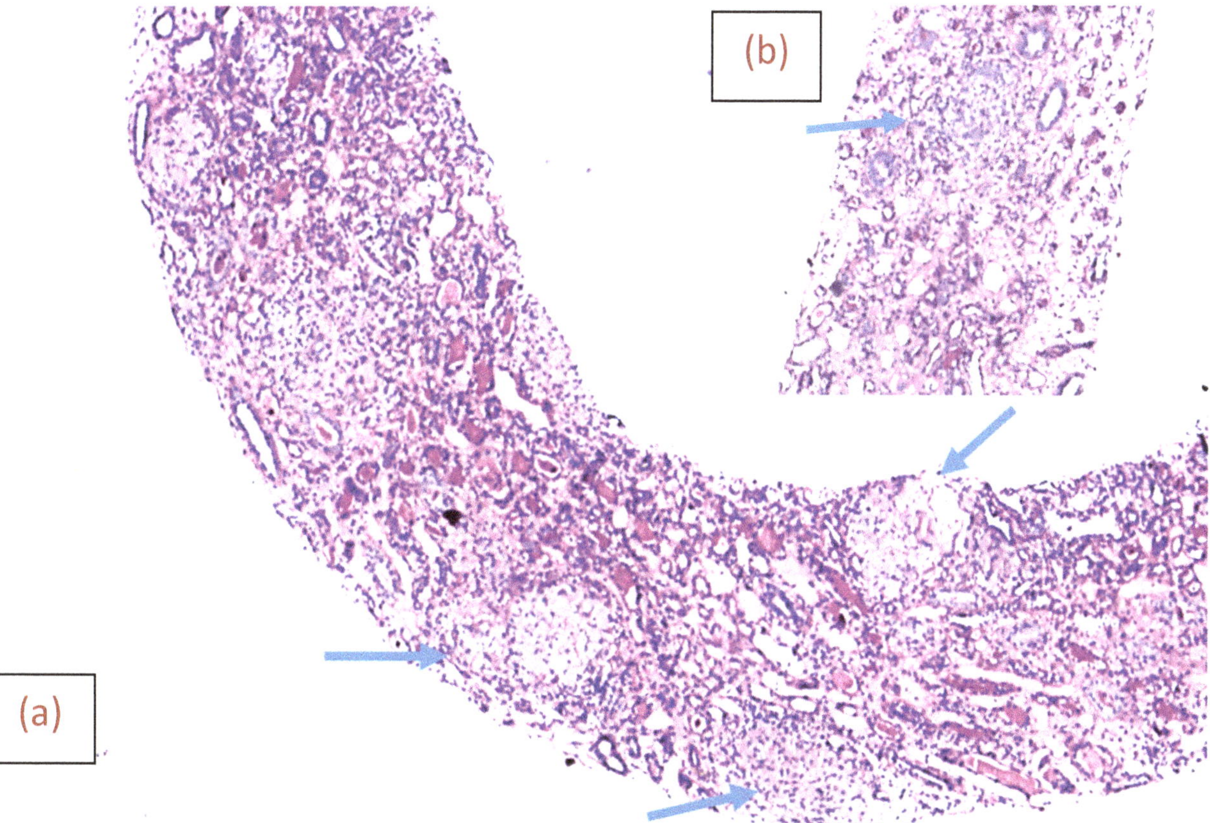

Figure 4:1.1: (a) PAS-stain: 4x: scanner view: There are numerous non-caseating, well formed, sharply defined granulomas seen in the renal cortex; comprising of epithelioid histiocytes and multinucleated giant cells. **(b)** Granulomas in renal medulla.

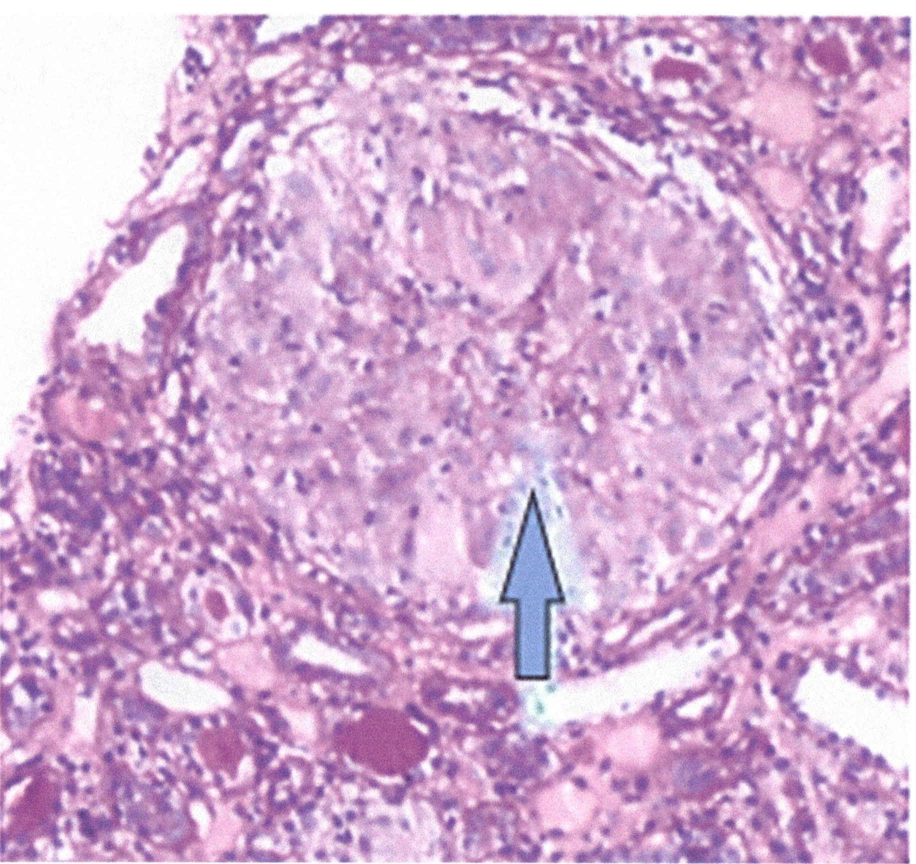

Figure 4:1.2: PAS Stain:10x: Non-caseating, well formed, sharply defined epithelioid cells granuloma.

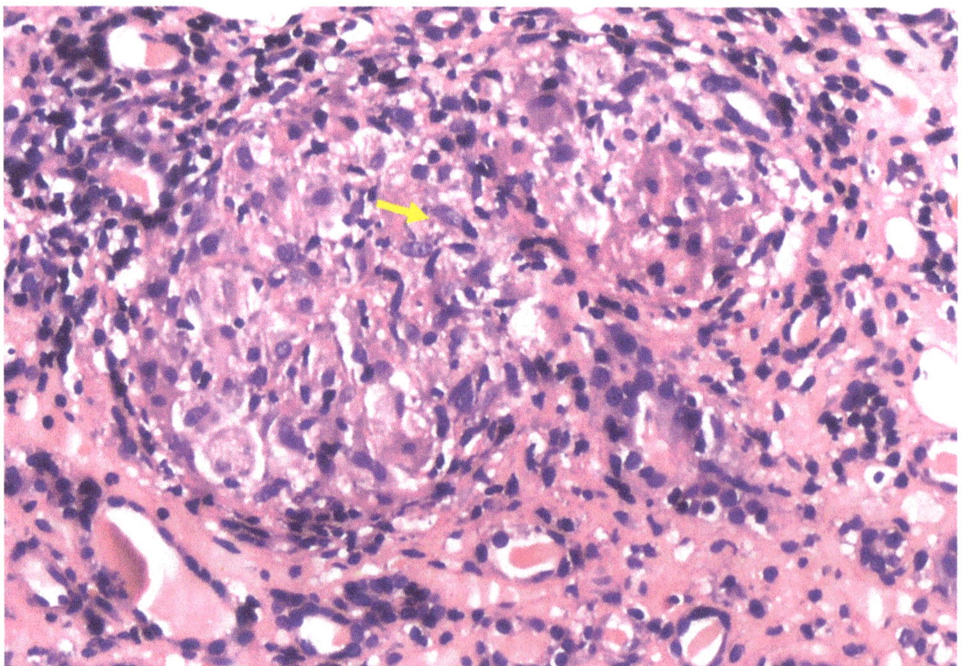

Figure 4:1.3: H&E Stain: 20 x: Granuloma with epithelioid cells (slipper shaped nuclei- shown by (yellow arrow).

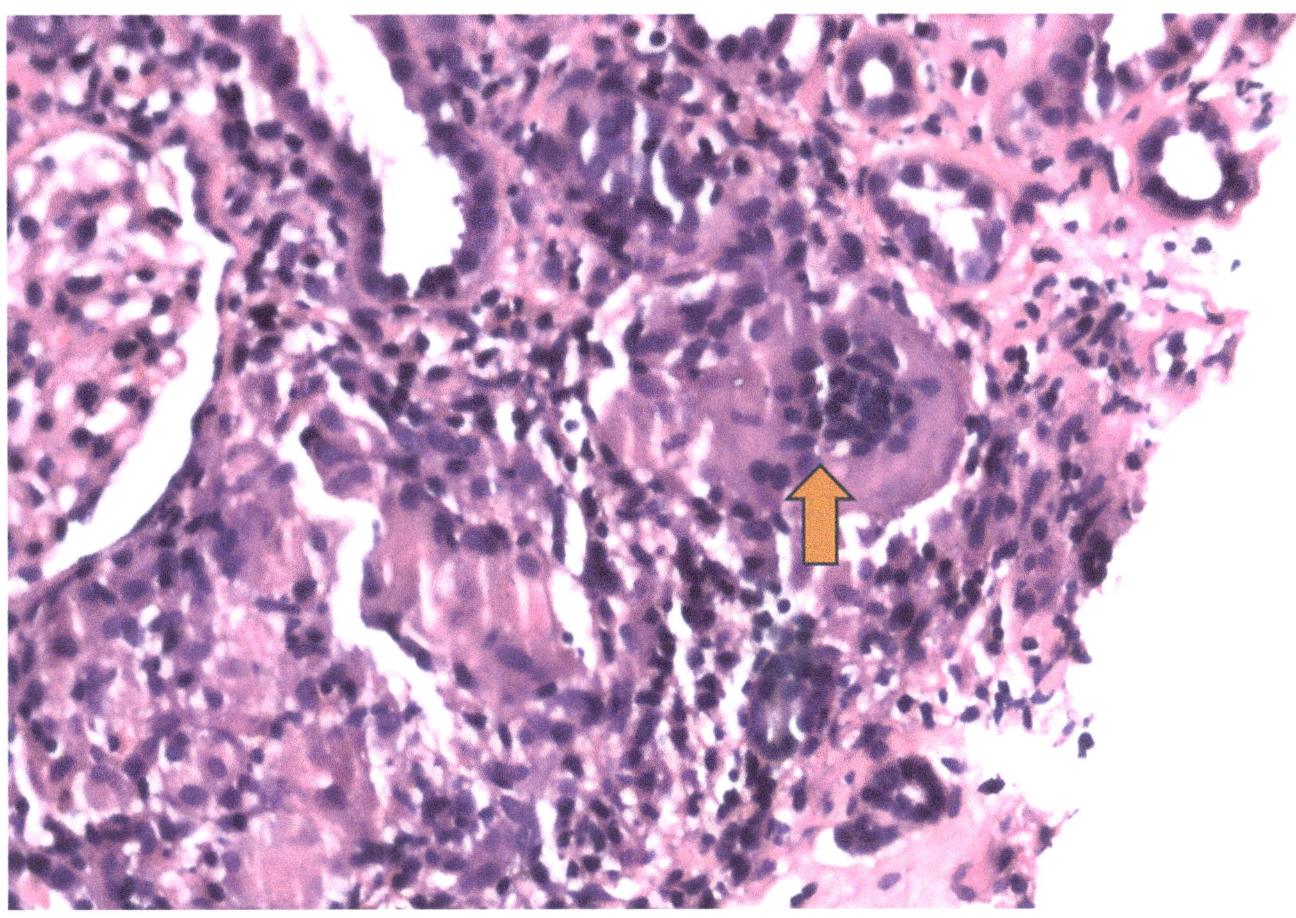

Figure 4:1.4: H&E Stain: 20 x: Multinucleated giant cells in Interstitium.

Interpretation: A non-caseating Granulomatous interstitial nephritis.? Allopurinol related.

Follow up: Serum creatinine came down to 1.6mg/dl after stopping Allopurinol after a week.

Final Diagnosis: A non-caseating Granulomatous interstitial nephritis: Allopurinol related.

Pathology Pearls

Other causes of Granulomatous interstitial Nephritis:

TB, Sarcoidosis, Fungi (histoplasmosis, coccidioidomycosis), Bacteria (Brucella, Chlamydia), Spirochetes (Treponema), Parasites (Lesihmania, Toxoplasma), Autoimmune diseases: Sjogrens disease, Lupus, ANCA associated Vasculitis, IgG 4 related tubulointerstitial disease, TINU (Tubulointerstitial nephritis and uveitis.

*In acute pyelonephritis, neutrophils appear first in peritubular capillaries. This is followed by capillary wall rupture, with leakage of fluid and cells into the interstitium.

CASE 2

History: 34-year-old male, non-hypertensive, non-diabetic, presented with loss of appetite, nausea, increased frequency of nighttime urination. No pedal edema. No frothyuria or hematuria. BP :110/70 mm of Hg. On routine check-up, he was found to have renal dysfunction. There is history of using NSAIDs for 3 days, 10 days back for an episode of gout involving right great toe. No family H/O renal disease.

Investigations: Serum creatinine:5.76mg/dl. Urine analysis: protein:2+, RBCs:4 to 6/HPF, WBCs:2 to 4/HPF, serum uric acid:9mg/dl, serum albumin:2.1gm/dl, UPCR:3.28, USG findings: Right kidney:11.9x5.6, Left kidney:10.7 x5.7cm.

Clinical Diagnosis: AKI-AIN probably NSAIDs induced.

Light microscopy:

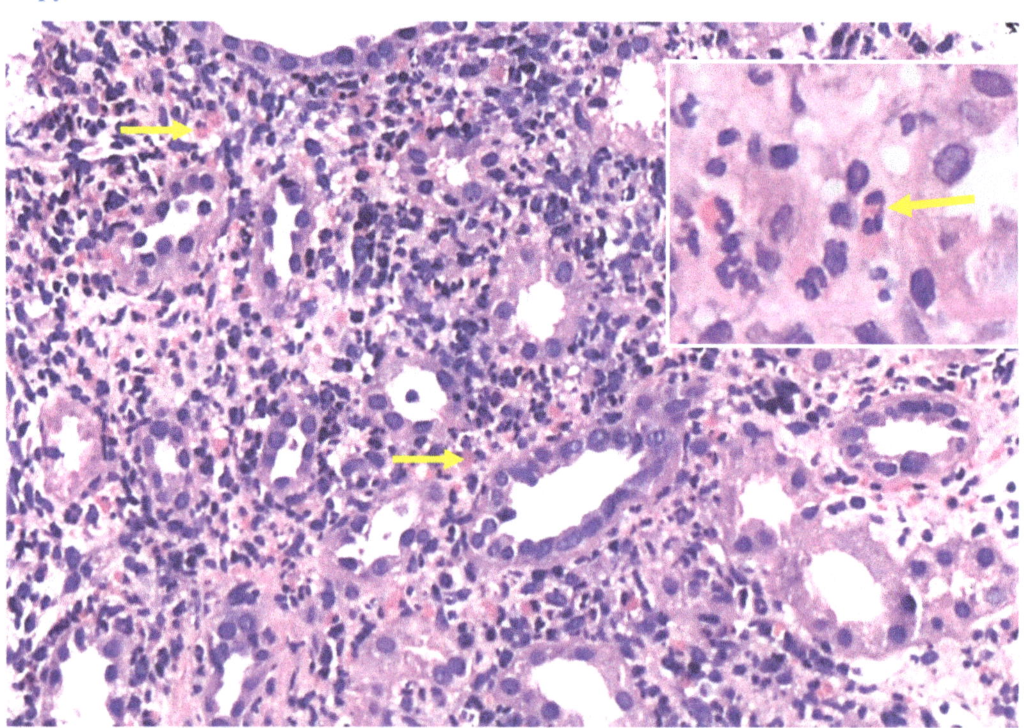

Figure 4:2.1: H&E Stain:10x: Diffuse interstitial infiltrate comprising of predominantly eosinophils (yellow arrows), few lymphocytes and occasional plasma cells. **(Inset Image)** Eosinophils: bilobed nuclei with orange coloured cytoplasmic granules.

Interpretation: Acute Tubulointerstitial Nephritis (ATIN).

Final Diagnosis: NSAIDs induced ATIN

History: 33-year female, non-diabetic and non-hypertensive, came with h/o loss of appetite, nausea, weight loss of 7 kg in last 6 months. There are night sweats and mild evening rise fever, pedal edema on & off for 4 months.

Investigations: Urine analysis: Urine Protein: 4+, RBCs: 30 to 40/HPF, serum creatinine:6.2mg/dl, serum albumin:3.3gm/dl, Hb: 10 gm/dl, Total leucocyte count: 20,300/cu mm, ESR = 102. USG findings: B/L Bulky kidneys.

Clinical Diagnosis: AKI or CKD due to underlying TB or Malignancy.

Differential diagnoses: AIN/CIN.

Light microscopy:

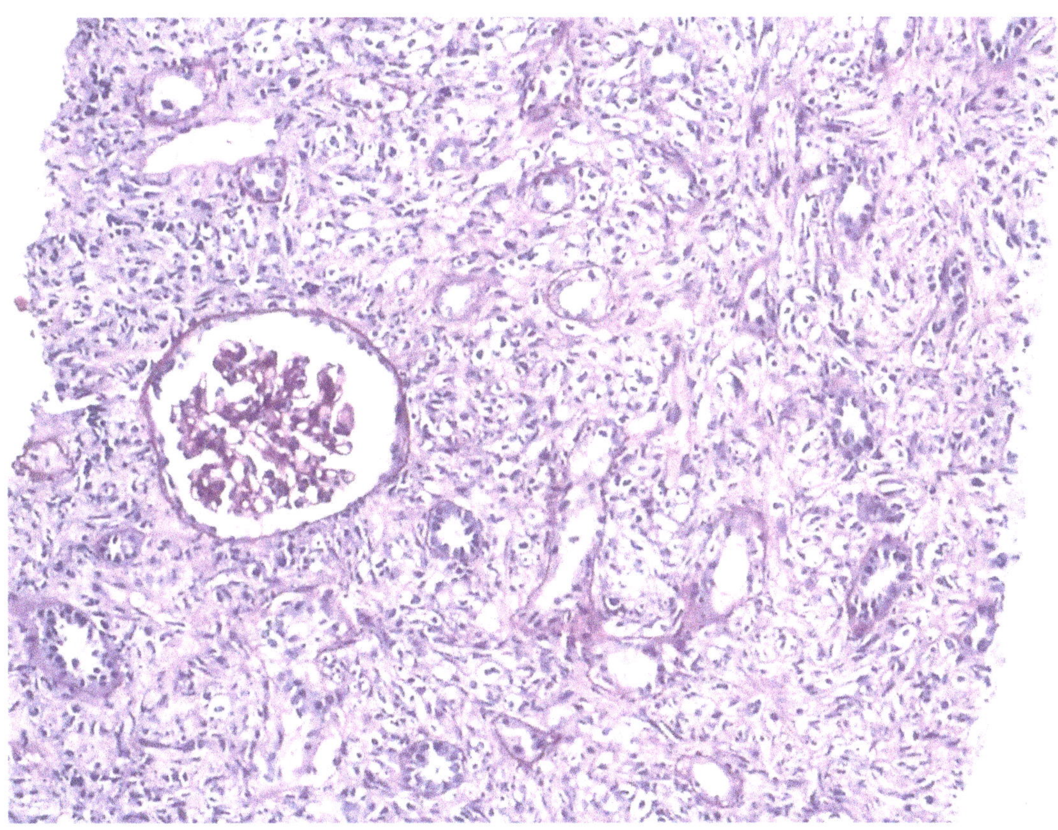

Figure: 4:3.1: PAS Stain:10x: Glomerulus appears normal, moderate tubulointerstitial changes of chronicity.

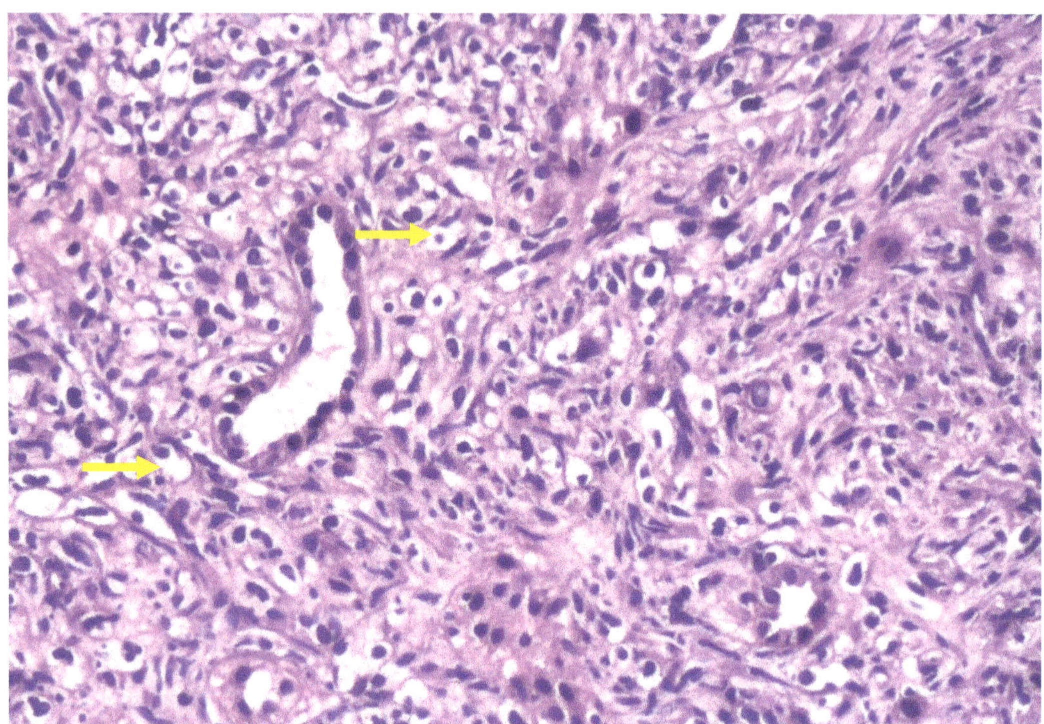

Figure: 4:3.2: H&E Stain:20x: The interstitium is widened and fibrosed around the atrophic tubules with a dense diffuse infiltrate predominantly of atypical cells (yellow arrows) forming nests and trabeculae.

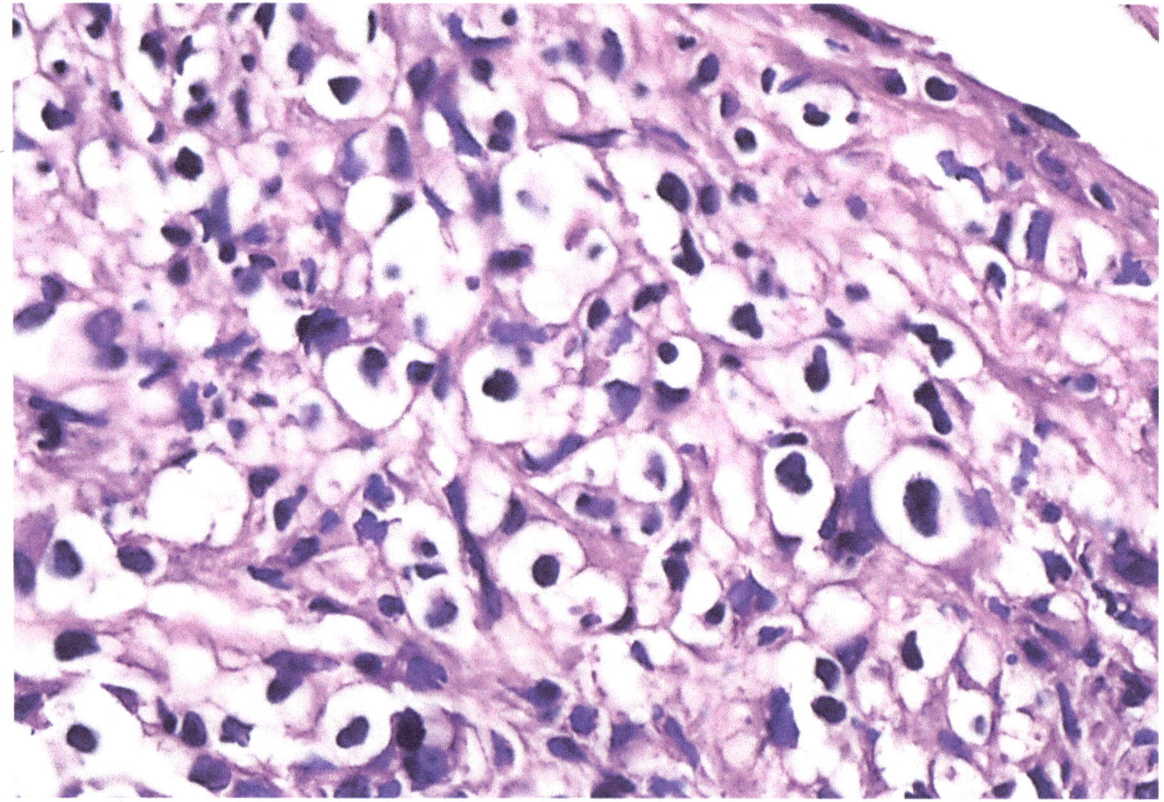

Figure: 4:3.3: H&E Stain:40x: These atypical cells have well-defined cell borders, clear cytoplasm and round to oval hyperchromatic nuclei.

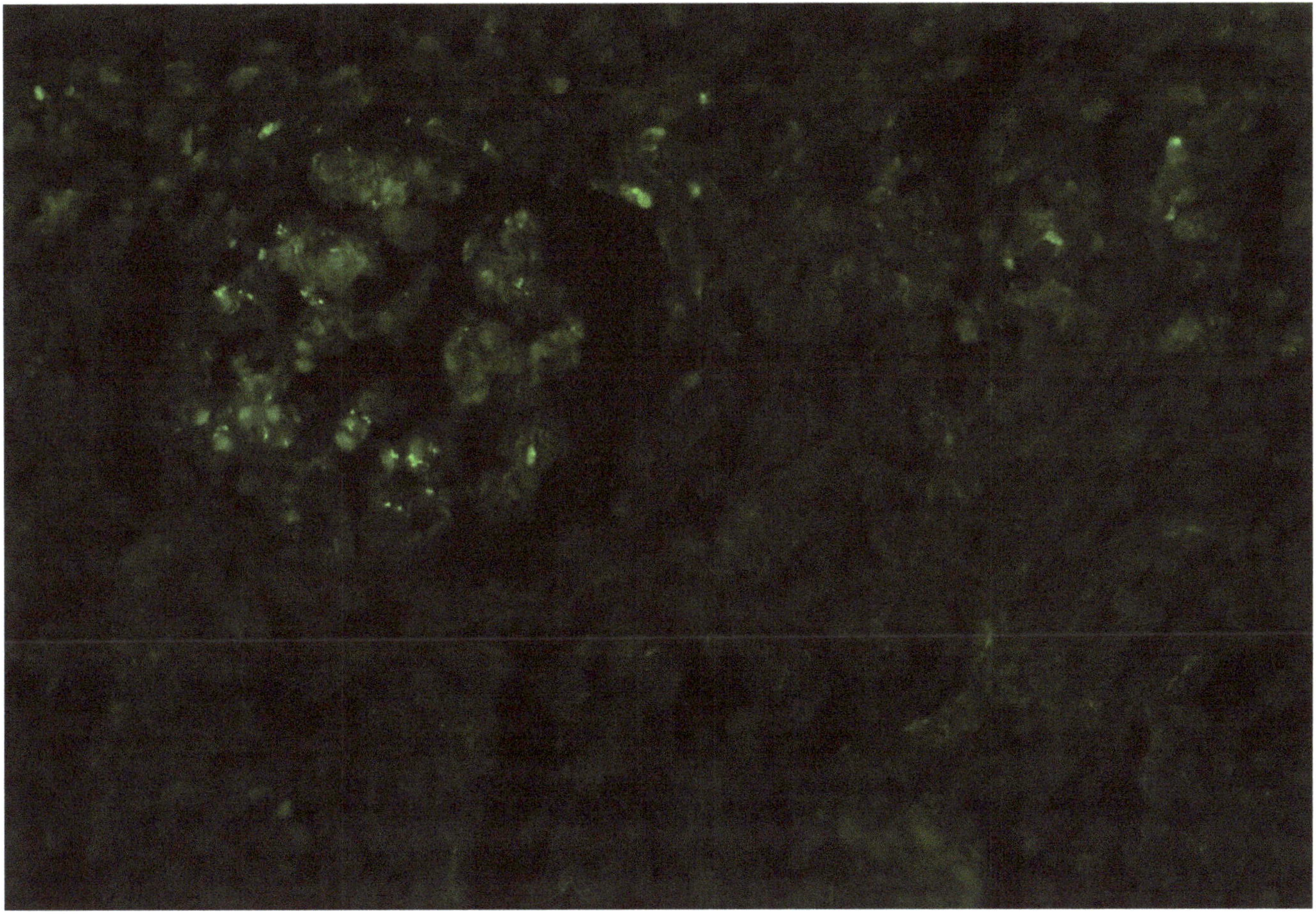

Figure: 4:3.4: Immunoflourensence: 20 x: Negative.

Interpretation: Normal glomeruli and moderate tubulointerstitial changes of chronicity (40%) with diffuse interstitial infiltrate comprising of predominantly atypical cells.

Follow-up: Later, the patient went for a PET scan, which showed an anterior mediastinal mass, the biopsy of which confirmed the diagnosis of Primary Mediastinal High-Grade Large B-cell Lymphoma with the help of the following IHC studies.

Immunohistochemistry: Atypical cells express LCA, CD20, CD 30, BCL2 with Ki proliferation index of 80% to 90%. There is negative reactivity for CD3, CD 10, Tdt, Cmyc& Ctyokeratin.

The kidney (needle) biopsy shows the same reactivity for the above mentioned IHC markers as the primary neoplasm.

Final diagnosis: Primary Mediastinal High-Grade Large B-cell Lymphoma with Renal Metastasis.

Vascular Diseases

Artery has 3 layers: from inside out: internal elastic lamina (Figure 5.1: B: yellow arrow); media (muscle layer: smooth muscle cells: Figure 5.1: B: orange arrow) and adventitia (outside the media blends with interstitium: Figure 5.1:C: yellow arrow).

For an artery: Internal elastic lamina should be present, and the media should have a thickness of at least two cell layers.

Endothelial cells (Figure 5.1 A): Line the luminal surface of the artery and show flattened to ovoid nuclei. Normally there is no space between the endothelial cells and internal elastic lamina.

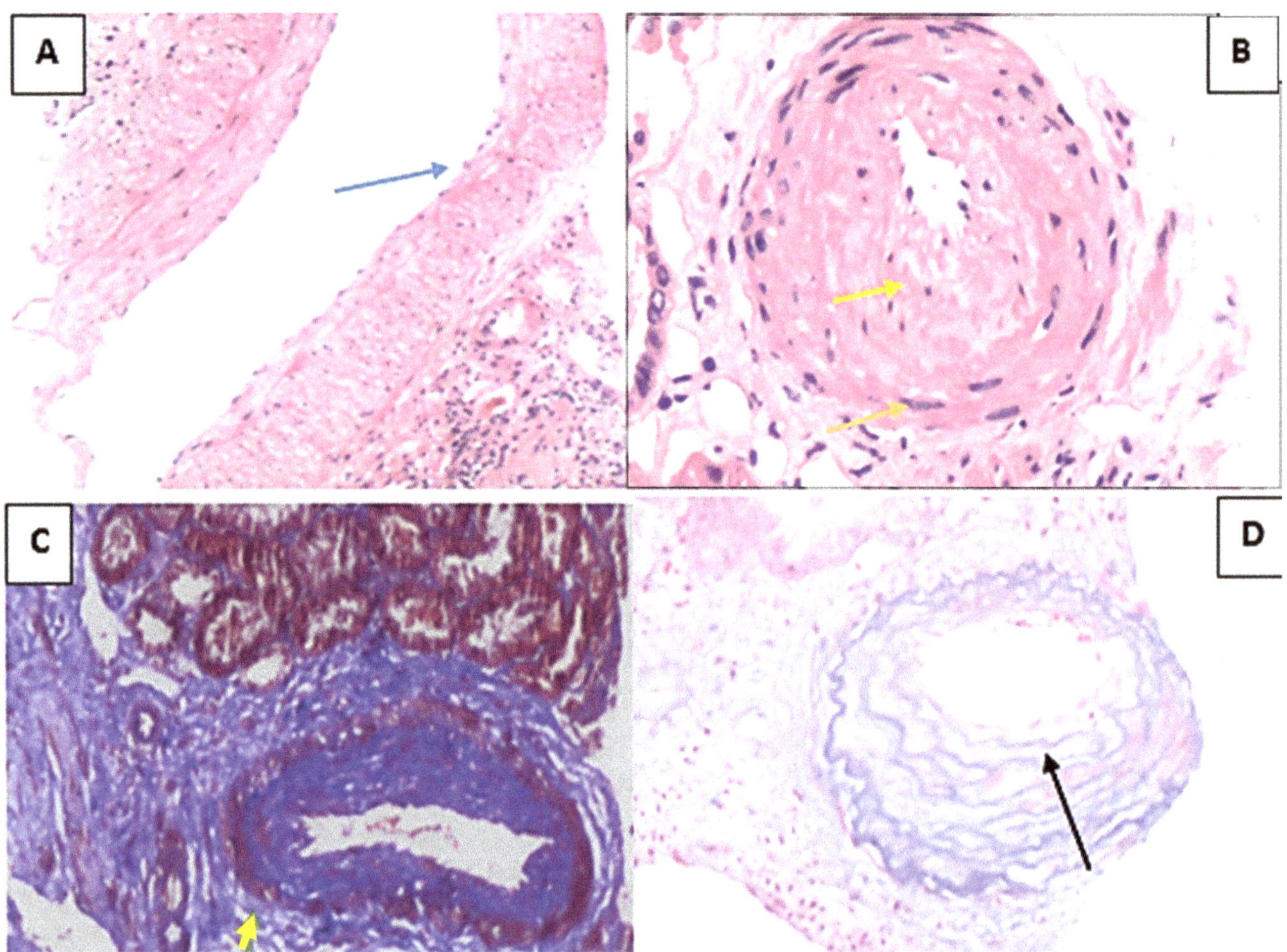

Figure: 5.1: Artery showing arteriosclerosis: A:H&E Stain:10x:arrow showing endothelial cells (blue arrow)lining the intima B:H&E Stain:20x:wavy internal elastic lamina(yellow arrow)which is showing intimal fibrosis with reduplicated internal elastic lamina, C: MT Stain: 10x, Arteriosclerosis: intimal fibrosis and yellow arrow showing adventitia layer which blends with interstitial tissue, D:MT Stain:20x: black arrow is showing intimal fibrosis with reduplication of internal elastic lamina.

1. **Arteriolar hyalinosis:** Hyaline is glassy, smooth, homogeneous and eosinophilic extracellular material. There is intimal hyalinosis in diabetic/hypertensive nephropathy (Figure 5.2).

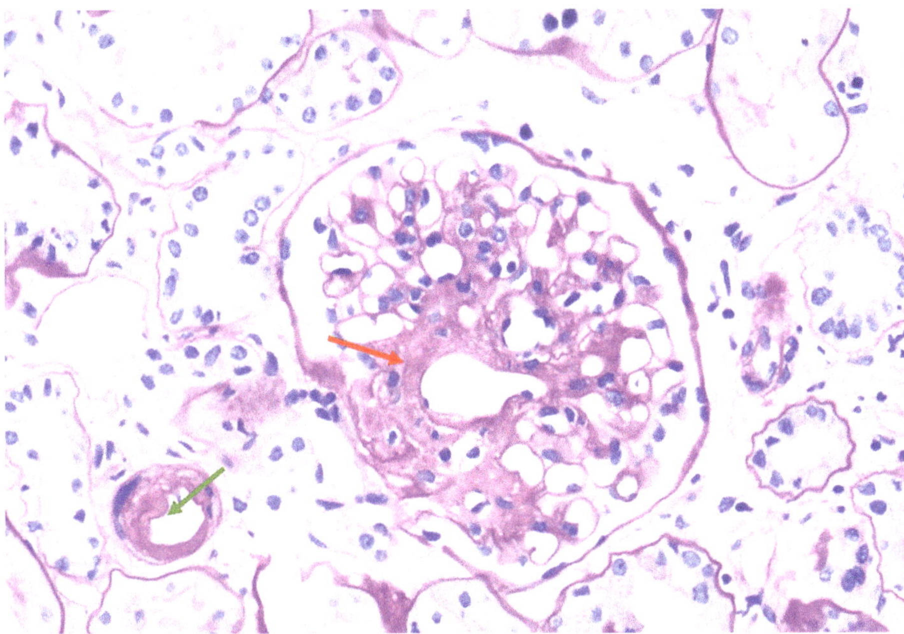

Figure 5.2: Both afferent (red arrow) and Efferent (green arrow) arteriolar intimal hyalinosis in a case of Diabetic nephropathy.

2. **CNI toxicity:** Nodular hyalinosis, involving the muscle layer (intramural hyaline deposits).

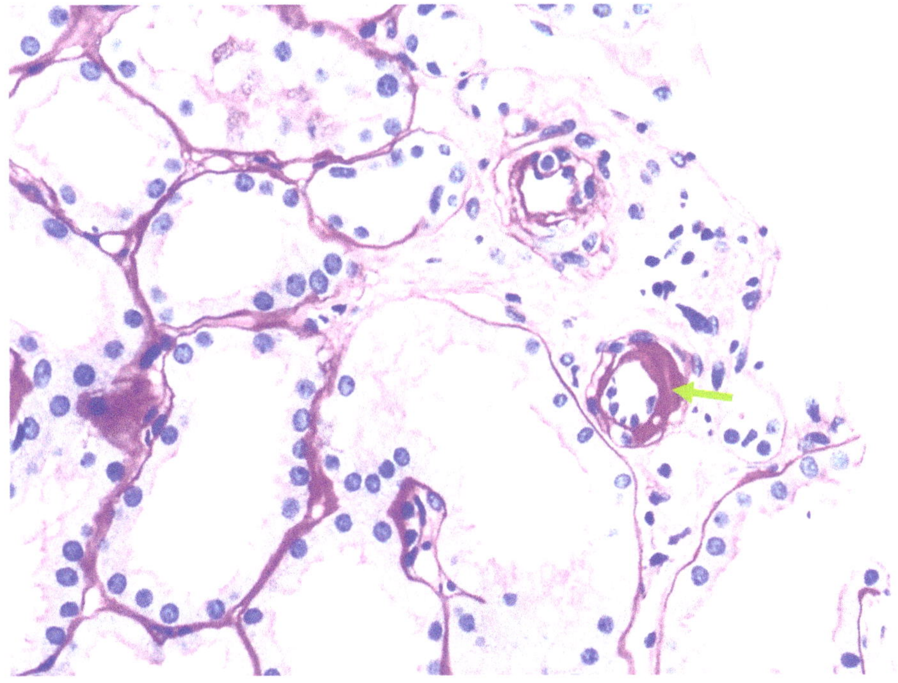

Figure 5.3: Arteriolar intramural hyalinosis (green arrow)in a case of CNI toxicity of an allograft (needle) biopsy.

3. **Onion skinning:** Myointimal hyalinosis of arteriole seen in Accelerated hypertension.
4. **Fibrin:** Seen in TMA (Thrombotic Microangiopathy): Fibrin is fuchsinophilic (reddish) on MT stain and fibrillar in appearance.
5. **Amyloid deposition:** Extracellular congophilic material seen in glomeruli or interstitium of vessels.

History: 47 years old male came with mild swelling on and off in feet for last one month. There is significant froth in urine. No hematuria. He is also having profound generalised weakness. BP is 110/60 mm of Hg. There is no h/o using NSAIDs or indigenous medicines. No history of skin rash, oral ulcers, or joint pains. He has no h/o using skin lightening creams. He is nonsmoker and non-alcoholic.

Investigations: Hb:9.6 gm/dl, TLC: 4,500/cu mm, Platelet count:1.3 lakhs/cu mm. serum creatinine: 2.5 mg/dl. Urine analysis: Protein 3+, Pus cells 4-5/HPF, RBCs: 5-6/HPF. Urine protein to creatinine ratio: 2.3 g/g. USG findings: bilateral bulky kidneys.

Clinical diagnosis: Renal dysfunction with sub-nephrotic range proteinuria without hypertension and with bicytopenia.

Differential diagnoses: Membranous nephropathy/Paraproteinemia associated renal disease.

Light microscopy:

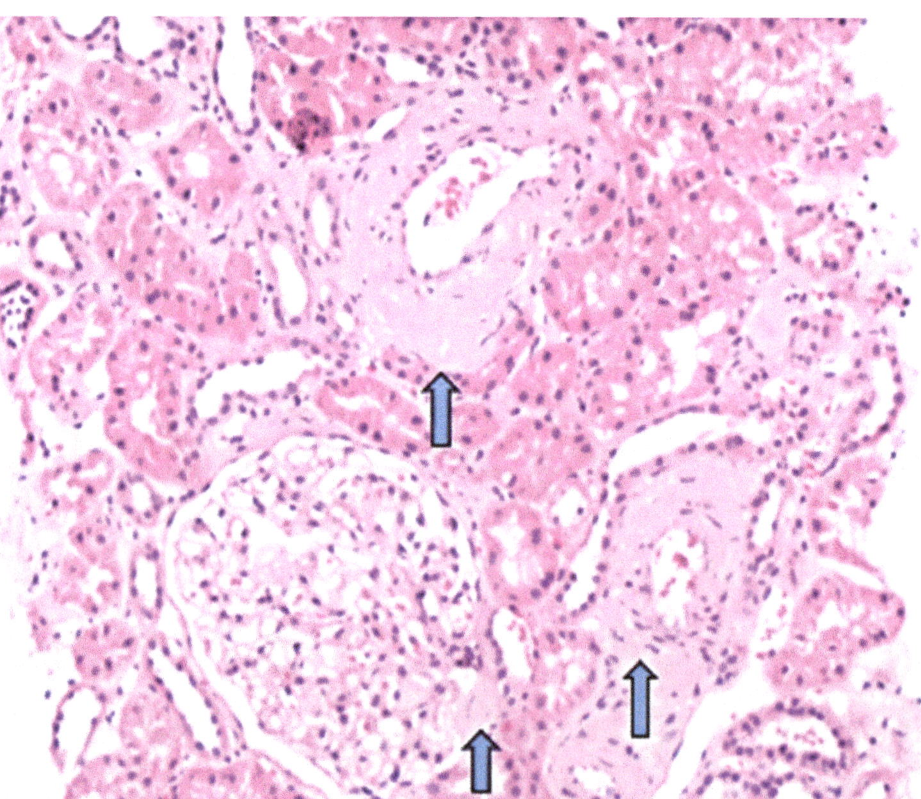

Figure 5:1.1: H&E Stain-10x: Pale eosinophilic waxy material around the vessels and glomerular hilar arteriole.

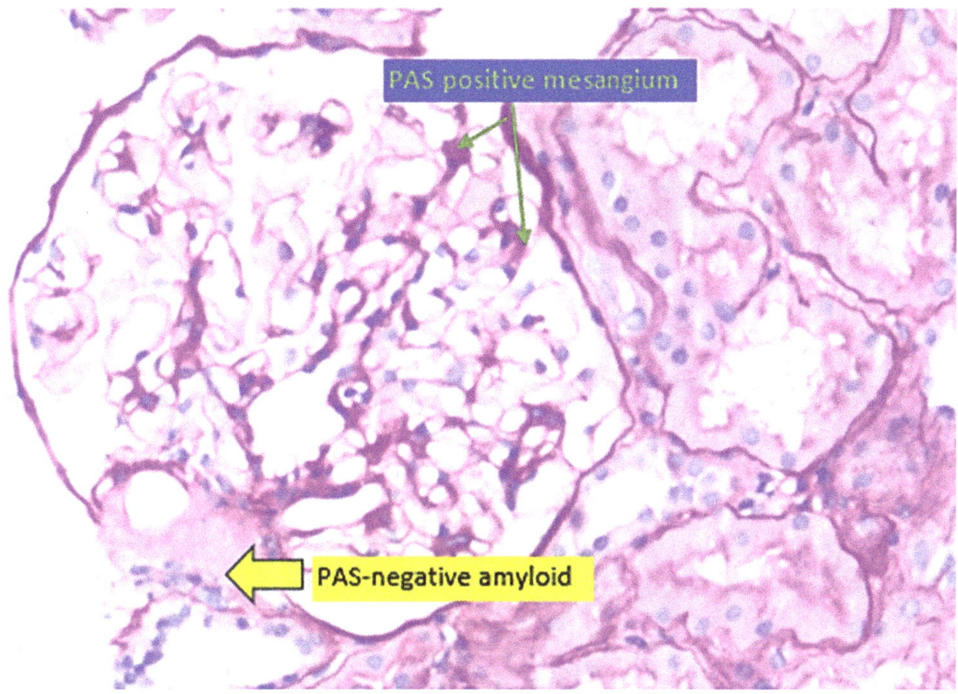

Figure 5:1.2: PAS Stain: 20x: Glomerulus with PAS positive mesangium(green arrow), Bowman capsule and Tubular basement membranes and PAS-negative Amyloid (yellow arrow)around the hilar arteriole.The glomerulus appears normal.

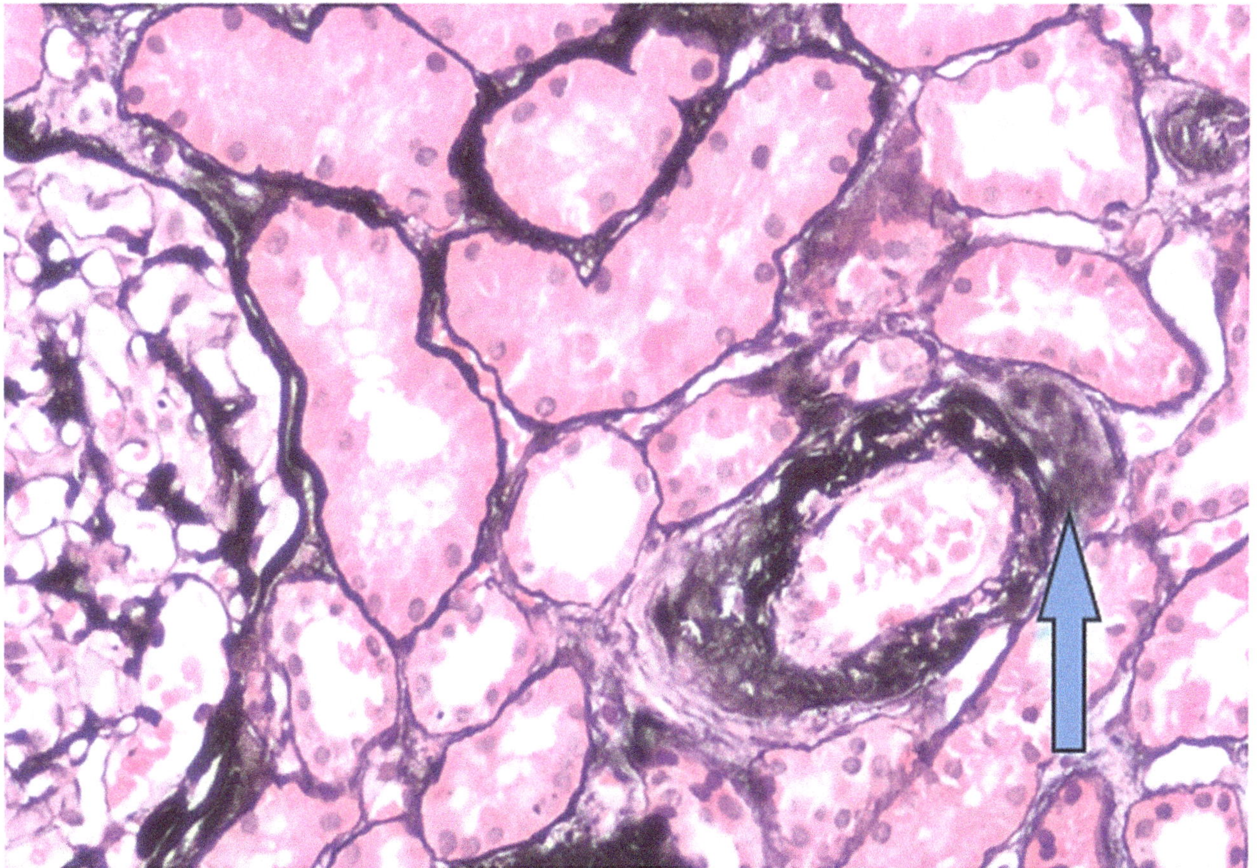

Figure 5:1.3: PASM Stain:20x: Silver -negative Amyloid around the arteriole.

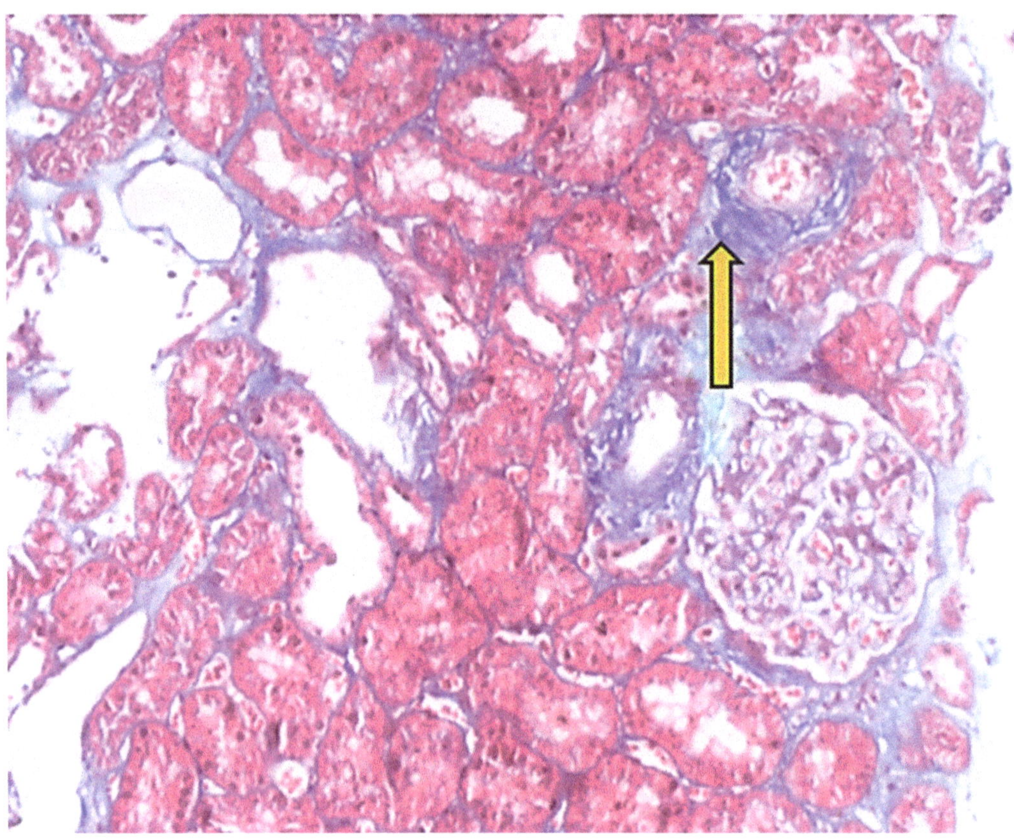

Figure 5:1.4: Masson Trichrome Stain:10x:Bluish Amyloid around the arteriole, glomerulus being normal with no amyloid deposits

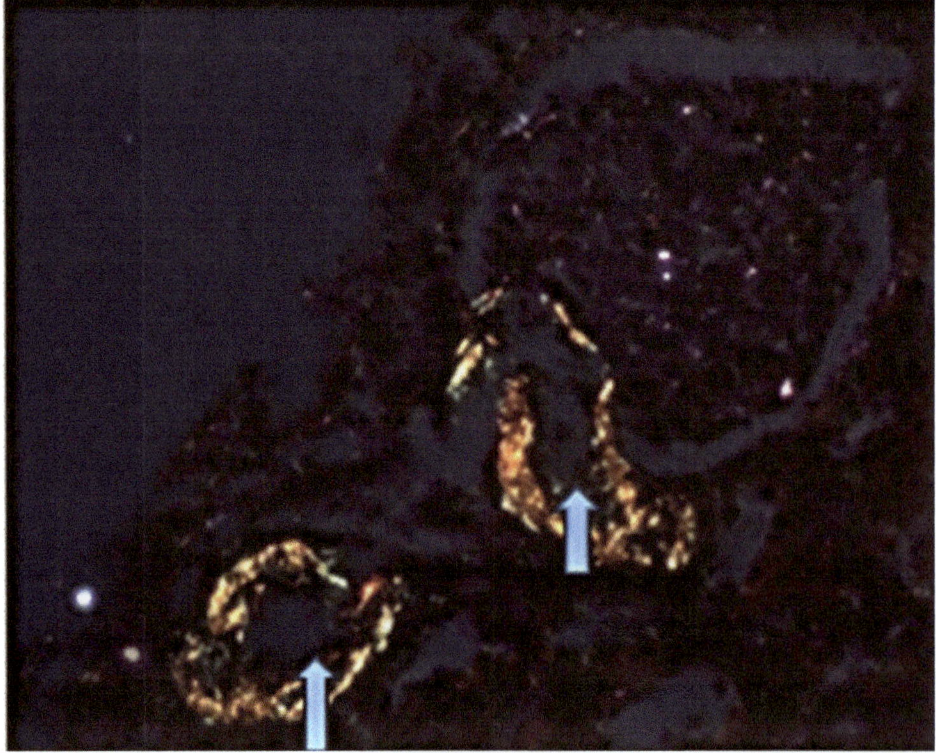

Figure 5:1.5: Congo Red stain:10x: Apple green birefringence under polarization; only in vessels and not in glomerulus.

Immunofluorescence:

Immunofluorescence:

There is lambda light chain restriction around the vessel walls (Figure:5:1.6,5:1.7) sparing the glomeruli/tubular casts/cytoplasm of tubular epithelial cells.

VASCULAR LIMITED AMYLOID

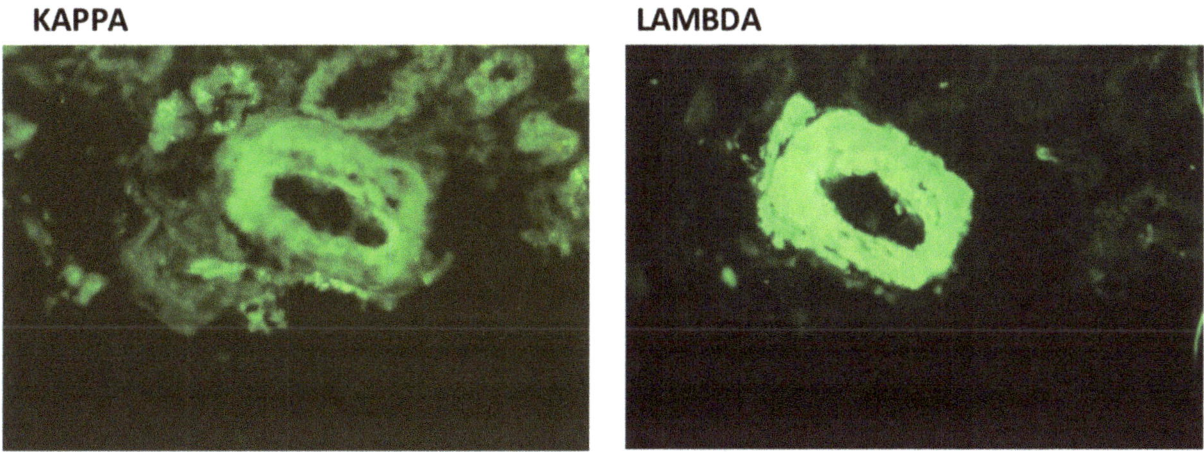

Figure 5:1.6: Immunofluorescence: 20x: Arteriole: LAMBDA LIGHT CHAIN RESTRICTION-The amyloid is positive for Lambda light chain and negative for Kappa Light chain.

ARTERY

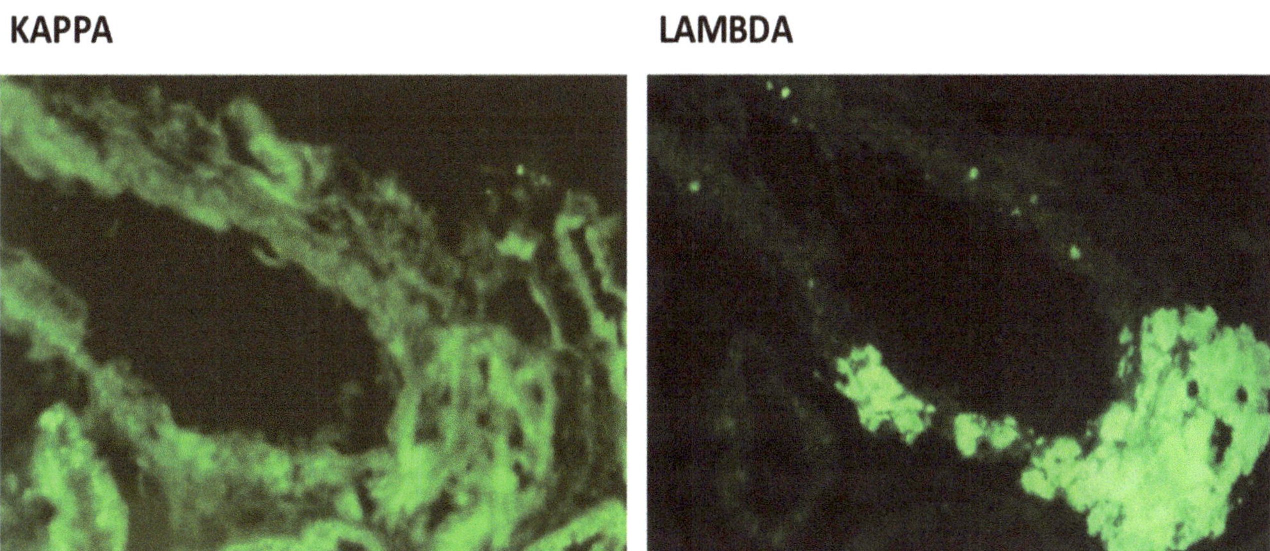

Figure 5:1.7: Immunofluorescence: 20x: Artery: The amyloid is positive for Lambda light chain and negative for Kappa Light chain: Lambda light chain restriction.

Interpretation:

Vascular limited AL Amyloidosis*

Suggested Reading:

*Clinical features of patients with immunoglobulin light chain amyloidosis (AL) with vascular-limited deposition in the kidney: Eirin A,et.al. Nephrol Dial Transplant. 2012 Mar;27(3):1097-101. Epub 2011 Nov 7.

Additional Investigations: Serum Immunofixation electrophoresis: IgG Lambda – M Band Present.

Final Diagnosis: Vascular limited AL Amyloidosis in a case of multiple myeloma.

History: 55 years old female, a known Hypertensive, non-diabetic, presented with progressive decrease in urine volume over last 2 weeks with increase in swelling starting from facial puffiness to a generalised edema all over body. There is no history of haematuria. No h/o over the counter medication use. No h/o indigenous medicines use. There is a palpable non pruritic rash over skin noted 4 weeks back and treated by dermatologist with topical steroids and topical CNI. No h/o arthritis. No redness or watering eyes.

Investigations: Serum creatinine:12mg/dl, UPCR:3.8 g/g, no active urinary sediment, USG findings: bilateral normal sized kidneys.

Clinical Diagnosis: Rapidly progressive glomerulonephritis with cutaneous vasculitis

Differential diagnoses: ANCA Vasculitis/ Cryoglobulinaemic glomerulonephritis

Light Microscopy:

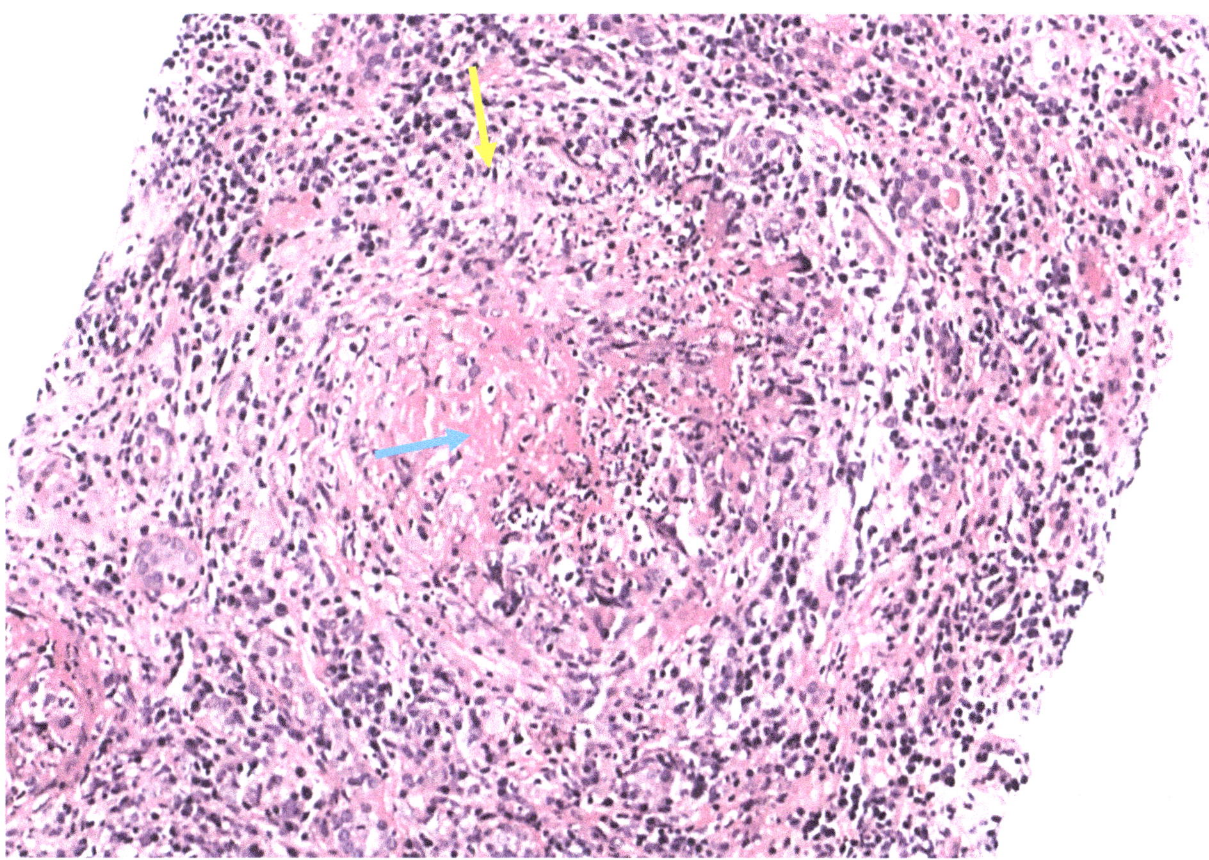

Figure 5:2.1: H& Stain:20x: Glomerulus: Fibrinoid necrosis (blue arrow) and an overlying circumferential cellular crescent (yellow arrow).

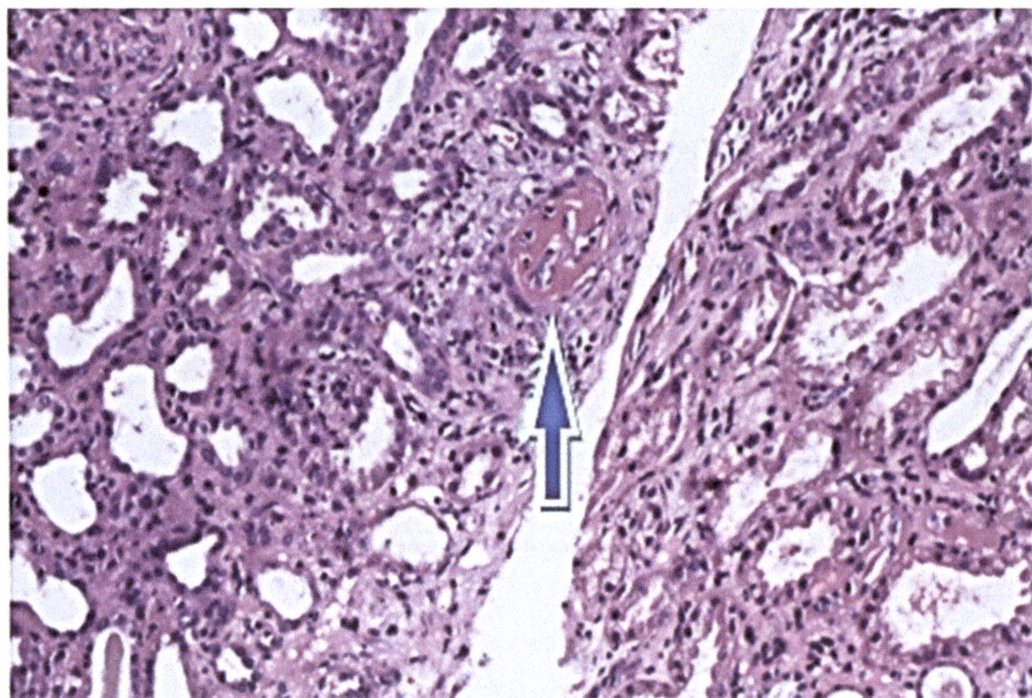

Figure 5:2.2: H&E Stain-10x: small artery (blue arrow): Necrotizing arteritis: fibrin is eosinophilic amorphous in appearance with karyorrhectic debris.

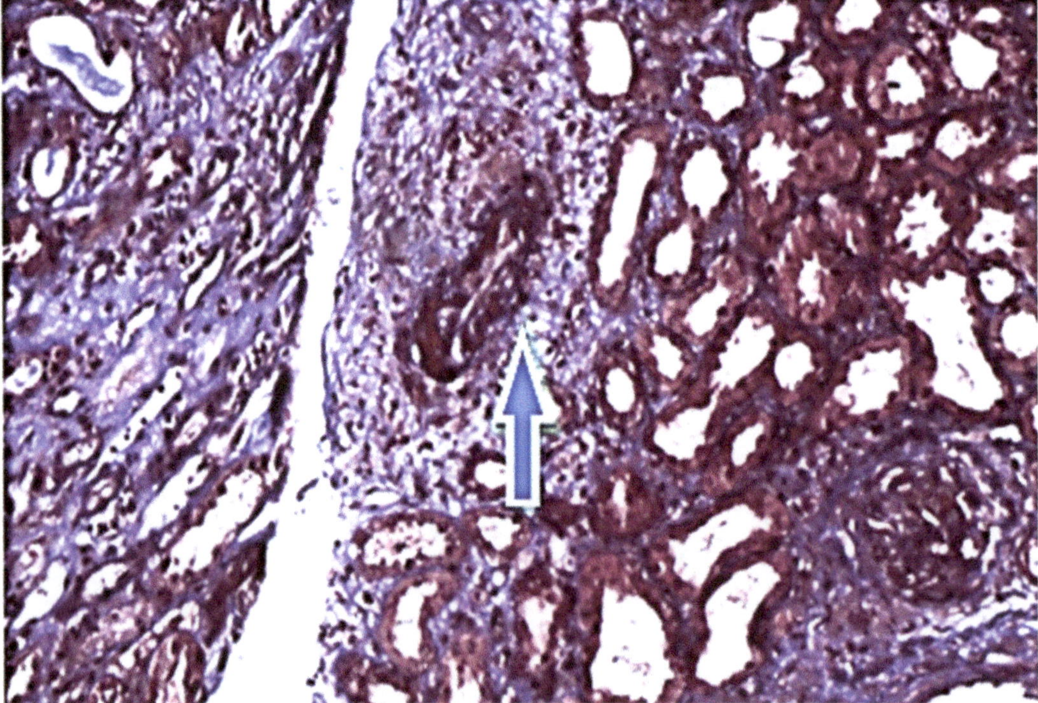

Figure 5:2.3: Masson Trichrome Stain 10x: small artery (blue arrow): Necrotizing arteritis: arrow: a small sized artery: fuchsinophilic (reddish) necrosis of muscle layer, with surrounding inflammation having granulomatous appearance.

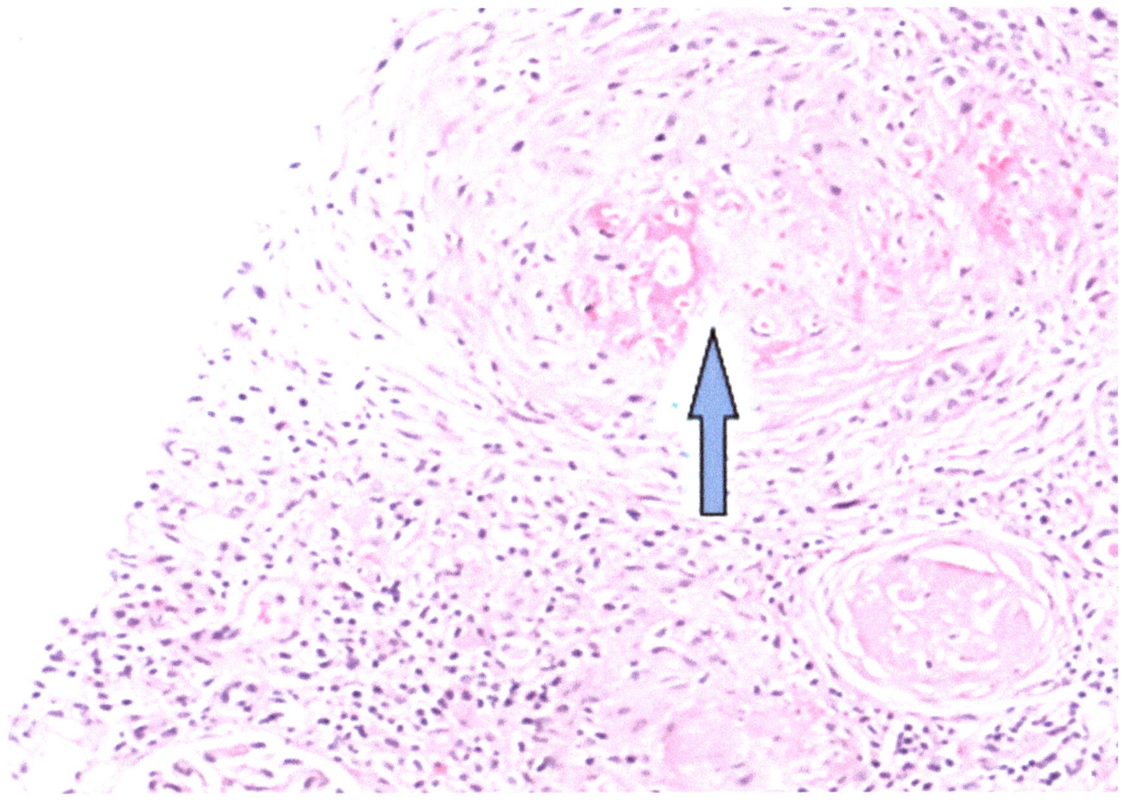

Figure 5:2.4: H&E Stain:20x: Large artery: Fibrinoid necrosis of the muscle layer of the artery, mimicking as necrotizing crescent in H&E Stain, but in serial sections with special stains it is diagnosed as necrosis of the artery.

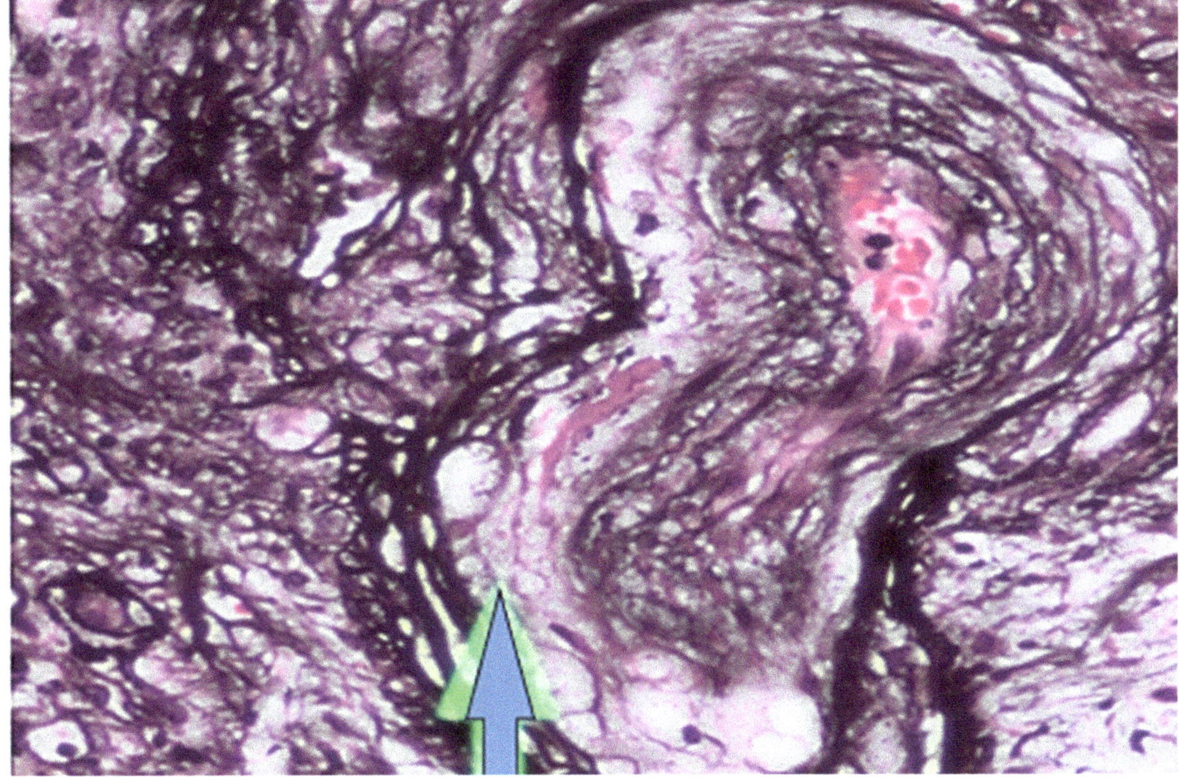

Figure 5:2.5: PASM Stain:40x: The same large artery: Fibrinoid necrosis of muscle layer of artery.

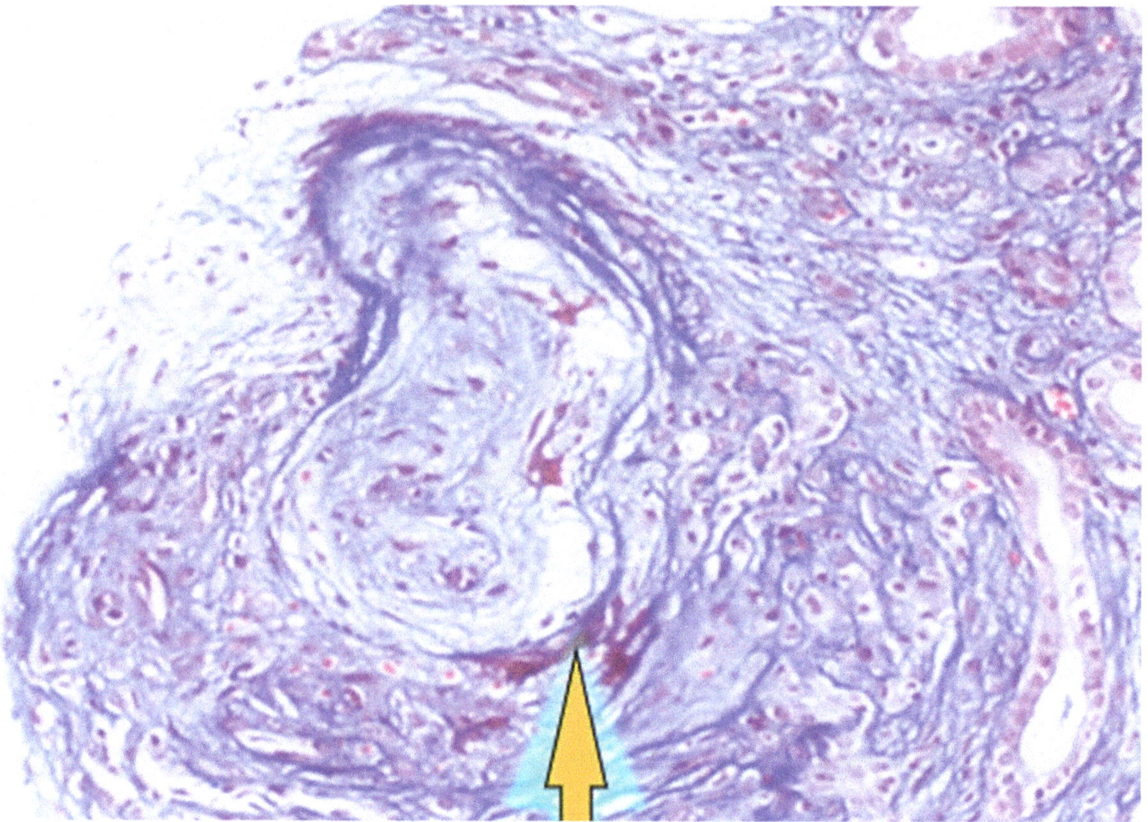

Figure 5:2.6: Masson Trichrome:20x: The same large artery: fuchsinophilic fibrin.

Immunofluorescence:

The IF study shows no immune deposits in glomeruli.

Interpretation: Necrotizing crescentic glomerulonephritis with necrotizing vasculitis.

Additional investigations: C3, C4 – Normal, ANA Profile – Negative, p-ANCA – Negative, c-ANCA Strongly positive.

Final diagnosis: ANCA-mediated pauci-immune crescentic glomerulonephritis with necrotizing vasculitis. (Berden's classification: Crescentic class).

CASE 3

History: 57 years old male, hypertensive, non-diabetic, presented with pedal edema for 2 weeks, decreased urine output since a week, polyarthritis and anaemia. BP 160/100 mm of Hg, pain and swelling in small and large joints of limbs for 3 weeks.

Investigations: Serum creatinine :5.57 mg/dl, Urine protein: creatinine ratio:6 g/g, urine protein: 3+, RBC casts: 3 to 4/HPF. viral markers: non-reactive, Hemoglobin:8.6gm/dl, TLC:6,000/cu mm, platelets:1.5lakhs/cu mm, ESR:110 mm at the end of one hour.

Clinical diagnosis: Rapidly progressive renal failure with hypertension & nephrotic range proteinuria along with polyarthritis and anemia.

Differential diagnoses: Immune-complex mediated glomerulonephritis / Pauci-immune crescentic glomerulonephritis.

Light Microscopy:

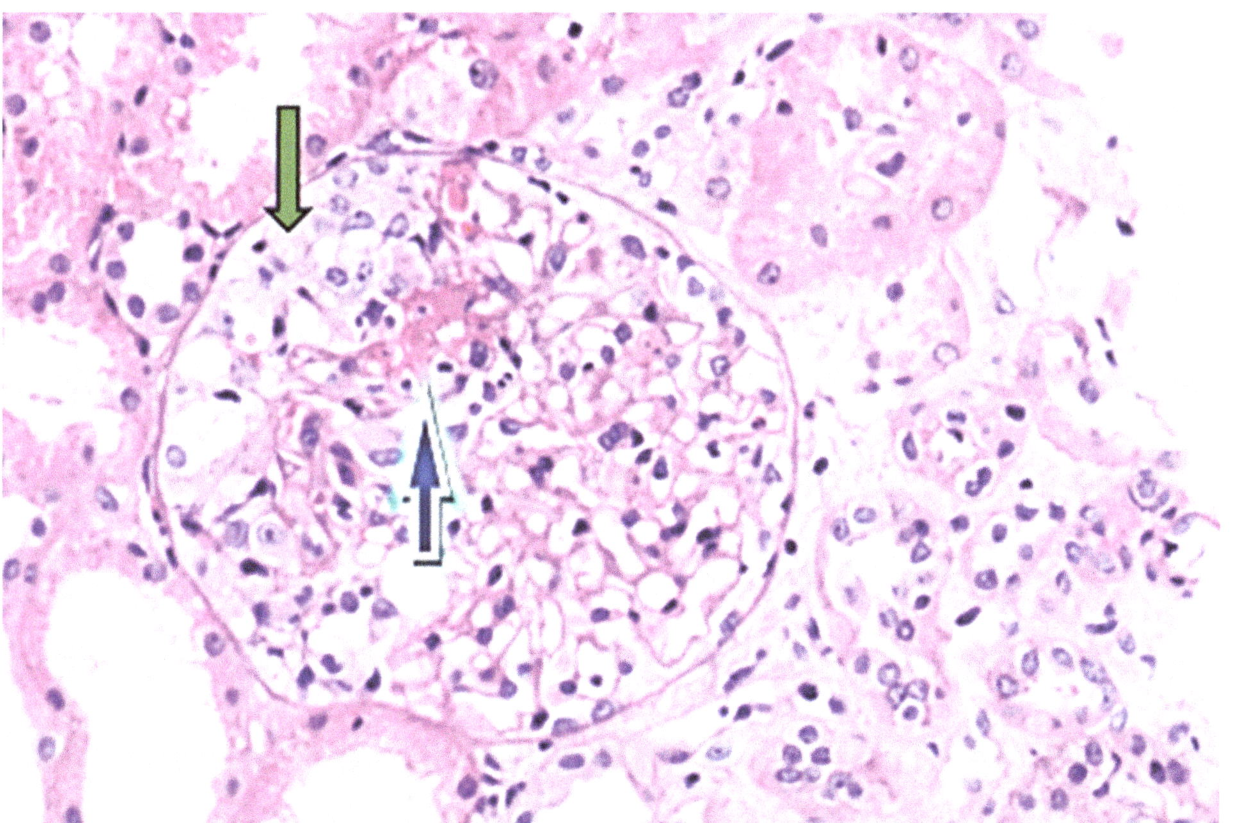

Figure 5:3.1: H&EStain:20x:Glomerulus:Segmental Fibrinoid Necrosis with karyorrhectic debris (blue arrow) and an overlying segmental cellular crescent (green arrow).

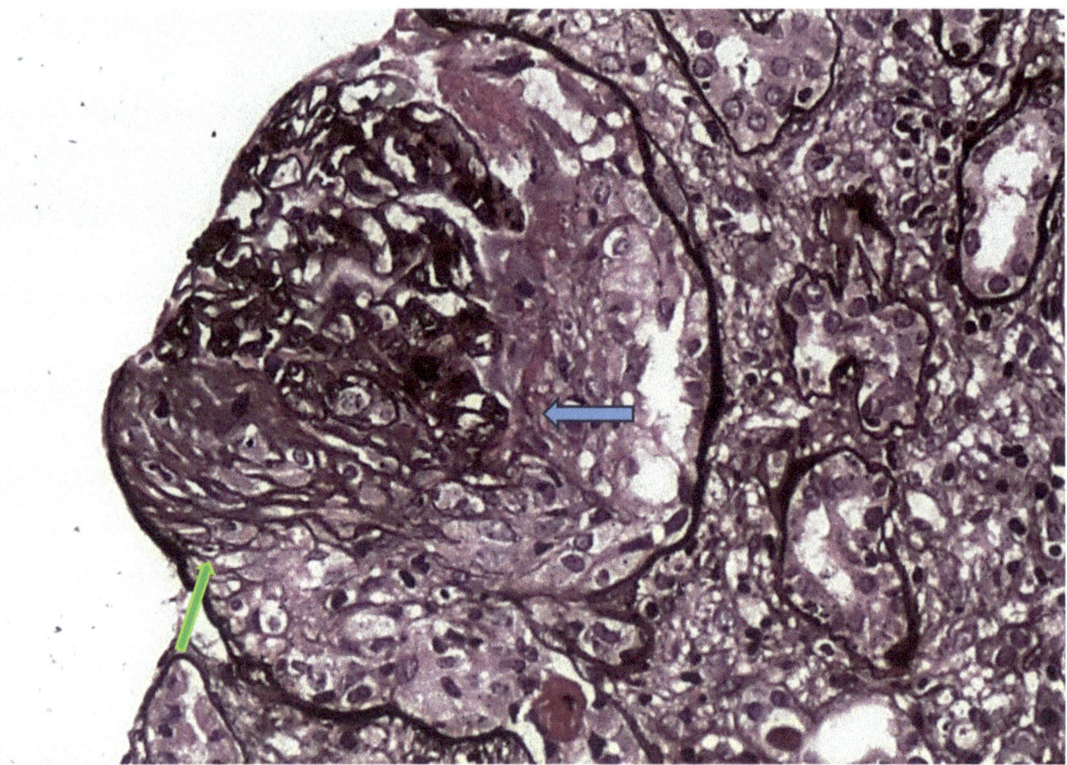

Figure 5:3.2: Silver stain: 20x: Glomerulus: Circumferential cellular crescent (green arrow) and fibrin strands interspesersed with cells of crescent (blue arrow).

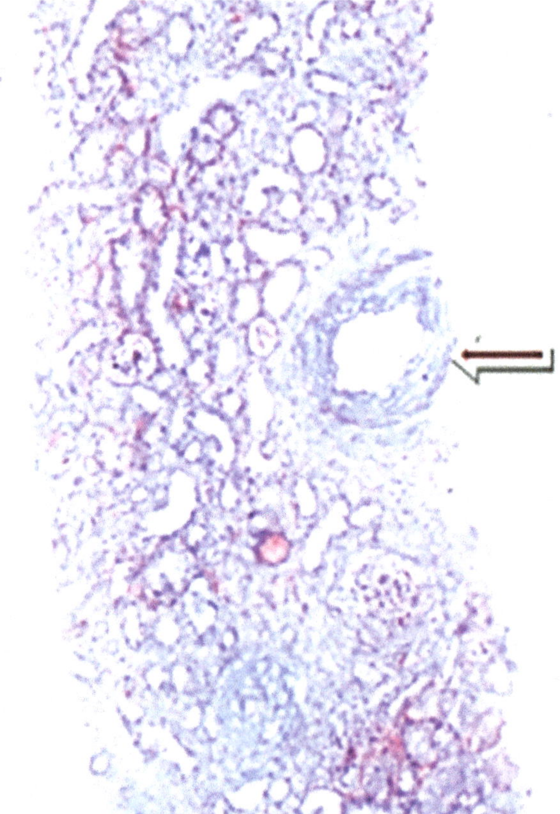

Figure 5:3.3: Masson Trichrome: 10x: Large artery: arteriosclerosis and no vasculitis.

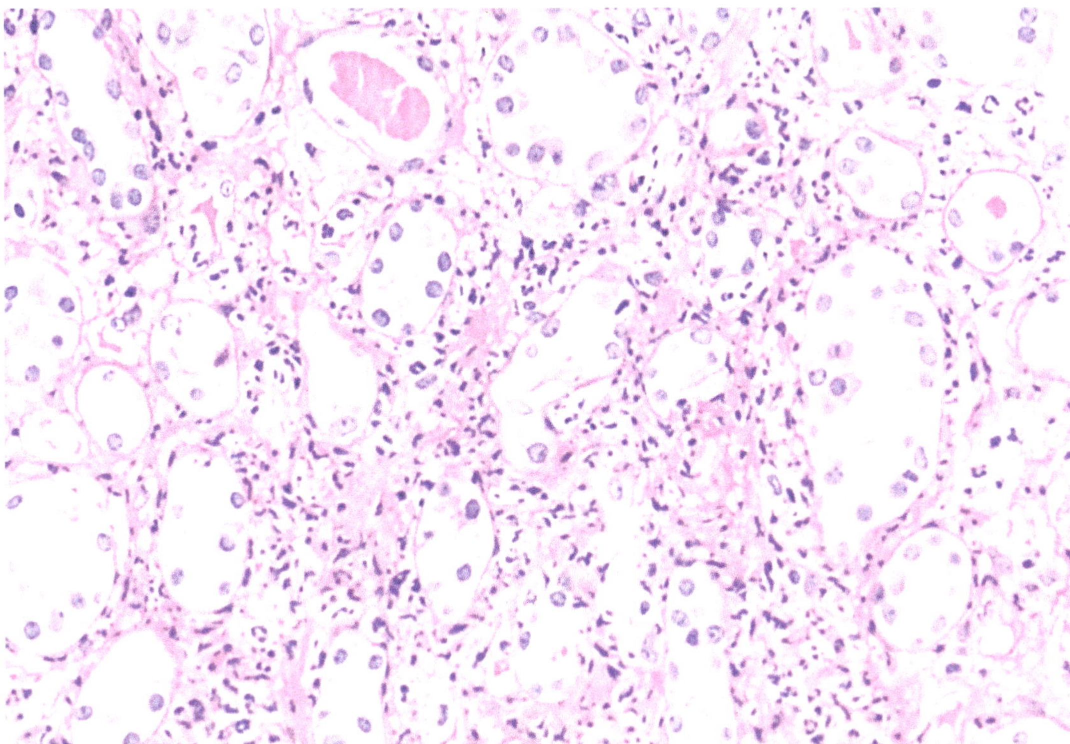

Figure 5:3.4: H&E Stain:20x: Medullary angiitis: Neutrophilic interstitial infiltrate and karyorrhectic debris. The neutrophilic infiltrate is limited to only renal medulla and no evidence of neutrophilic tubular casts.

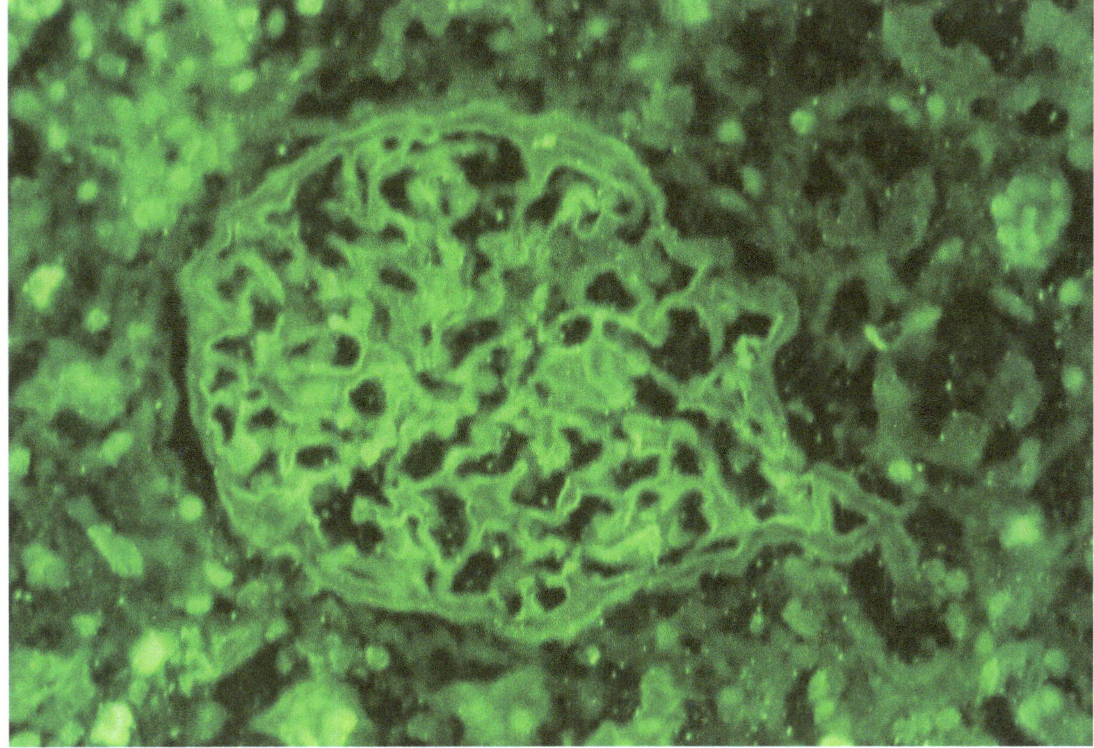

Figure 5:3.5: Immunofluorescence IgG:20x:glomerulus: negative.

Interpretation: Necrotizing & Crescentic glomerulonephritis.

Additional investigations: Urine for culture and sensitivity: sterile, cANCA serology came strongly positive with high titres.

Final diagnosis: ANCA-mediated pauci-immune crescentic glomerulonephritis with medullary angiitis. (Berden's classification: Crescentic class).

Pathology Pearls

Medullary angiitis: 3 features seen in renal medulla:

1.   Interstitial haemorrhage

2.   Karyorrhectic debris

3.   Neutrophilic infiltrate

Medullary angiitis can also be seen in:

1.   ANCA mediated GN

2.   IgA Nephropathy

CASE 4

History: 55 years old male K/C/O type 2 Diabetes mellitus, hypertension, reformed smoker(chronic), coronary artery disease with PCI and stenting twice – most recent 3 weeks back. Two months back patient had an episode of Left hemiparesis for which he had undergone Right Internal Carotid Artery -stenting. Two months back baseline serum creatinine was 1.4mg/dl, last 3 weeks there has been progressive rise in creatinine post cardiac intervention. There is discrepancy in BP in his both arms of 30 mm of Hg. Right BP: 135/90 mm of Hg, Left arm BP :165/100 mm of Hg. Bilateral lower limbs pulses were equally felt.

Investigations: Serum creatinine :3.5 mg/dl, Urine analysis: Protein :2+, RBCs:5 to 6/HPF, pus cells:3 to 4/HPF. Urine Protein to creatinine ratio:2.7 g/g. MR renal angiogram without contrast - no significant stenosis.

Clinical DD: AKI on CKD, AKI post vascular intervention in the background of extensive atherosclerotic disease.

Differential Diagnoses: 1. Contrast induced nephropathy 2. Atheroembolic AKI 3. ATN- Ischemic 4. CKD – related to diabetic / Ischemic Nephropathy.

Light microscopy:

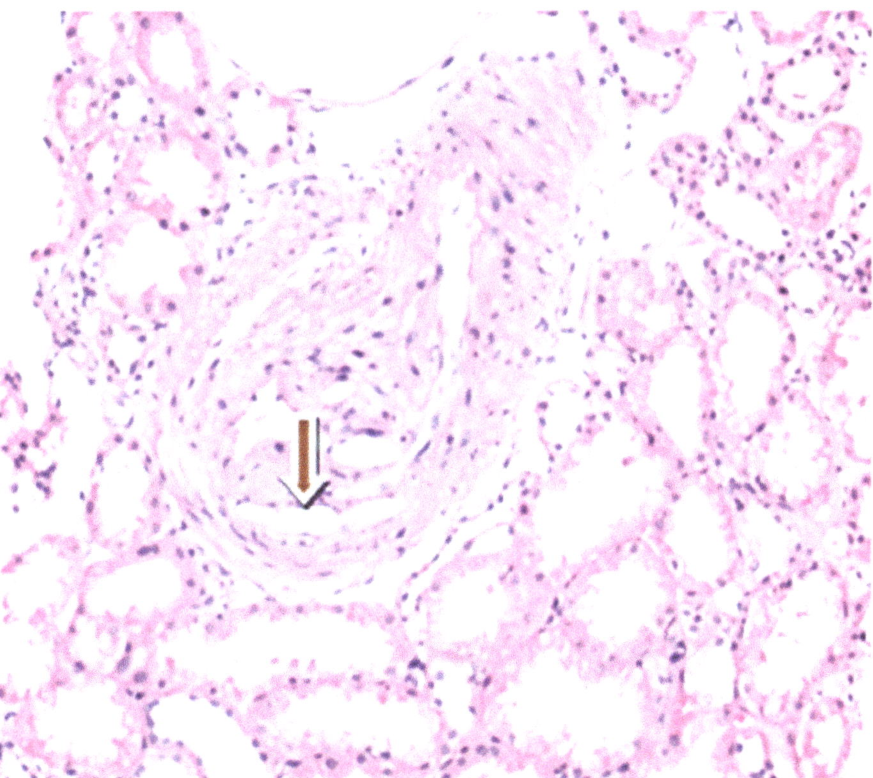

Figure 5:4.1: H&E Stain:10x: The large artery shows mild intimal fibrosis and elongated, convex shaped, empty, needle-like clefts/spaces lodged within the artery, occluding the lumen –characteristic of cholesterol emboli, inciting a fibrous reaction around it.

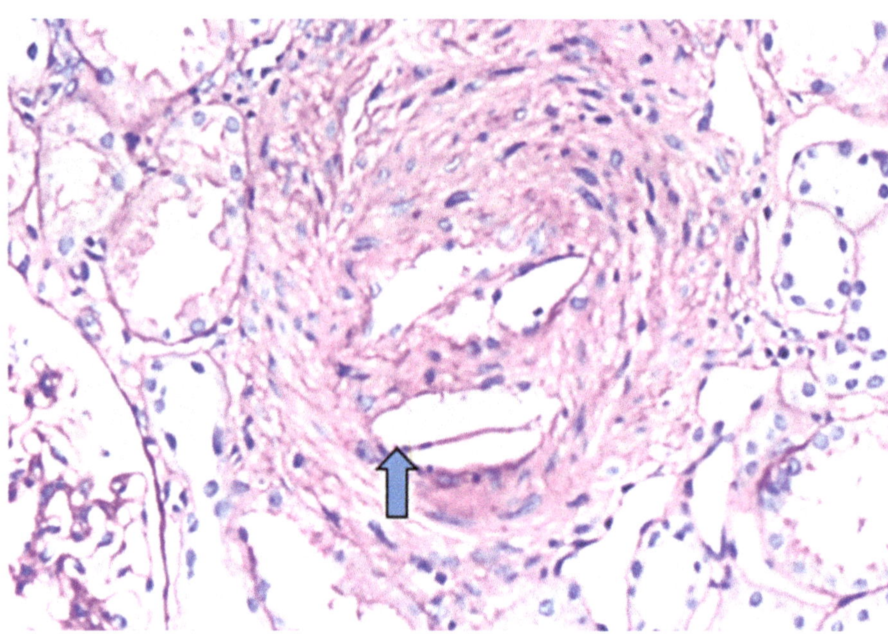

Figure 5:4.2: PAS-Stain:20x: cholesterol emboli: cholesterol gets dissolved during the processing and leaves characteristic clefts.

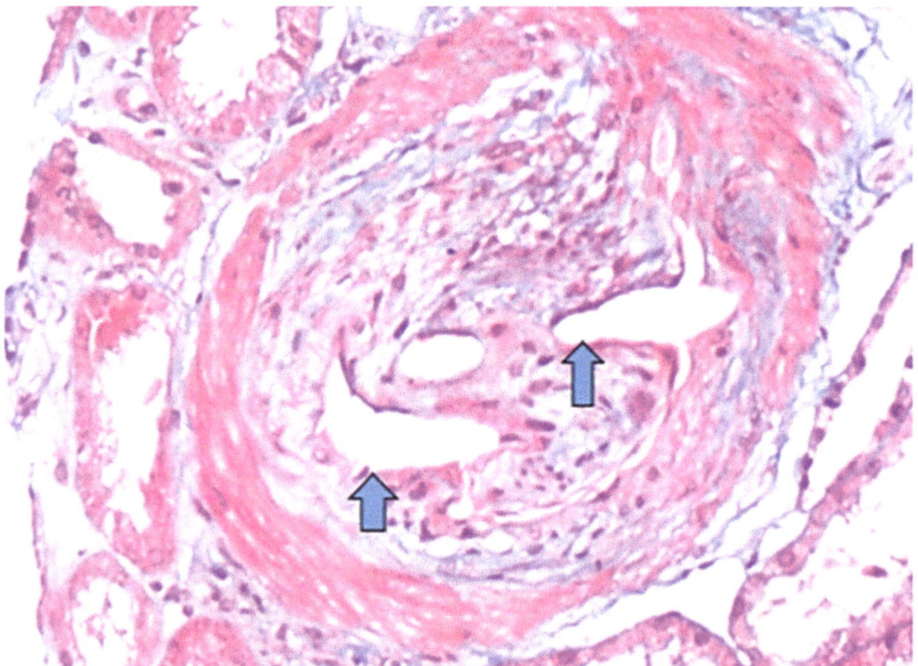

Figure 5:4.3: Masson Trichrome Stain:20x: cholesterol emboli, inciting a fibrous reaction around it.

Interpretation: Atheroembolic Renal disease

Final Diagnosis: AKI due to atheroembolic renal disease.

Pathology Pearls

Cholesterol emboli have also been observed in nephrectomy done for Renovascular Hypertension.

History: 38 years old male, non-diabetic, chronic smoker, hypertensive for 10 years, with past h/o transient ischemic attack 2 years back, on regular medication, detected to have mild renal dysfunction with serum creatinine 1.5 mg/dl one year back, now came with headache and blurring of vision with malignant hypertension. On admission BP 210/110 mm of Hg. There is no history of vascular intervention like angiogram, in recent past. No h/o NSAIDs use. There is no h/o indigenous medication use. There is no h/o any preceding infection. No h/o rash or joint pains.

Investigations: Serum Creatinine:5 mg/dl, Urine protein: 3+ Urine RBCs: 20-25/HPF, Pus cells: 4-6/HPF. 24 Hour urine volume:750ml, 24 Hour Urine protein: 3gm. Serum albumin: 3.5g/dl. ANA: Negative, ANCA: Negative, Viral screen: Negative. Hemoglobin: 9.8g/dl, TLC: 8,400/cu mm, Platelet count: 1.8lakhs/cu mm, LDH:256 U/L.

Clinical diagnosis: Malignant hypertension with AKI-AKIN Stage 3 with underlying CKD & background atherosclerotic disease.

Differential diagnoses: 1. AKI due to malignant hypertension or atheroembolic disease. 2. CKD with rapid worsening due to chronic uncontrolled hypertension. 3. Secondary hypertension: Renal parenchymal disease/ renal artery stenosis/Primary hyperaldosteronism/Pheochromocytoma.

Light Microscopy:

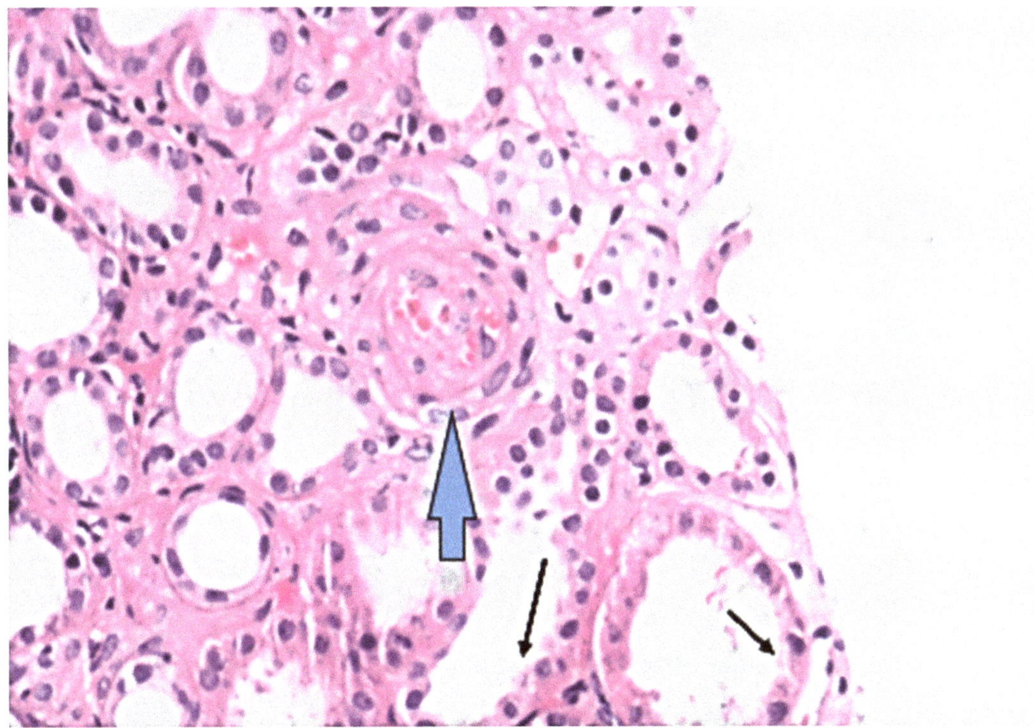

Figure 5:5.1: H&E Stain:20x: Onion skinning of an arteriole with fragmented RBCs (blue arrow) and mild tubular injury with loss of the brush border in tubules (**black** arrows).

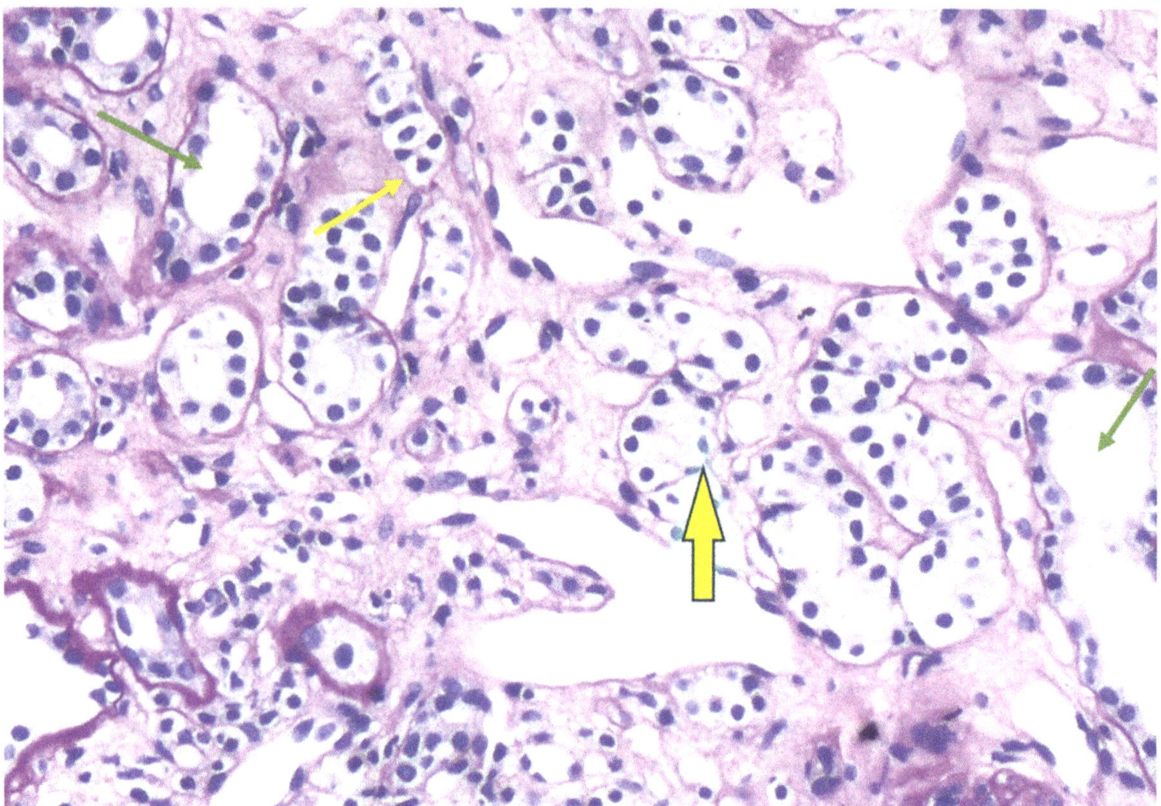

Figure 5:5.2: PAS Stain:10x: *Endocrine type tubular atrophy (yellow arrows): small in size and narrow or no tubular lumina, cuboidal epithelial cells and little or no basement membrane thickening, normal tubules (green arrows).

Interpretation: Hypertensive nephropathy.

Other findings in this case: Focal global glomerulosclerosis (01/10), focal ischemic changes (03/10), moderate tubulointerstitial changes of chronicity (30%), and focal small vessel changes of accelerated hypertension.

Additional investigations:

1. CT Renal angiogram/ MR Renal angiogram without contrast

2. Serum aldosterone and Plasma Renin activity

3. Serum Free Metanephrine levels

Follow up: CT-renal angiogram showed Left renal artery stenosis.

Final Diagnosis: AKI-AKIN stage 3 due to malignant hypertension secondary to unilateral left renal artery stenosis with underlying CKD due to chronic hypertension.

Pathology Pearls

The endocrinization pattern of tubular atrophy is caused by stenosis of the main renal artery.

Reference

*Heptinstall's Pathology of Kidney, Seventh edition, Chapter 03: Primer on the Pathologic Classification and Diagnosis of Kidney Disease: Tubular atrophy: page no.;109.

Chapter 6
Allograft Renal Pathology

EVALUATION OF DONOR BIOPSY ON FROZEN SECTION

1. **Sample adequacy:**
   - ≥25 glomeruli and ≥2 arteries should be present.

2. **Percentage of globally sclerosed glomeruli:**
   - No universally accepted cutoff but if >20%: higher the incidence of delayed graft function (DGF)
   - Strong correlation with donor age
   - Sample taken from subcapsular cortex show many numbers of sclerosed glomeruli and can be overestimated in wedge biopsies.

3. **Arteriosclerosis:**
   Moderate: ≥25% luminal narrowing predictive of worst graft outcome.

4. **IF/TA: Not consistently predictive**

5. **Thrombi: in glomeruli&/ arteries:**
   - Head trauma in donor can precipitate TMA.
   - If<50%of glomeruli show thrombi: good outcome is possible.
   - Cholesterol emboli: contraindication.

Four scoring systems can be used for deceased-donor kidney quality before transplantation.

1. Maryland Aggregate Pathology Index (MAPI)**
2. Banff
3. Remuzzi
4. Leuven

MAPI as predictor of graft survival considered slightly better***.

Deceased Donor Kidney Biopsy Scoring System for predicting graft survival: MAPI: Maryland Aggregate Pathology Index:

Score of predictive graft survival:	Present	Absent
Periglomerular fibrosis	4 points	0 points
Arteriolar hyalinosis	4 points	0 points
Scar (focus of scar or atrophy in 10 tubules)	3 points	0 points
Global glomerulosclerosis ≥15%	2 points	0 points
Wall to lumen ratio of interlobular arteries ≥ 0.5	2 points	0 points

MAPI=Sum of points

	Aggregate score	Graft survival at 5 years
1	0-7: Low MAPI	90%
2	8-11: Intermediate MAPI	63%
3	12-15: High MAPI	53%

***Reference**

Colvin/Chang: Diagnostic Pathology: Kidney Diseases: Second edition: Evaluation of the donor kidney: page no.945.

**Munivenkatappa, R. B. , Schweitzer, E. J. , Papadimitriou, J. C. , Drachenberg, C. B. , Thom, K. A. , Perencevich, E. N. , Haririan, A. , Rasetto, F. , Cooper, M. , Campos, L. , Barth, R. N. , Bartlett, S. T. & Philosophe, B. (2008). The Maryland Aggregate Pathology Index. American Journal of Transplantation, 8 (11), 2316-2324.

*** Deceased-Donor Kidney Biopsy Scoring Systems for Predicting Future Graft Function: A Comparative Study Kevin Chen,et.al, Trnsplantation Proceedings Volume 53, Issue 3, April 2021, Pages 906-912

Reporting of Allograft Renal Biopsies:

Banff Classification of Renal Allograft Pathology is used.

- Initial conception -1991
- Every 2 years-review
- Recent update-2022.

Banff specimen adequacy criteria on light microscopy:

10 glomeruli and 02 arteries.

Minimal adequacy criteria:

07 glomeruli and single artery.

BANFF LESIONS, DEFINITIONS AND SCORES

Lesion	Definition	Abbreviation	Score 0	Score 1	Score 2	Score 3
Glomerulitis (number of glomeruli involved)	Endothelial swelling with an infiltration of mononuclear cells and/or neutrophils within a capillary lumen of the tuft	g	None	≤ 25%	25-50%	≥ 50%
Interstitial inflammation	Percentage of the non-scarred area of cortex with inflammatory cells	i	None	≤ 25%	25-50%	≥ 50%
Tubulitis	Number of mononuclear cells between tubular epithelial cells or between the tubular lining and basement membrane. Very atrophic tubules to be excluded.	t	None	1-4	5-10	>10
Tubulitis in areas of interstitial fibrosis	Tubulitis in mildly (<25% of diameter of normal tubules) & moderately atrophic tubules (<50% of diameter of normal tubules) and not to score in severely atrophic tubules.	t-IFTA	None	1-4	5-10	>10
Endarteritis	Percentage of lumen occluded by subendothelial inflammation	v	None	<25%	≥25%	Transmural necrosis
Transplant glomerulopathy	GBM double contours in the maximally involved glomerulus	cg	None	1a: only scored by *EM 1b: ≤25% by LM	25-50%	>50%
Interstitial fibrosis	Percentage of cortical interstitial fibrosis	ci	≤5%	6-25%	26-50%	>50%
Tubular atrophy	Percentage of atrophic cortical tubules involved	ct	None	≤25%	26-50%	≥50%
Fibrous intimal thickening	Percentage narrowing of luminal area by intimal fibrosis without elastosis; may have inflammatory cells away from the intima	cv	None	<25%	26-50%	>50%

Lesion	Definition	Abbreviation	Score 0	Score 1	Score 2	Score 3
Mesangial matrix widening	Intercapillary width is more than two cell diameters in at least two lobules; graded according to the percentage of non-sclerosed glomeruli involved	Mm	None	<25%	26-50%	>50%
Total inflammation	Percentage of entire cortex, scarred and non-scarred occupied by inflammatory cells	Ti	<10%	10-25%	26-50%	>50%
Inflammation in scarred cortex	Percentage of scarred area occupied by inflammatory cells	i-IFTA	<10%	10-25%	26-50%	>50%
Peritubular capillaritis	Maximum leucocytes in a capillary with ≥10% of PTCs having at least one leucocyte	ptc	<3	3-4	5-10	>10
Arteriolar hyalinosis	PAS positive arteriolar hyaline thickening	ah	None	Mild to moderate in ≥1	Moderate to severe in >1	Severe in many
Hyaline arteriolar thickening	Peripheral nodular hyalinosis	aah	None	Non circumferential in 1 vessel	Noncircumferential – many vessels	Circumferential in 1 vessel
C4d	Percentage of PTCs with circumferential linear staining, cortex and medulla	C4d	None	<10%	10-50%	>50%

*By EM, duplication observed in more than one loop is scored 1a. GBM: Glomerular basement membranes, PTC: Peritubular capillary, PAS: Periodic acid-Schiff

* Banff classification: Diagnostic categories:

Category 1: Normal biopsy or non-specific changes

Category 2: Antibody Mediated Rejection (AMR) and Microvascular inflammation/Injury (MVI):

Diagnostic features of AMR/MVI:

Active lesions:		
	(i)	g > 0 in the absence of glomerulonephritis
	(ii)	ptc > 0 in the absence of acute TCMR or borderline (suspicious) for acute TCMR
	(iii)	v > 0
	(iv)	acute thrombotic microangiopathy (TMA) in the absence of any other cause.
Chronic lesions:	(i)	cg > 0 (by LM or EM), if no evidence of chronic TMA and if absence of recurrent or de novo glomerulonephritis
	(ii)	severe ptcml: ≥7 in one cortical peritubular capillary and 5 or more in 2 additional capillaries.
MVI at or above threshold: AMR	At least moderate MVI (g + ptc ≥ 2) and	
	And/Or Biopsy-based transcript diagnostics for AMR/MVI above a defined threshold and	
	C4d positive and	
	DSA positive.	

MVI at or above threshold: **Microvascular inflammation/injury (MVI)**	At least moderate MVI (g + ptc ≥ 2) and
	And/OR Biopsy-based transcript diagnostics for AMR/MVI above a defined threshold and
	C4d negative and
	DSA negative.
MVI below threshold: **AMR**	(g + ptc< 2) and
	And Biopsy-based transcript diagnostics for AMR/MVI below a defined threshold and
	C4d positive and
	DSA positive/negative.
MVI below threshold : **Probable AMR:**	(g + ptc < 2) and
	And Biopsy-based transcript diagnostics for AMR/MVI below a defined threshold and
	C4d negative and
	DSA positive.
Active AMR:	g, ptc, C4d positivity, cg = 0, ptcml = 0
Chronic active AMR:	g, ptc, C4d positivity, cg> and or severe ptcml
Chronic AMR:	Probable AMR with chronic lesions and prior documented diagnosis of active or chronic active AMR, or documented prior evidence of DSA.

A. Active AMR: All 3/3 criteria must be met for diagnosis:

Criteria I: Light microscopic findings of at least one:	(a) Microvascular inflammation : (b) glomerulitis (g≥0) with peritubular capillaritis (ptc ≥0), in the absence of recurrent or de novo glomerulonephritis, although in the presence of acute TCMR, borderline infiltrate, or infection.; then (ptc≥1) alone is not sufficient, (g≥1) is required.
	(c) Transplant endarteritis (v > 0).
	(d) TMA, on excluding other causes
Criteria II: Evidence of one or more:	(a) By IHC: C4d > 0: linear and continuous positivity in peritubular capillaries or medullary vasa recta. By IF: C4d > 1; as IF is very sensitive C4d 1 is not considered positive.
	(b) (g + ptc) ≥2,with none of the two is zero(0), in the absence of recurrent or de novo glomerulonephritis, although in the presence of acute TCMR, borderline infiltrate, or infection.
	(c) There is increased expression of gene transcripts associated with AMR/MVI above a defined threshold in the kidney tissue. The assay should be thoroughly validated for use as substitute for MVI and available.
Criteria III:	Presence of donor-specific antibodies (DSA) to HLA or Non-HLA antigens in the serum. C4d positivity may substitute for DSA, but still it is strongly advised to look for DSA in serum whenever criteria I and II are met. If HLA DSA is negative, then look for non-HLA DSA.

B. Chronic active AMR: All 3/3 criteria must be met for diagnosis:

Criteria I: Chronic lesions of AMR: One or more:	(a)	Transplant glomerulopathy (cg > 0) by excluding other causes of chronic TMA and diagnosed by electron microscopy (EM) alone (cg1a),by LM as (cg1b) onwards
	(b)	Severe peritubular capillary basement membrane multilayering (ptcml1; requires EM)):≥ 7 layers in one capillary and ≥ 5 layers in two others.

Criteria II: Same as Criterion II as active AMR

Criteria III: Same as criterion III for active AMR.

C. Chronic AMR (Probable AMR +Chronic lesions):

1. cg > 0 and/or severe ptcml
2. C4d being negative
3. Prior documented diagnosis of active or chronic active/Chronic active AMR and/or documented prior(post-transplant) and/or current positive DSA.

D. C4d staining without evidence of rejection:

All 4 /4 features must be met for diagnosis:

1.	**C4d positivity:** By IHC: C4d > 0: linear and continuous positivity in peritubular capillaries or medullary vasa recta. By IF: C4d > 1; as IF is very sensitive C4d 1 is not considered positive
2.	Criterion I for active or chronic active AMR not met
3.	Biopsy-based transcript diagnostics for AMR/MVI as in criterion 2 for active and chronic active AMR: Negative
4.	No acute or chronic active TCMR, or borderline changes

E. Microvascular inflammation/injury (MVI), DSA-negative and C4d-negative:

All 3/3 criteria must be met for diagnosis:

1.	At least moderate microvascular inflammation ([g + ptc] ≥2) in the absence of recurrent or de novo glomerulonephritis, although in the presence of acute TCMR, borderline infiltrate, or infection, ptc ≥ 2 alone is not sufficient and g must be ≥1
2.	C4d negative by IF /IHC
3.	DSA is negative.

F. Probable AMR:

All 4 /4 criteria must be met for diagnosis:

1. glomerulitis (g≥1) with peritubular capillaritis (ptc≥1)
2. Cg & ptcml: absent
3. C4d negative
4. DSA: positive.

G. C4d staining with acute tubular injury (ATI):

All 3 criteria must be met for diagnosis:

1. Presence of Acute tubular injury (ATI)
1. C4d positivity
2. Cg & ptcml: absent
Clinical scenarios: (i)   Probable AMR: Early posttransplant in crossmatch positive DSA sensitised patient (ii) Accommodation: ABO-incompatibility (iii) No AMR:DSA negative in conventional transplants.

Category 3: Suspicious for borderline TCMR:

t1, i1 or ; t2, i1 or ; t3, i1 or t1, i2 or t1, i3.

Category 4: T-Cell Mediated Rejection (TCMR):

A. Acute TCMR:	
Acute TCMR, Grade I A:	t2, i2 or i3
Acute TCMR, Grade I B:	t3, i2 or i3
Acute TCMR, Grade II A:	v 1 regardless of scores t & i
Acute TCMR, Grade II B:	v 2 regardless of scores t & i
Acute TCMR, Grade III:	v 3 regardless of scores t & i
B. Chronic Active TCMR:	
Chronic Active TCMR, Grade IA:	t 2 or t-IFTA 2, i-IFTA $\geq$ 2, ti $\geq$ 2
Chronic Active TCMR, Grade I B:	t 3 or t-IFTA 3, i-IFTA $\geq$ 2, ti $\geq$ 2.
Chronic Active TCMR, Grade II : Transplant arteriopathy	Artery with neointima formation without elastic fibres and mononuclear cell infiltration. It is seen in chronic TCMR/ABMR. This may also be a manifestation of chronic active or chronic ABMR or mixed ABMR/TCMR.

Category 5: Polyomavirus Nephropathy (PVN).

References:

*A 2018 Reference Guide to the Banff Classification of Renal Allograft Pathology Candice Roufosse, et.al, Transplanation2018;102: 1795–1814).
*The Banff 2019 Kidney Meeting Report (I): Updates on and clarification of criteria for T cell– and antibody-mediatedrejection Alexandre Loupy et.al : Am J Transplant. 2020;20:2318–2331

*The Banff 2022 Kidney Meeting Report: Reappraisal of microvascular inflammation and the role of biopsy-based transcript diagnostics :Maarten Naesens, et.al, American Journal of Transplantation, 24(2024)338-349.

Evaluation of an allograft renal biopsy:

Important clinical information:

1. Donor source: live related/deceased/swap
2. Duration: post-transplant
3. Drug Therapy
4. Native Kidney Disease
5. Anti-donor HLA antibodies
6. Renal function
7. Proteinurea

CASE 1

History: 34 years old male, nondiabetic, and non-hypertensive, ESRD on dialysis for last one year.59-year-old mother as donor. No induction apart from Methylprednisolone. Uneventful perioperative course. Nadir Creatinine 0.9 on Post op Day 5. Post operative day:10, creeping rise in serum creatinine :1.5mg/dl while on triple immunosuppression, Valgancyclovir and Cotrimoxazole prophylaxis. No fever/Vomitings/diarrhea/decrease in urine output. Decreased oral intake and BP is 100/70 mm of Hg.

Urine analysis: Protein Trace, RBCs: 10-15/HPF, Pus cells: 3-4/HPF. Tacrolimus trough level 9ng/ml.

Clinical DD: Tacrolimus toxicity/Pre renal AKI / Allograft Rejection.

Light microscopy:

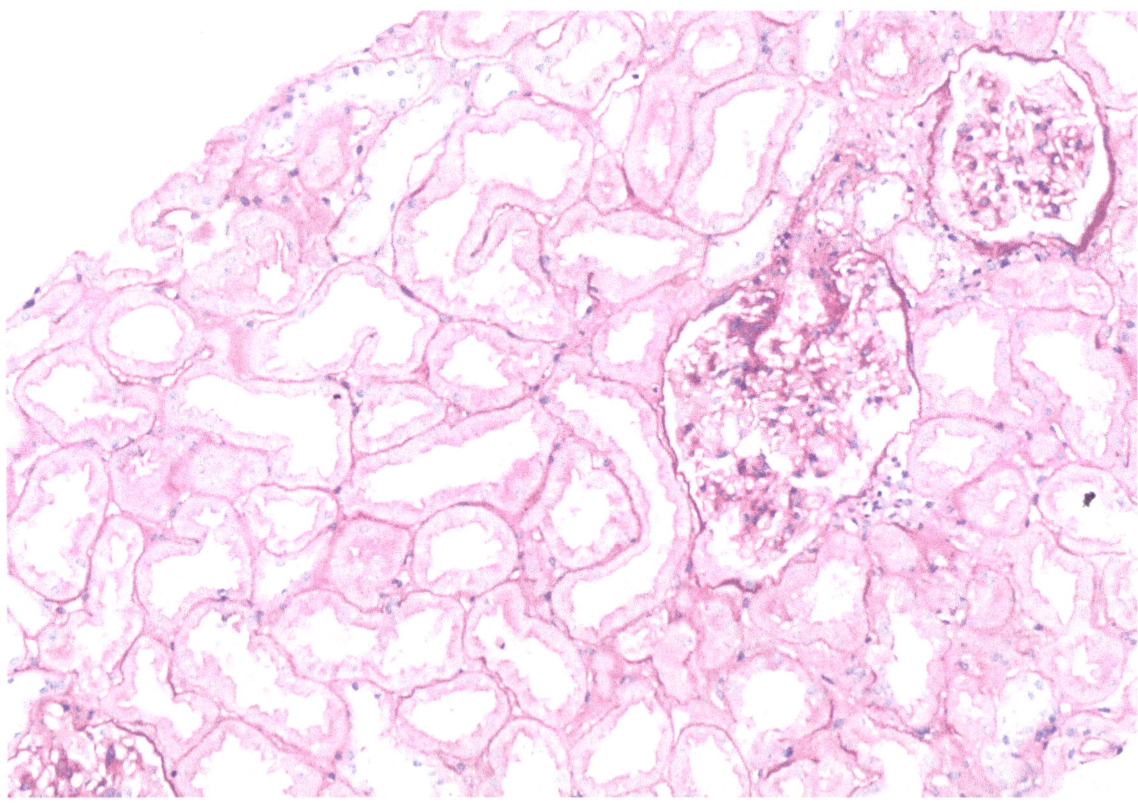

Figure 6:1.1: PAS Stain:10x: Mild Acute Tubular Injury: Normocellular glomeruli with mild variable PAS positive mesangial matrix expansion, loss of the brush border and no significant IF/TA or inflammation

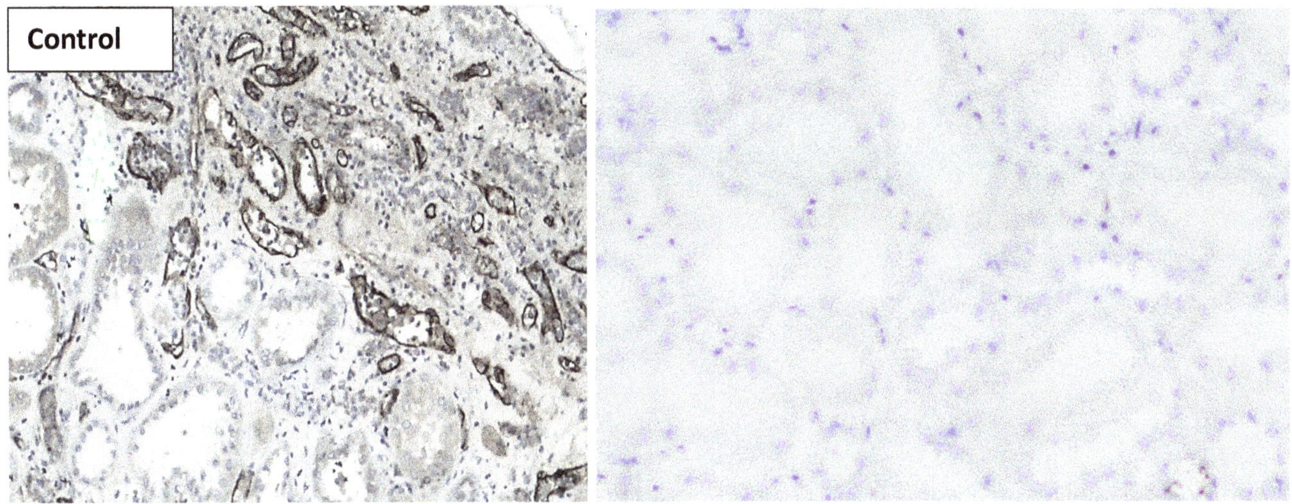

Figure 6:1.2: Immunohistochemistry C4d Stain:20x: It does not show positivity around the peritubular capillaries.

Interpretation: Mild Acute tubular injury.

There is no evidence of rejection in the biopsy studied.

Banff score: g0, t0, i0, v0, cg0, ct0, ci0, cv0, aah0, mm1,C4d0,ptc0,ti0,i-IFTA 0.

Case 2

History: 17 years old male, non-diabetic, hypertensive, ESRD due to unknown etiology, on Haemodialysis for last 2 months, underwent live related renal transplantation. Donor:49-yearsold father. Donor normotensive/nondiabetic. Induction agent: Anti-Thymocyte Globulin (ATG): 1 gm/Kg total dose along with Methylprednisolone followed by triple drug maintenance immunosuppression (Tac/MMF/Steroid). Uneventful peri operative and post operative one month course.DJ Stent removed at 2 weeks. Nadir creatinine reached 0.9 mg/dl. One-month post-transplant there is an asymptomatic rise in serum creatinine. BP 150/90mm of Hg. No pedal edema. No fever/diarrhoea/urinary complaints.

Investigations: Serum Creatinine :1.8 mg/dl, Potassium 5.0mEq/L, Chloride:110mEq/. Tacrolimus level:3.36ng/ml. Urine Protein 1+, RBC: 6-8/HPF, Pus cells: 4-5/HPF, USG : Normal, No Renal artery stenosis.

Clinical DD: Allograft Rejection/ Recurrence of native renal disease.

Light Microscopy:

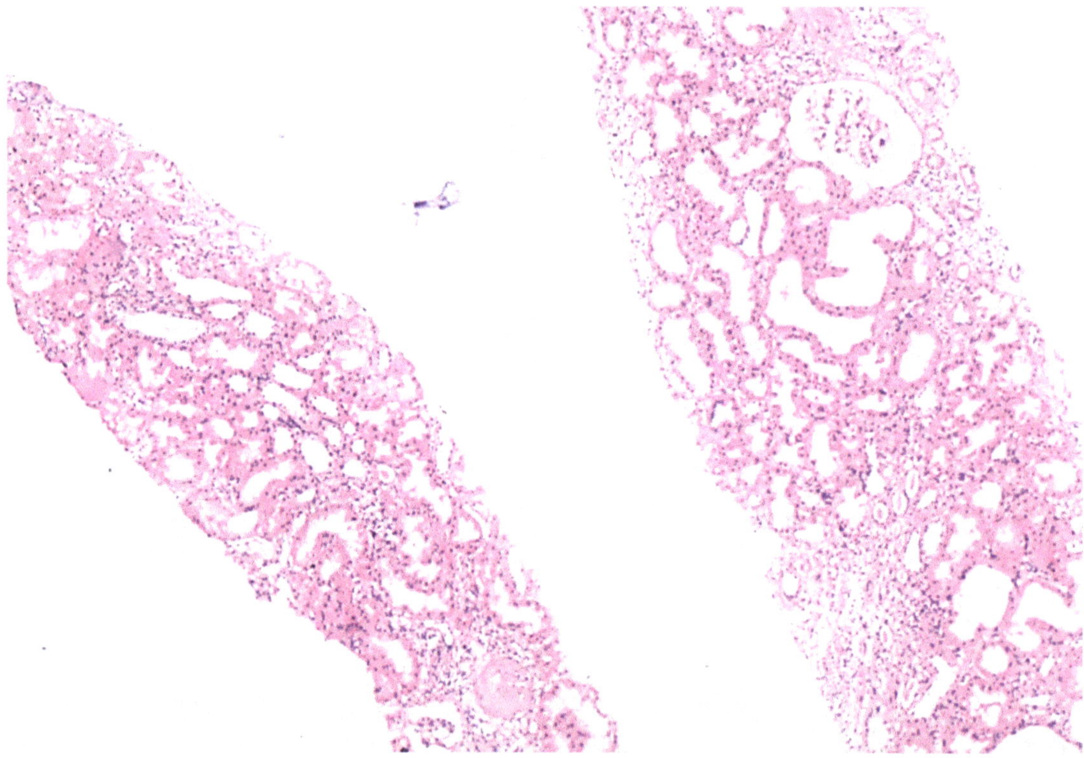

Figure: 6:2.1: H&E Stain:4x: Mild interstitial inflammation involving up to 20% of the cortex sampled.

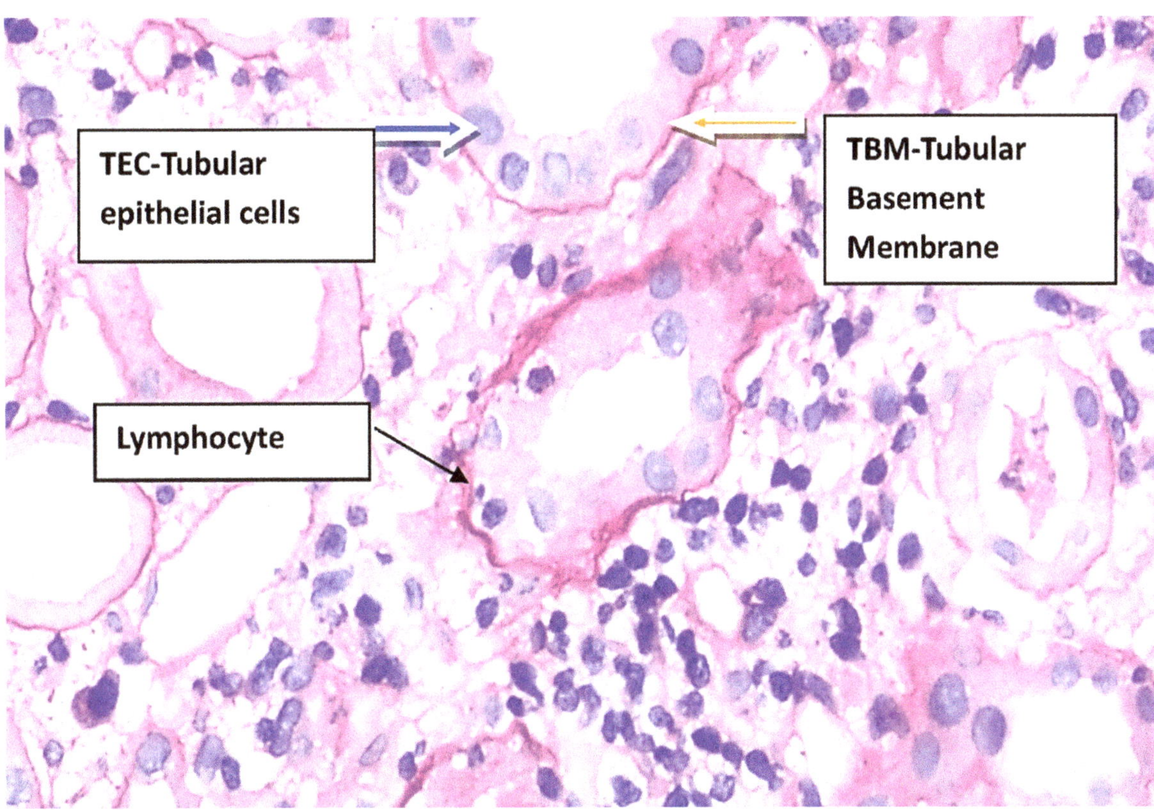

Figure 6:2.2: PAS Stain:40x: Tubules: Mild Tubulitis: smaller, darker mononuclear cell -lymphocyte (**black** arrow)along the basolateral aspect of tubular basement membrane(Yellow arrow)and inside TBM with a perinuclear halo and mild interstitial inflammation. The Tubular epithelial cells (blue arrow) are faint in colour as compared to lymphocytes.

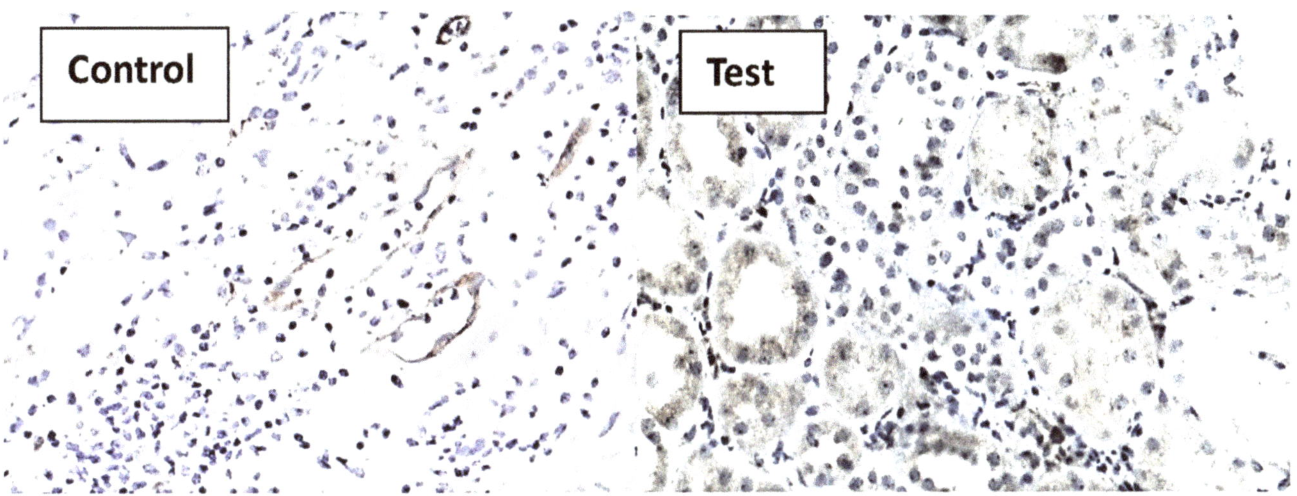

Figure 6:2.3: Immunohistochemistry C4d Stain: 20x: It does not show positivity around the peritubular capillaries.

Interpretation: Borderline changes suspicious of an acute T-cell mediated rejection.

Banff score: g0, **t1, i1**, v0, cg0, ct0, ci0, cv0, aah0, mm0, C4d0, ptc0, ti1, i-IFTA 0.

Pathology Pearls

Table 6:2.1: Identifying Tubulitis.

Sr. No.	Features	Mononuclear inflammatory infiltrate	Tubular Epithelial cell (TEC)
1.	Cell alignment	Basolateral aspect of TEC	Apical to tubular lumen
2.	Size	Smaller than TEC	Larger than mononuclear inflammatory cell
3.	Nucleus	Darker than TEC	Faint than mononuclear inflammatory cell
4.	Perinuclear halo	Present	Absent

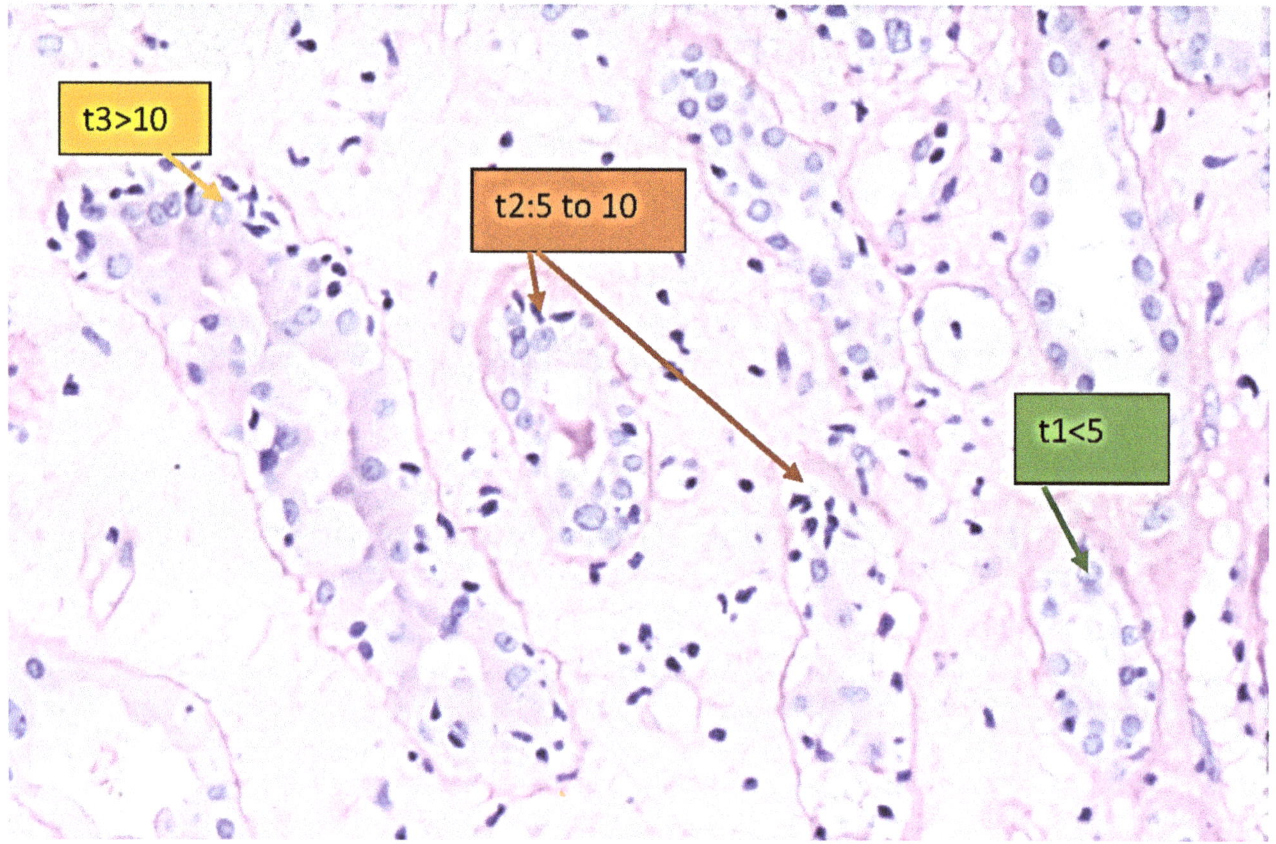

Figure 6:2.3: PAS Stain:20x: Tubulitis:

t1: Foci of 1 to 4 mononuclear cells /tubular cross section (or 10 tubular cells)

t2: Foci with 5 to 10mononuclear cells /tubular cross section (or 10 tubular cells)

t3: Foci with >10 mononuclear cells /tubular cross section (or 10 tubular cells) or the presence of 2≥areas of tubular basement destruction accompanied by i2/i3 inflammation and t2 elsewhere.

CASE 3

History: 40 years old male, non-diabetic, non-hypertensive, ESRD of unknown etiology, on dialysis for 2 years underwent Kidney transplant , wife being donor. HLA match:2/6. Induction agent ATG :1.5 g/kg given divided over 2 days. Nadir creatinine reached 1 mg/dl. Uneventful peri and post operative course. On triple drug immunosuppression (Tac/MMF/Steroid). 5 months post-transplant came with a serum creatinine of 2.5 mg/dl. Mild graft tenderness and feverish sensation. No history of diarrhea/vomiting/urinary complaints/pedal edema/ shortness of breath.

Investigations: Serum Creatinine 2.5 mg/dl. Urine Protein: 2+, RBCs:5-8/HPF, pus cells: 5-6/HPF. Tacrolimus trough level:5ng/ml. USG findings: Raised parenchymal echotexture and Resistive Index (RI) of the Graft, No Renal artery stenosis.

Clinical DD: Allograft Rejection/ Native kidney disease recurrence / Pyelonephritis/ CMV infection / BKV Nephropathy.

Light microscopy:

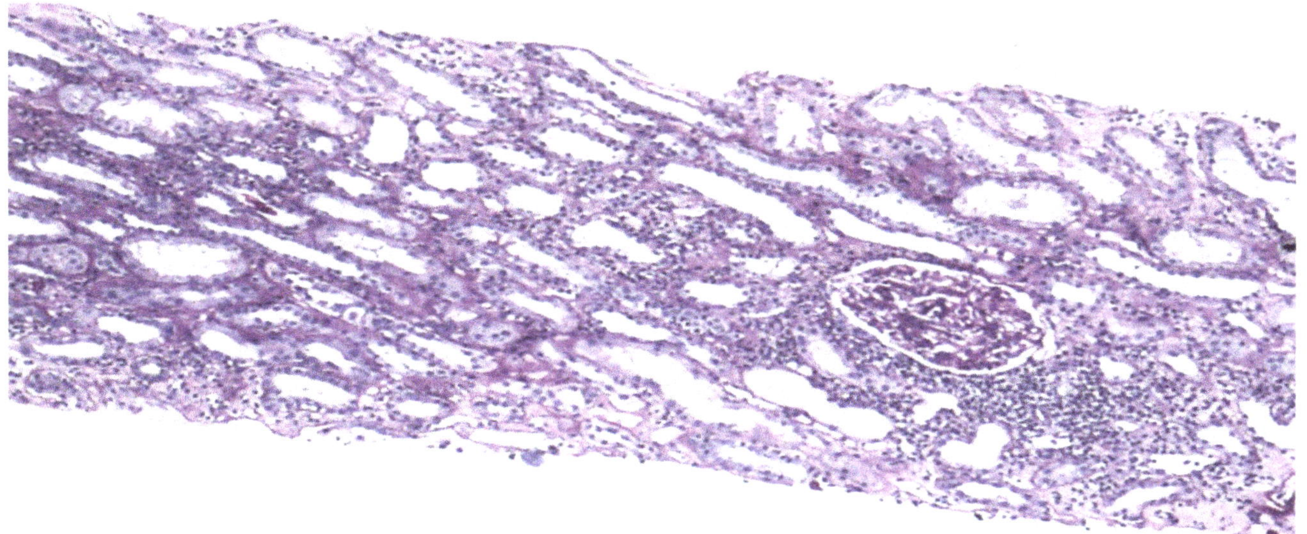

Figure 6:3.1: PAS Stain: 4x:Moderate interstitial inflammation involving about 30% of the cortex.

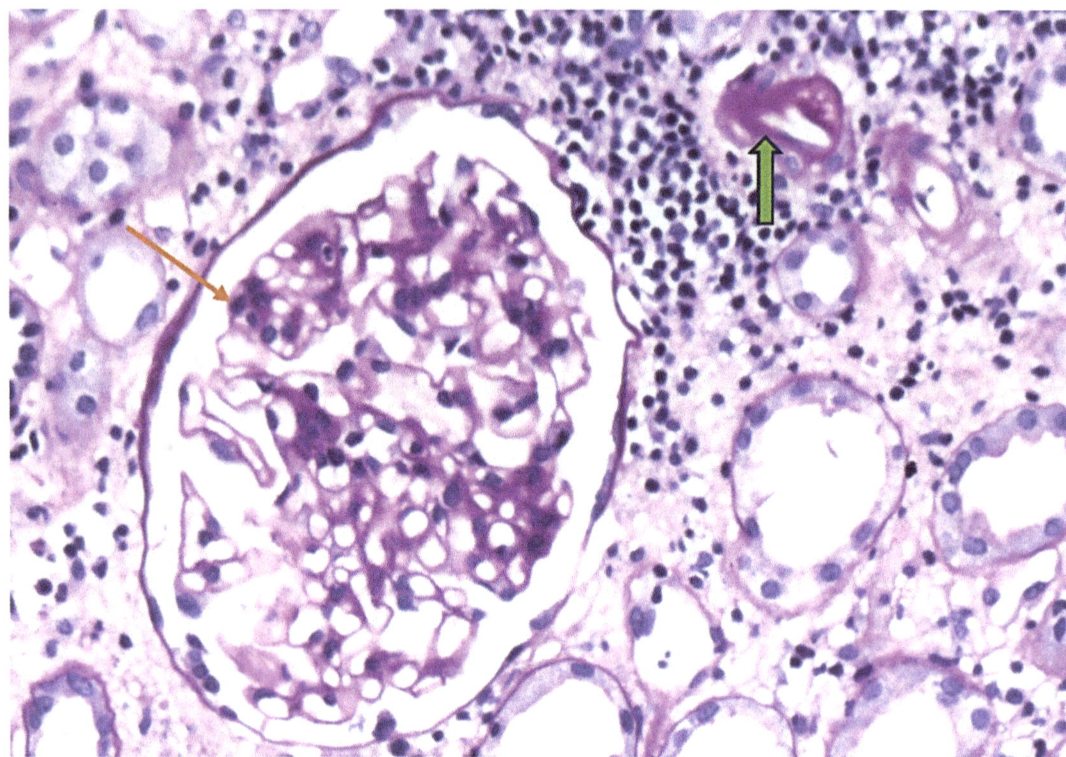

Figure 6:3.2: PAS Stain: Glomerulus: Mild mesangial hypercellularity (orange arrow) and small arteriole mild arteriolar hyalinosis (green arrow).

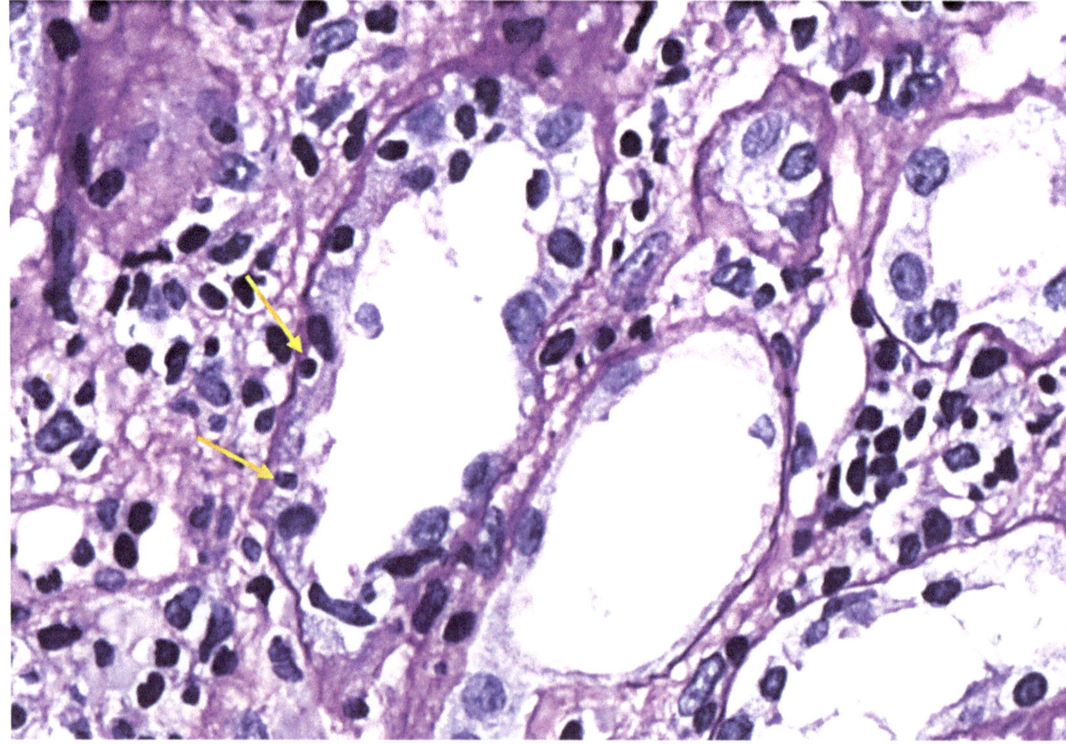

Figure 6:3.3: PAS Stain: ModerateTubulitis:about 6 mononuclear cells are seen inside the tubular basement membrane at the basolateral aspect of tubular epithelial cells (yellow arrows).

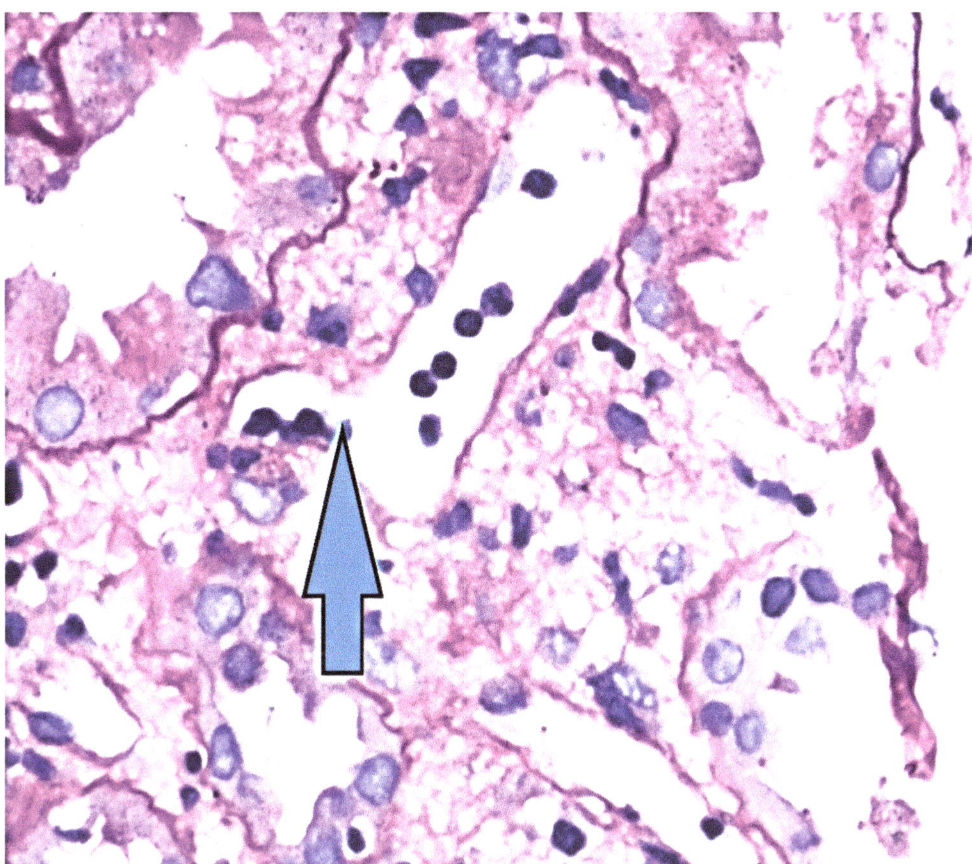

Figure 6:3.4: PAS Stain:40x: Moderate peritubular capillaritis: 09 inflammatory cells in the peritubular capillary (blue arrow) involving about 30% of peritubular capillaries of the cortex sampled.

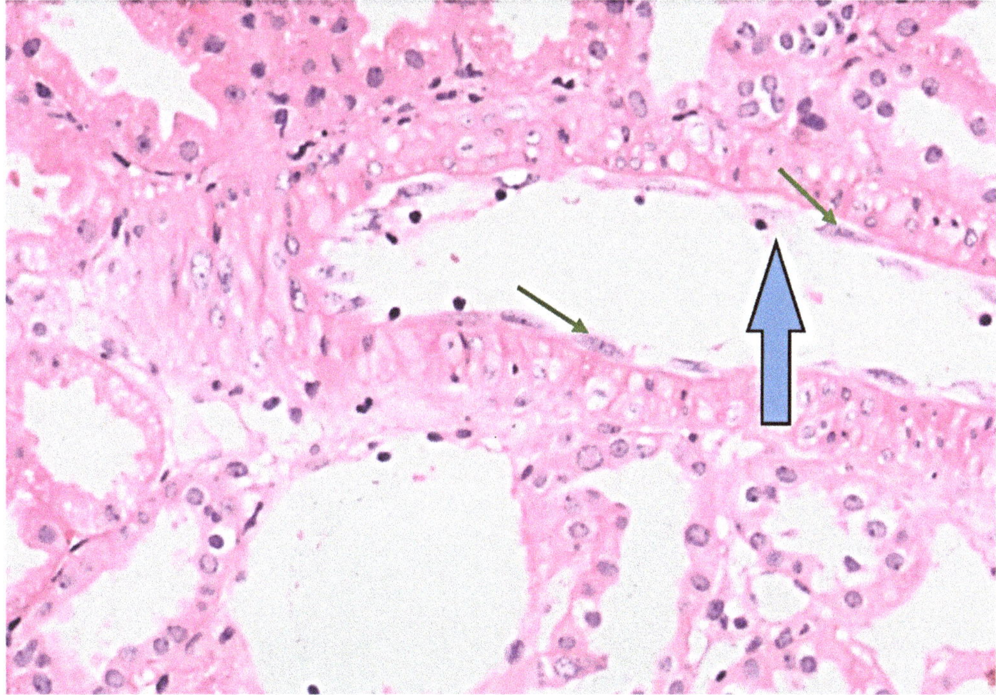

Figure 6:3.5: H&E Stain:Artery: Small dark blue mononuclear cells (blue arrow) sticking to endothelial cells (elongated nuclei-green arrows)of an artery but not lifting it up.No evidence of endarteritis.

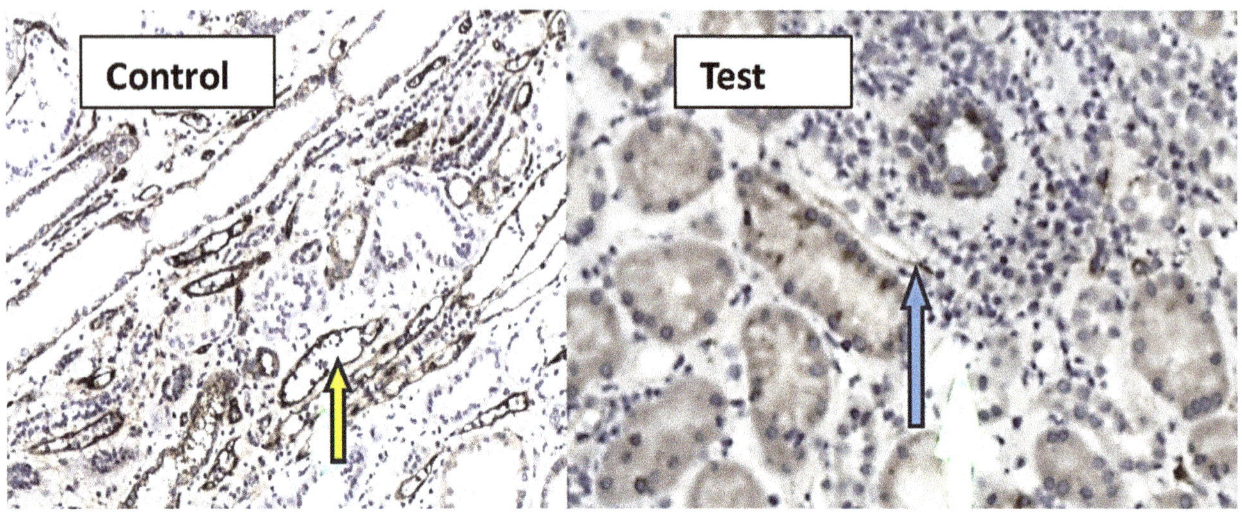

Figure 6:3.6: Immunohistochemistry C4d Stain: 20x: It shows focal irregular positivity (blue arrow) around few of the peritubular capillaries, which is not significant to consider it as positive.

Interpretation: Acute T-cell mediated rejection, Banff grade IA.

Banff score: g0, t2, i2, v0, cg0, ct1, ci0, cv0, aah0, mm0, C4d0, ptc2, ti2, i-IFTA 0.

Case 4

History: 54years old male, ESRD of unknown etiology, on Maintenance haemodialysis (MHD) for 3 years, underwent living donor renal transplant with brother as donor. No induction agent except Methyl prednisolone. Maintenance on triple drug immunosuppression (Tacrolimus + Mycophenolate Mofetil(MMF) + Steroid) . CMV status D+/R+. Uneventful intraoperative and post operative course. Nadir creatinine = 1 mg/dl. 4 months post-transplant graft dysfunction. No fever or any other systemic symptoms of infection or nephritis except rise in BP and mild pedal edema. BP: 160/100 mm of Hg.

Investigations: Creatinine 3.3mg/dl, Urine protein: 2+, RBCs: 5 to 6/HPF, LDH:150U/L. Hemoglobin:12 gm/dl, TLC:7, 500/cu mm, Platelet count: 1,50,000/cu mm. CMV PCR – Negative, BKV PCR – Negative. Urine culture: sterile. Tac level :7ng/ml. USG: Raised parenchymal echotexture and RI of the Graft, No Renal artery stenosis.

Clinical Diagnosis: Allograft Rejection / Native kidney disease recurrence / Tacrolimus toxicity.

Light microscopy:

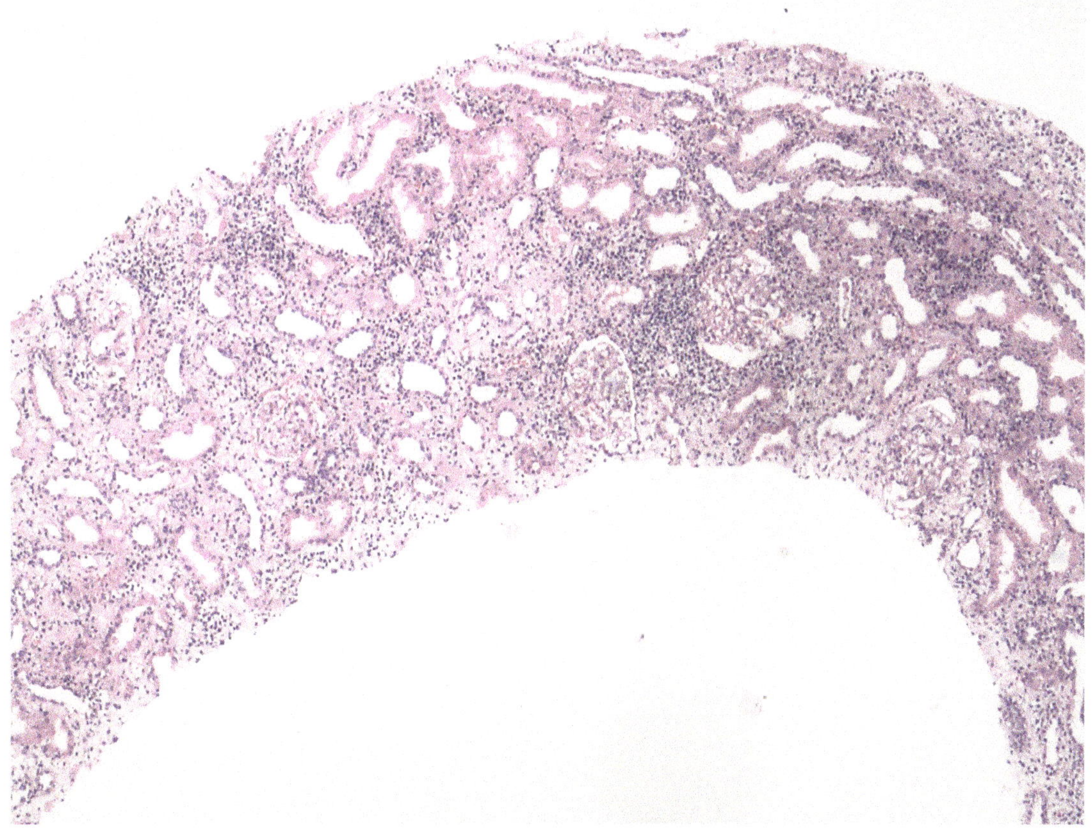

Figure 6:4.1: H&E Stain: 4x: Marked interstitial infiltrate involving almost the entire cortex.

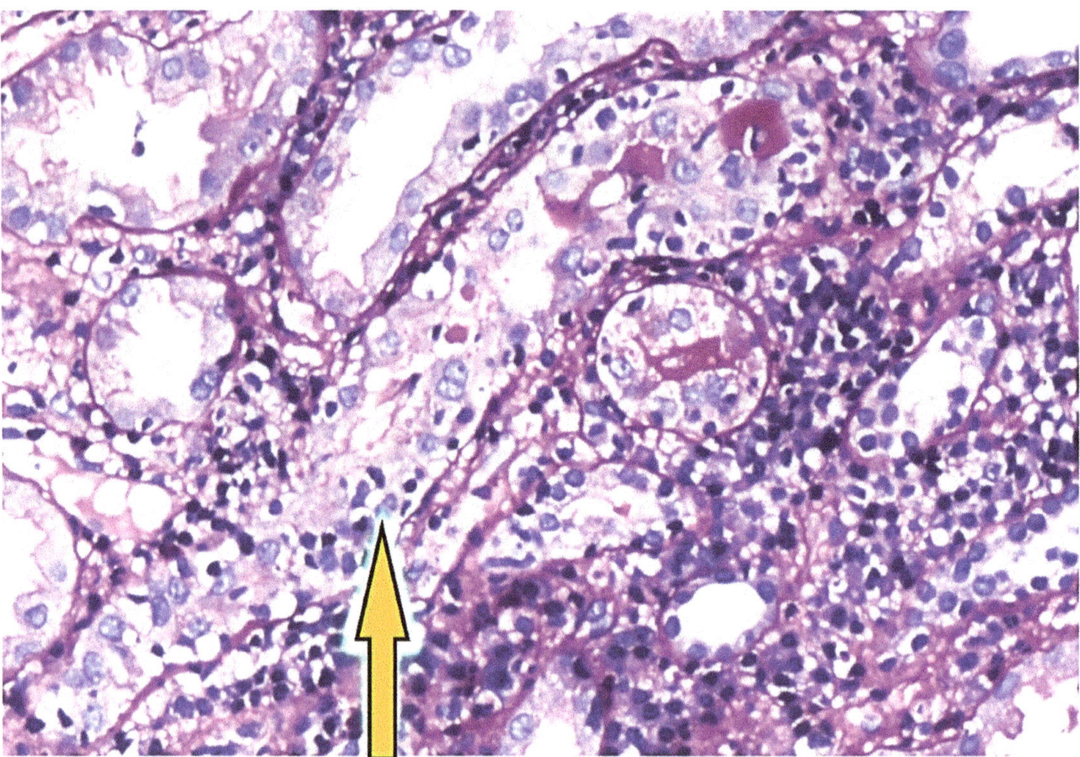

Figure 6:4.2: PAS Stain:20x:Tubules: Marked Tubulitis(yellow arrow) with > 10 mononuclear cells at the basolateral aspect of tubular epithelial cells inside the tubular basement membranes.

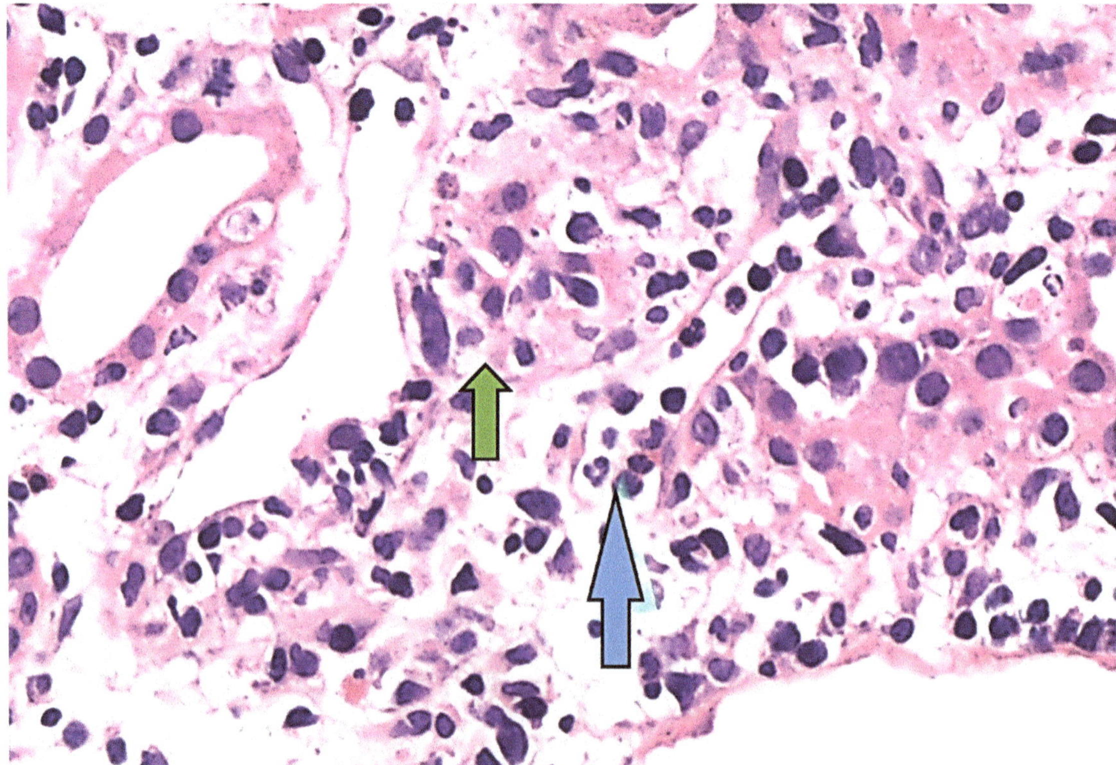

Figure 6:4.3: H&E Stain: 40x: Marked peritubular capillaritis (>10 inflammatory cells) comprising of few lymphocytes and occasional neutrophils (blue arrow) and adjacent tubules showing marked tubulitis (green arrow).

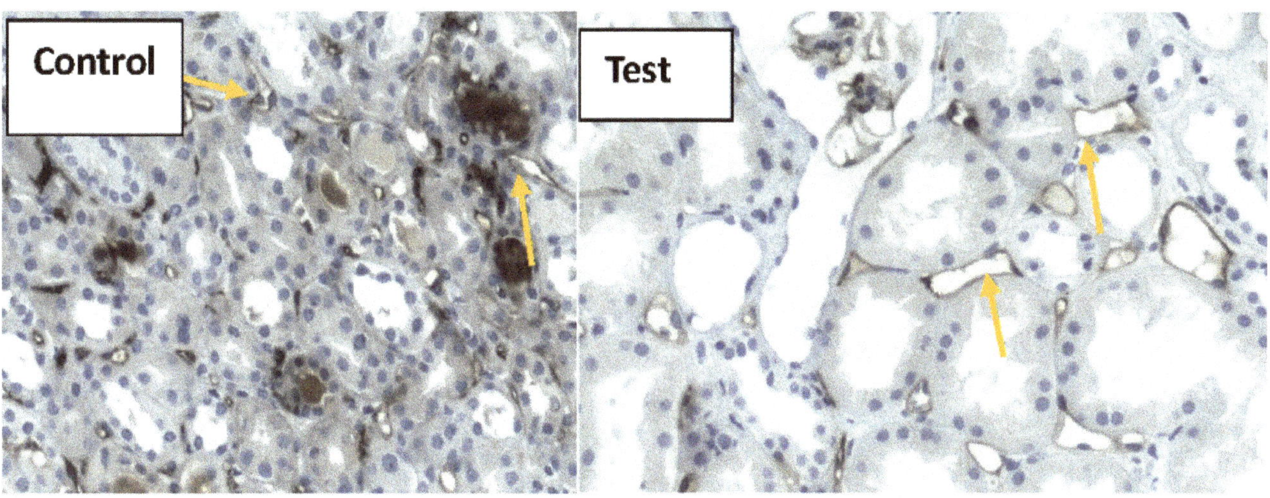

Figure 6: 4.4: Immunohistochemistry C4d Stain:20x: Diffuse linear circumferential positivity around the peritubular capillaries.

Interpretation:

Features of marked tubulitis with marked inflammation, mild tubulointerstitial changes of chronicity (05%), marked peritubular capillaritis and mild arteriolar hyalinosis. These changes are consistent with features of **an Acute T-cell mediated rejection, Banff Type IB.**

In view of diffuse C4d positivity, mild acute tubular injury and marked peritubular capillaritis with presence of occasional neutrophils too, a possibility of concurrent **Active Antibody mediated rejection (AMR),** is considered.

Banff score: g0, t3, i3, v0, cg0, ct1, ci0, cv0, aah1, mm0, C4d3, ptc3, ti3, i-IFTA 0.

Additional Investigation: Serum Donor specific antibody (DSA) : Positive ; confirming AMR.

Final diagnosis: Acute T-cell mediated rejection, Banff grade IB with concurrent AMR.

CASE 5

History: 45 years old male, ESRD of unknown aetiology, on MHD for one year, underwent living donor renal transplant with wife as donor. Induction with ATG 3 mg/kg and Methyl prednisolone. Maintenance triple immunosuppression. CMV status D+/R+. Uneventful intraoperative and post operative course. Nadir creatinine : 1 mg/dl.Now 6 months post-transplant graft dysfunction. No fever or any other systemic symptoms of infection or nephritis except rise in BP and mild pedal oedema. BP :150/90 mm of Hg.

Investigations: Serum creatinine: 3.3mg/dl, Potassium:4.8mEq/L, Urine protein:1+, RBCs:3-4/HPF, Pus cells: 5-6/HPF. 24 hr Urine Protein:1.2 g/day. LDH :200 IU/L,Hb: 11 gm/dl,TLC :8,500/HPF, Platelet count:1,75,000/cu mm. CMV PCR – Negative, BKV PCR – Negative. DSA:Negative. Urine culture: sterile. Tacrolimus drug level:6 ng/dl.

Clinical Diagnosis: Acute allograft Rejection / Native Kidney disease recurrence.

Light microscopy:

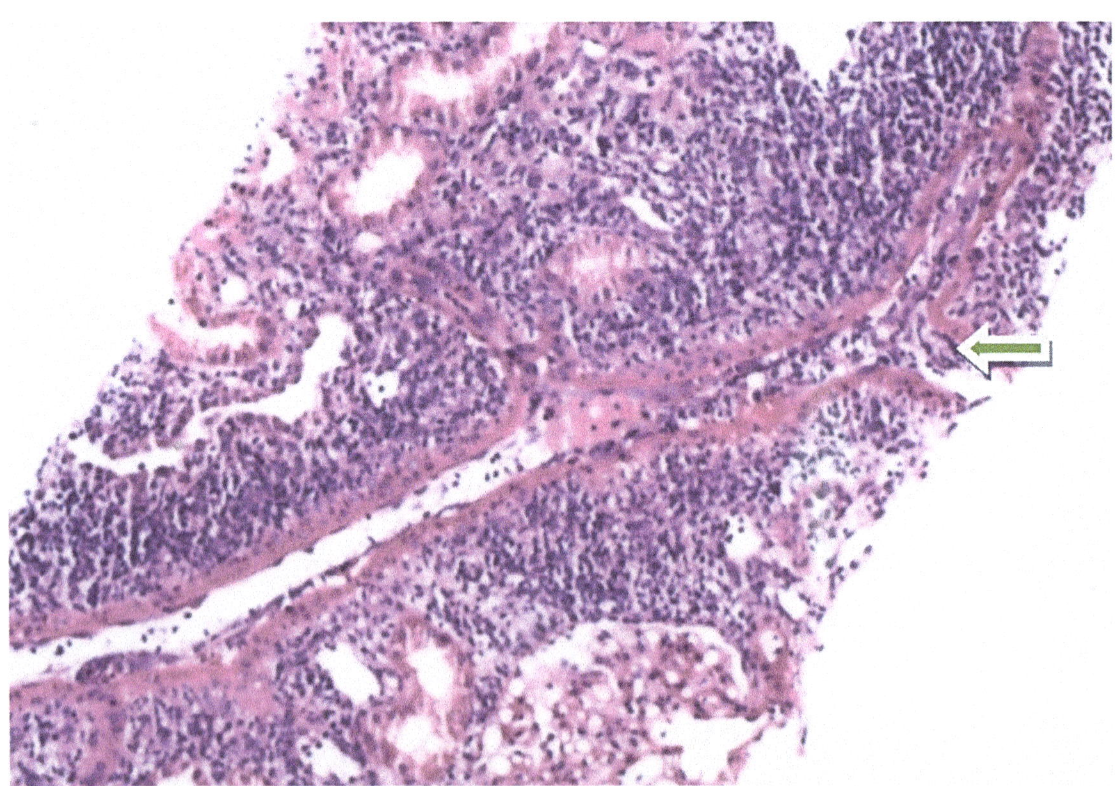

Figure 6:5.1: H&E Stain:10x: Marked interstitial inflammation and Endarteritis: lifting of the endothelium and mononuclear inflammatoery cells underneath it (green arrow). Few of the surrounding tubules show tubulitis.

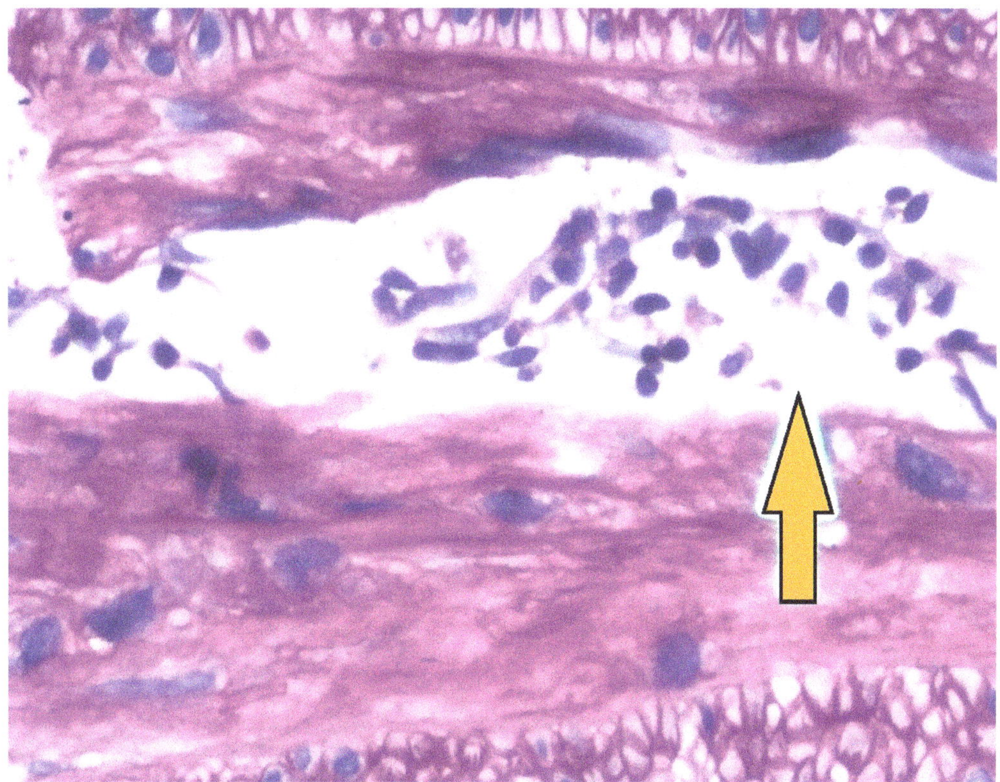

Figure 6:5.2: H&E Stain:40x:Endarteritis: other large artery: Lifting of the endothelial cells and presence of inflammatory cells underneath it.

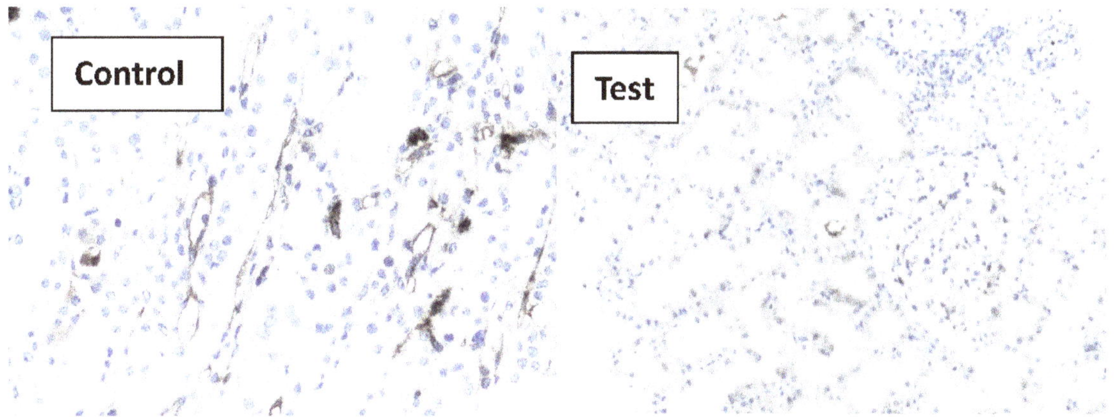

Figure 6:5.3: Immunohistochemistry C4d Stain 20x: Test is negative.

Interpretation:

Features of marked interstitial inflammation, marked tubulitis and endarteritis, consistent with an **Acute T-cell mediated rejection, Banff grade IIB.**

Banff score: g0, t3, i3, v2, cg0, ct1, ci0, cv0, aah0, mm0, C4d0, ptc3, ti3, i-IFTA -0.

History: 43 years old male, Hypertensive and ESRD of unknown etiology, on MHD for 6 months, underwent living donor renal transplant with mother as donor. No induction except Methyl prednisolone. Maintenance with triple immunosuppression-Tacrolimus, MMF and Steroid. CMV status D+/R+. Uneventful intraoperative and post operative course. Nadir creatinine:0.9 mg/dl. Now 4 years post-transplant, with no follow up for last 1 year. Noncompliant with medication. Came with pedal edema of last 1 month duration. No fever or any other systemic symptoms of infection or nephritis. BP 160/100.

Investigations: Serum creatinine :6.7mg/dl, Sodium :136mEq/L, Potassium:5.6mEq/L, Chloride: 111mEq/L, Urine protein: 2+, RBCs: 5-6/HPF, LDH :200 IU/L, Hb:8 gm/dl, TLC:5,500/cu mm, Platelet count: 1,50,000/cu mm. CMV PCR – Negative, BKV PCR: Negative. DSA: Negative. Urine culture: sterile. Tacrolimus level :2.2ng/ml.

Clinical DD: CKD 5 T / Allograft Rejection

Light microscopy:

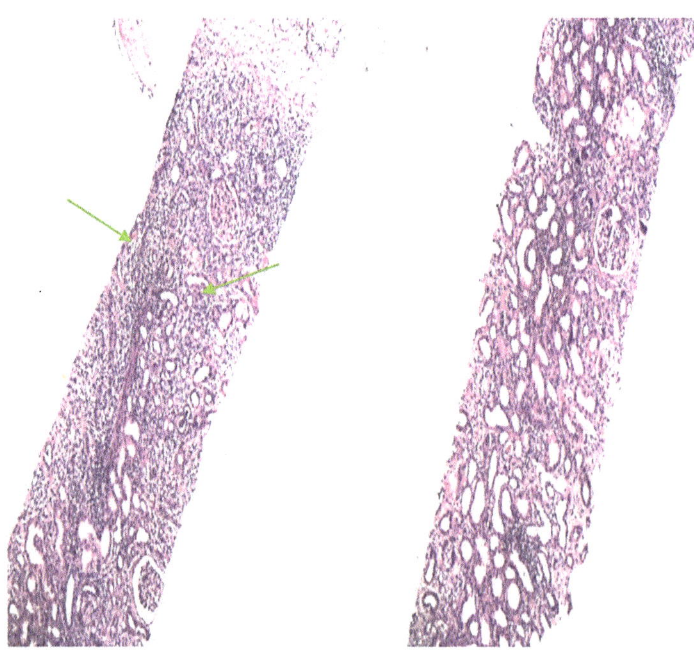

Figure 6:6.1: H&E Stain:10x: Allograft renal biopsy showing moderate tubular atrophy (ct2) and moderate interstitial fibrosis (ci2) (green arrows), marked tubulitis (t3) and (t-IFTA:3) and diffuse interstitial inflammation in the fibrosed(i-IFTA:3) and entire cortical area(ti:3).

Interpretation: Chronic Active T-cell mediated Rejection, Banff grade IB.

Banff score: g0, t3, i2, v0, cg0, ct2, ci2, cv0, aah1, mm0, C4d0, ptc3, ti3, t-IFTA 3, i-IFTA -3.

Pathology Pearls

Table 6:6.1: Differential diagnoses of tubulointerstitial chronicity in allograft biopsy.

Sr. No	Features	Chronic active TCMR	Chronic /active ABMR	CNI Toxicity	PVN	Recurrent/ denovo Glom disease
1.	Glomerulitis	-/+	+	-	-	-
2.	Tubulitis (t)	+	-	-	+	-
3.	Peritubular capillaritis	+	+	-	-	-
4.	Endarteritis	+	+	-	-	-
5.	C4d	-	+	-	-	-
6.	i-IFTA	+	+	+	+	+
7.	Transplant glomerulopathy (TG)	-	+	TMA	-	+
8.	PTCML	-	+	-	-	-
9.	Transplant Arteriopathy	+	+	-	-	-
10.	Striped fibrosis	-	-	+	-	-
11	AAH	-	-	+	-	-
12.	IHC: SV 40: Positivity	-	-	-	+	-
13.	Immunofluorescence	-	-	-	-	+

TMA: Thrombotic Microangiopathy, PTCML: Peritubular Capillary Multilayering

CASE 7

History: 32 years old male, hypertensive and ESRD of unknown etiology, underwent pre-emptive living donor renal transplant with brother as donor 5 years ago. The first graft failed with allograft biopsy suggesting Chronic allograft nephropathy. He was not compliant with medication and follow ups were irregular. On hemodialysis for last 1 year and registered for cadaver transplant. PRA-I: 60% PRA-II :30%. Received an offer for deceased donor kidney transplant. Donor is 35-year female non hypertensive, non-diabetic, brain death due to road traffic accident. Donor creatinine 0.7mg/dl and good urine output before harvesting organ. CDC cross match negative. Underwent transplant with ATG induction 1 mg/kg started intraoperative and Methylprednisolone 500 mg given before shifting to or and another 500 mg pulsed at time of anastomosis. Kidney colour not pink and bit cyanotic after arterial anastomosis and no urine flow in ureter at anastomosis. Intraoperative biopsy of the graft taken.

Investigations: Serum creatinine 6.8 mg/dl.

Clinical Diagnosis: Hyperacute graft rejection

Light microscopy:

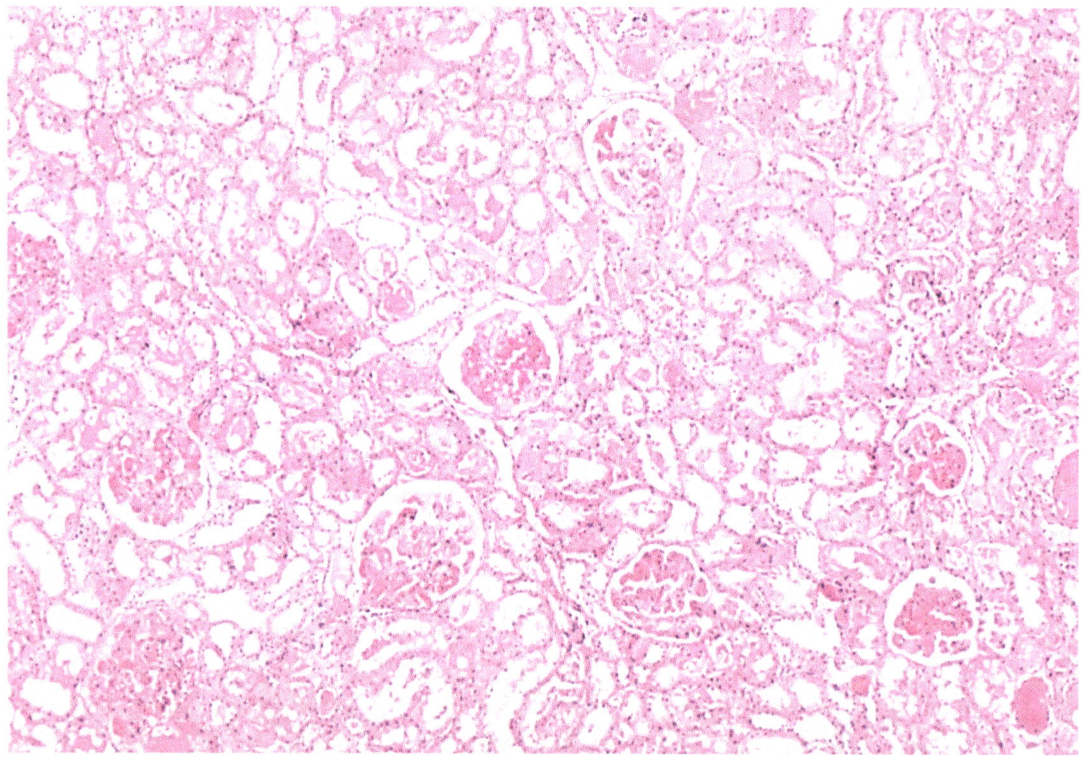

Figure 6:7.1: H&E Stain:4x: Congested glomeruli and mild tubular injury

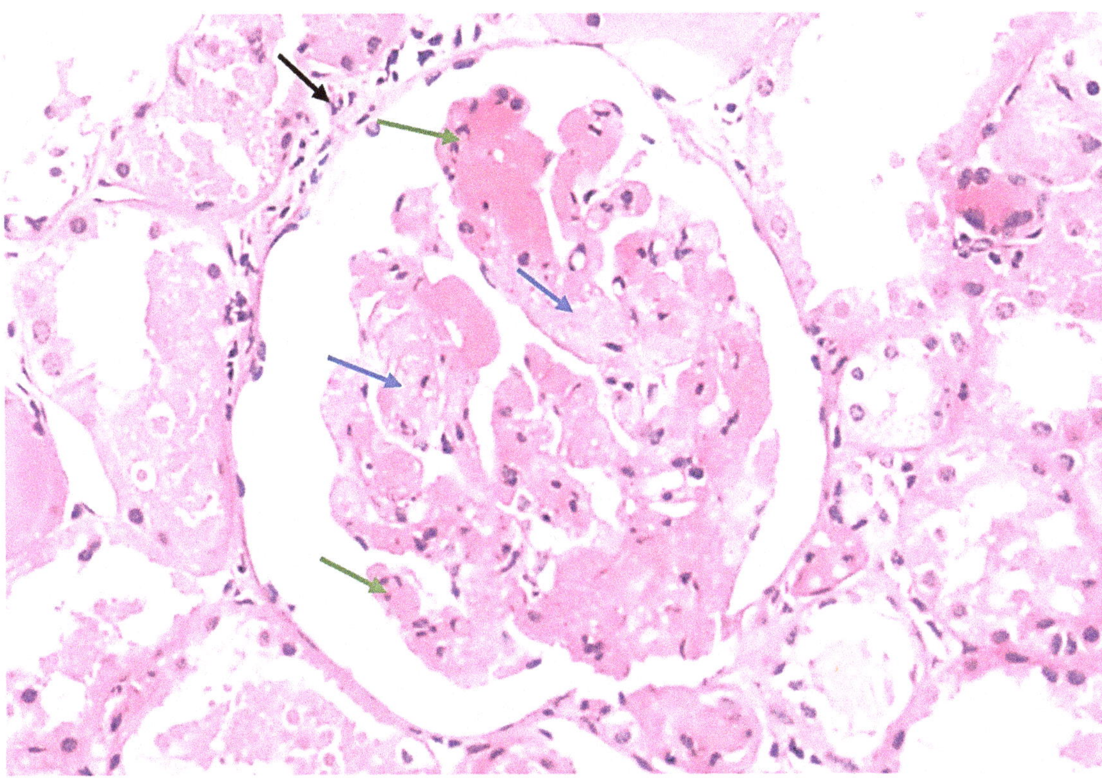

Figure 6:7.2: H&E Stain:20x: Glomerulus: Mesangiolysis (blue arrows), glomerulitis with neutrophils (green arrows) and periglomerular neutrophils around Bowman capsule (black arrow).

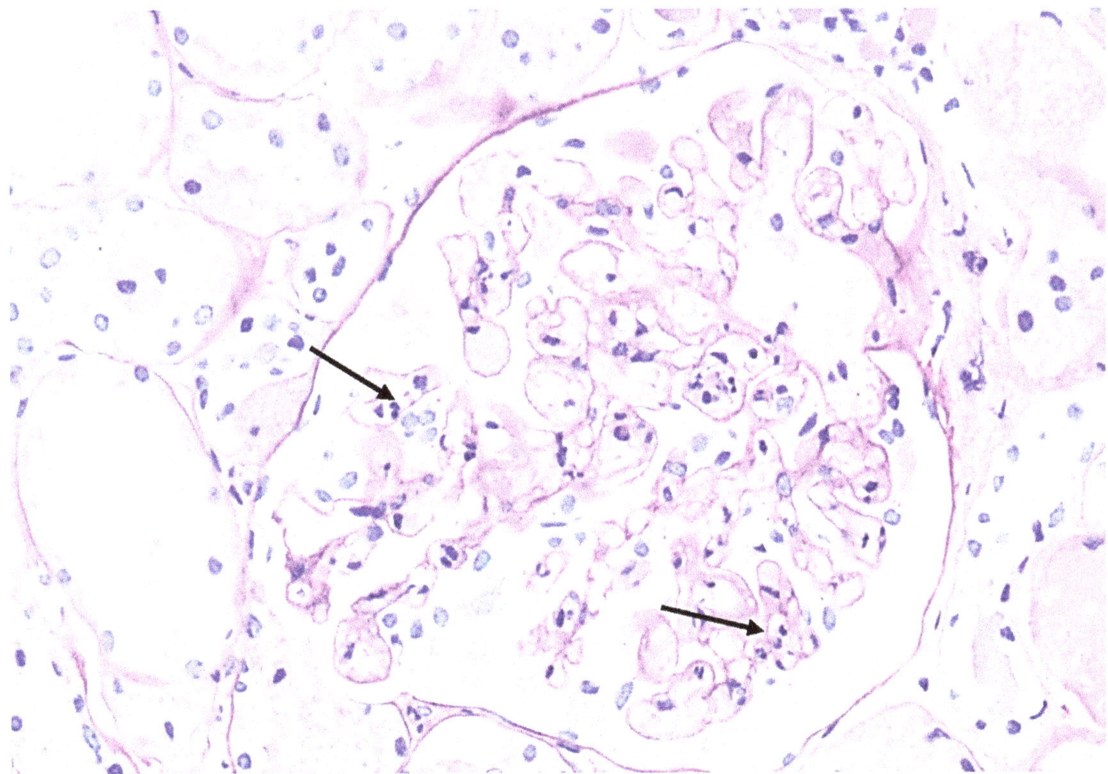

Figure 6:7.3: PAS Stain:20x: Glomerulitis (black arrows), few neutrophils and mononuclear cells obliterating the capillary lumina.

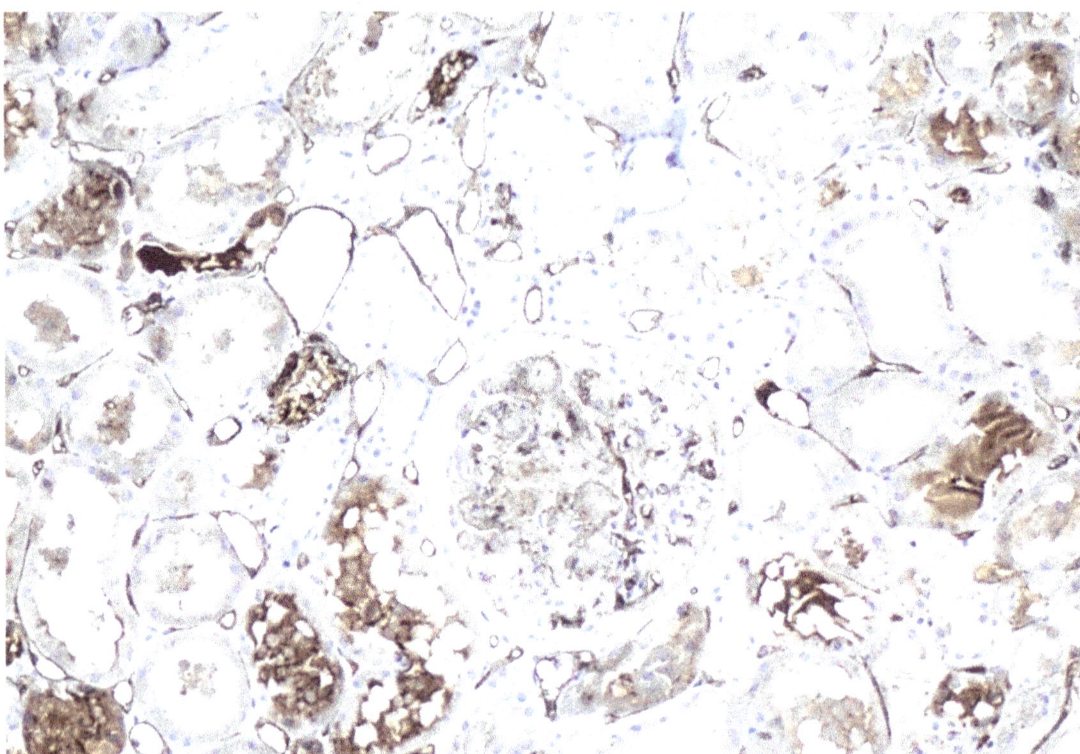

Figure 6:7.4: Immunohistochemistry:C4d stain:20x: Diffuse strong linear circumferential C4d positivity along the peritubular capillaries and around the GBM.

Interpretation:

Features of diffuse glomerulitis, acute tubular injury, peritubular capillaritis with diffuse C4d positivity; consistent with **Hyperacute Antibody mediated Rejection**.

History: 40 years old male, ESRD due to ADPKD, on MHD for one year, underwent living donor renal transplant with wife as donor. HLA match:3/6. Induction with ATG 3 mg/kg and Methyl prednisolone. Maintenance on triple immunosuppression with Tacrolimus, MMF, steroid. CMV status D+/R+. Uneventful intraoperative and post operative course. Nadir creatinine: 1 mg/dl. One-month post-transplant asymptomatic graft dysfunction. BP :150/90 mm of Hg.

Investigations: Serum creatinine :1.6 mg/dl, Potassium: 4.8mEq/L, Urine protein :1+, RBCs: 3-4/HPF, Pus cells: 5-6/HPF. LDH :100 IU/L, Hb:9.7gm/dl, TLC:12,500/cu mm, Platelet count: 1,20,000/cu mm. CMV PCR – Negative, BKV PCR – Negative. Graft doppler: Perfusion is good, but RI increased. Urine culture sterile. Tacrolimus drug level:9ng/ml.

Clinical DD: Acute graft rejection / ATN / CNI toxicity.

Light microscopy:

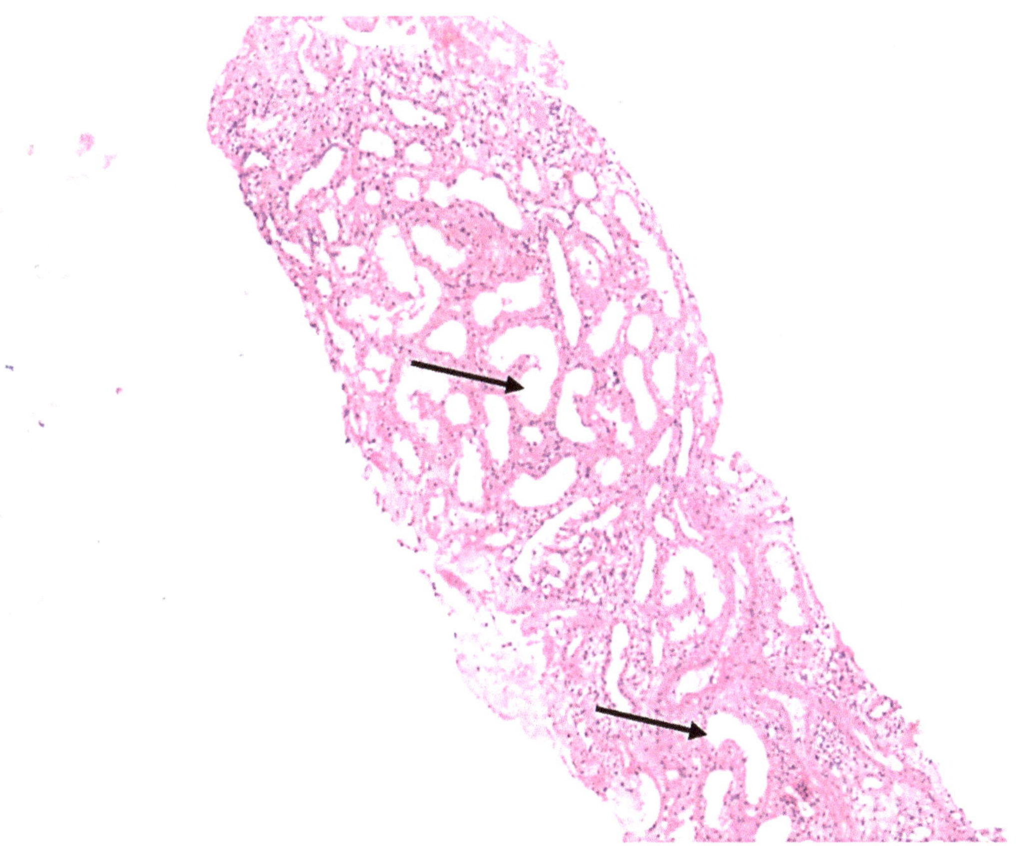

Figure 6:8.1: H&E Stain :4x: Mild tubular injury with loss of the brush border (**black** arrows).

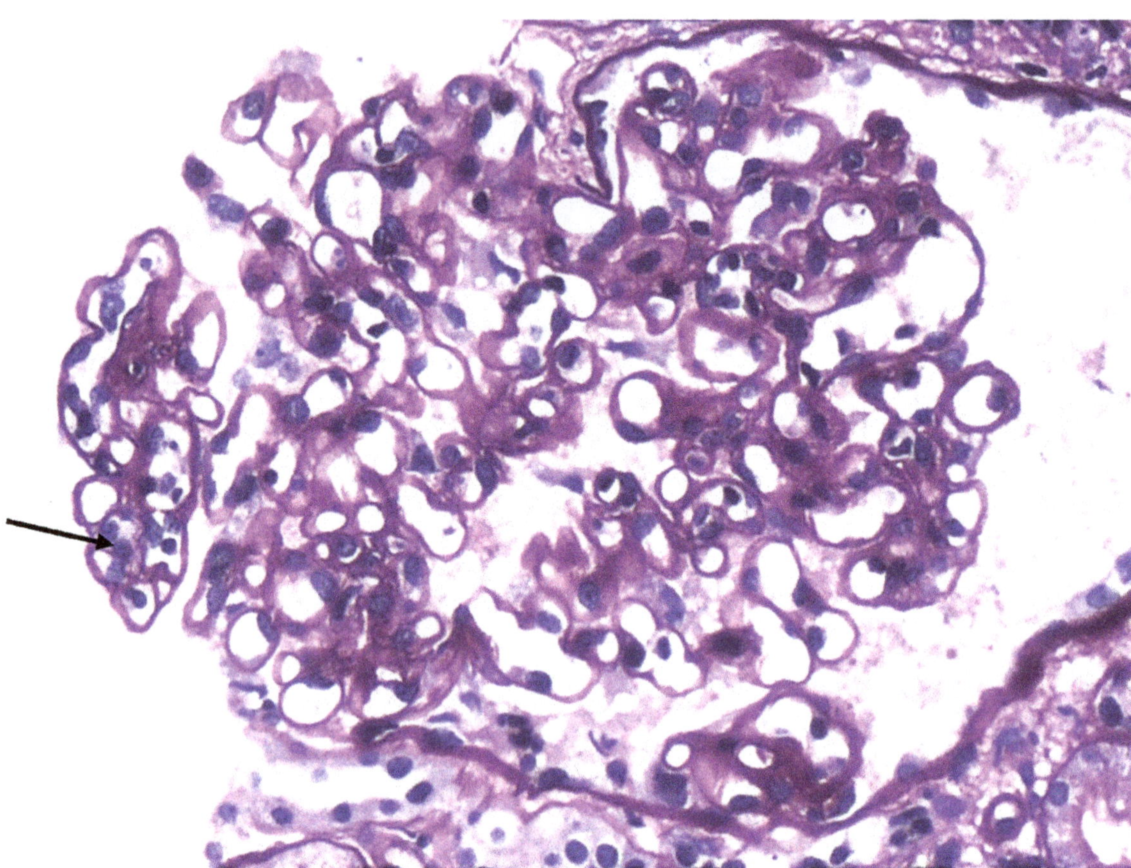

Figure 6:8.2: PAS Stain:20x: Segmental glomerulitis (**black** arrow).

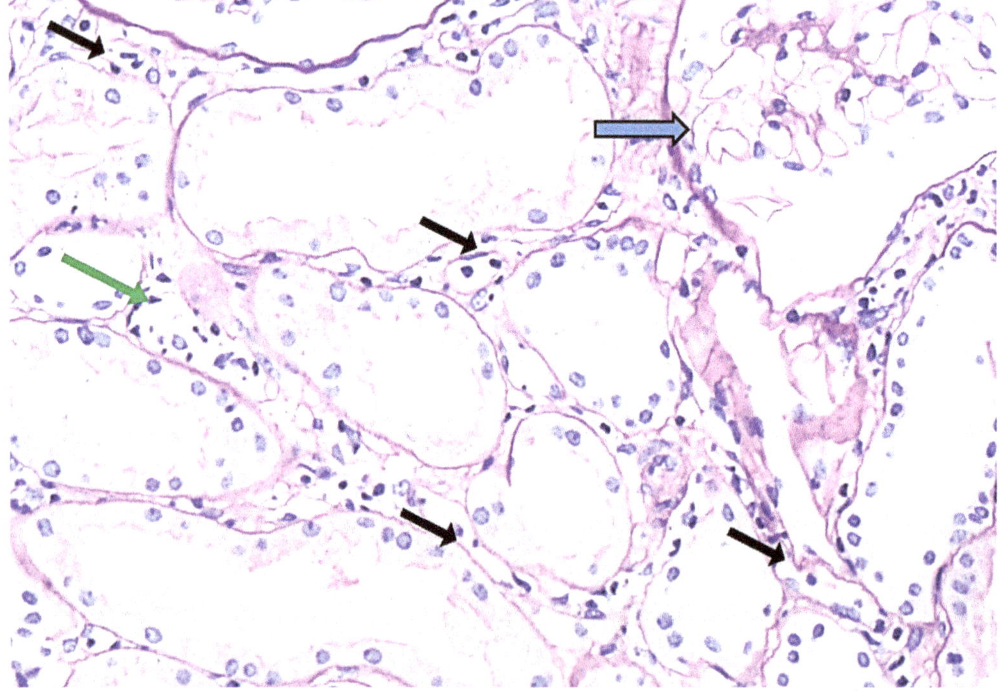

Figure 6:8.3: PAS Stain:20x: Mild peritubular capillaritis (**black** arrows), moderate peritubular capillaritis (**green** arrow), mild tubular injury with loss of the brush border and portion of a glomerulus (**blue** arrow) appears normal.

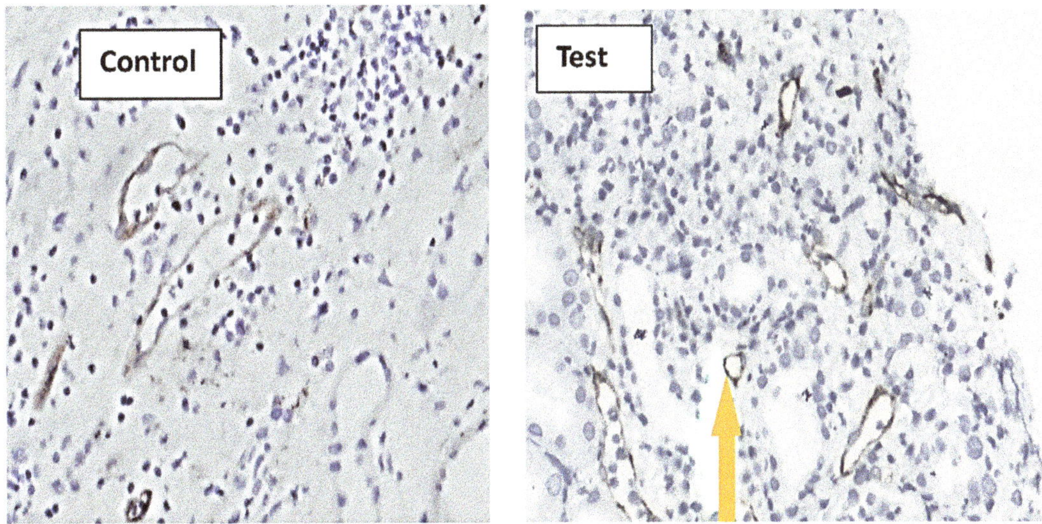

Figure 6:8.4: IHC:C4d stain:20x:C4d shows diffuse strong linear circumferential positivity around the peritubular capillaries (PTCs) involving about 80% of the PTCs.

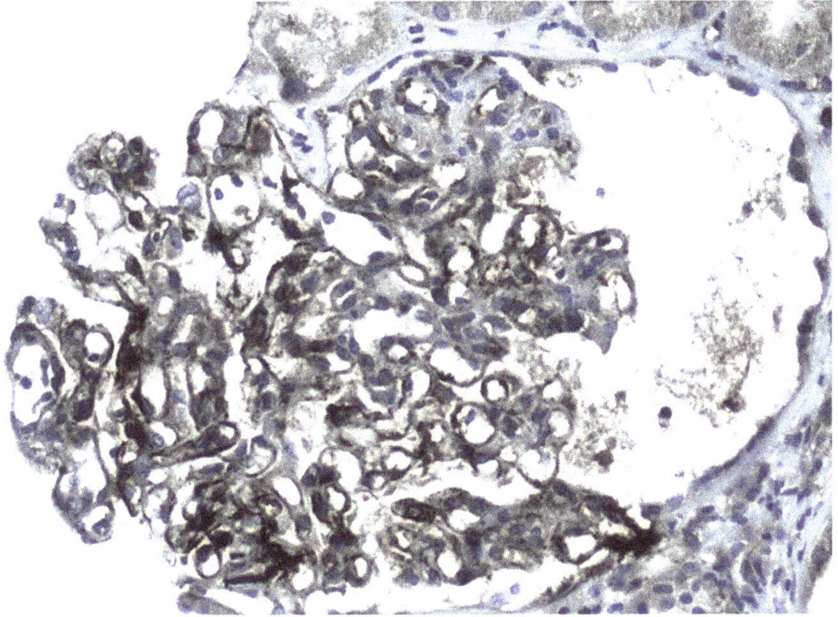

Figure 6:8.5: IHC:C4d Stain:20x: Diffuse linear circumferential positivity along the glomerular basement membranes.

Interpretation:

Features of focal glomerulitis, mild tubular injury, moderate peritubular capillaritis and diffuse C4d positivity are suggestive of an active antibody mediated rejection.

Banff score: g1, t0, i0, v0, cg0, ct0, ci0, cv0, aah1, mm0, C4d3, ptc2, ti0, i-IFTA 0.

Further evaluation: Serum DSA: Positive.

Final diagnosis: An active antibody mediated rejection.

CASE 9

History: 24 years old male, non-diabetic, hypertensive, ESRD of unknown aetiology, on MHD for 6 months, underwent living donor renal transplant with mother as donor. Induction with Methyl prednisolone. Maintenance triple immunosuppression. CMV status D+/R+. Uneventful intraoperative and post operative course. Nadir creatinine :0.8 mg/dl. Uneventful course for 5 years post-transplant. Lost to follow up for last one year. Compliance to medication is questionable in last one year. Now has graft dysfunction.

Investigations: Serum creatinine: 2.1 mg/dl, Potassium: 4.8mEq/L, Urine protein: 1+, RBCs: 3-4/HPF, Hb: 11g/dl, TLC :8,500/cu mm, Platelet count; 1,75,000/cu mm. CMV PCR – negative, BKV PCR – negative, Urine culture sterile. Tacrolimus drug level:2.2 ng/ml, USG findings: Raised parenchymal echotexture.

Clinical DD: Allograft rejection / Native kidney disease recurrence.

Light Microscopy:

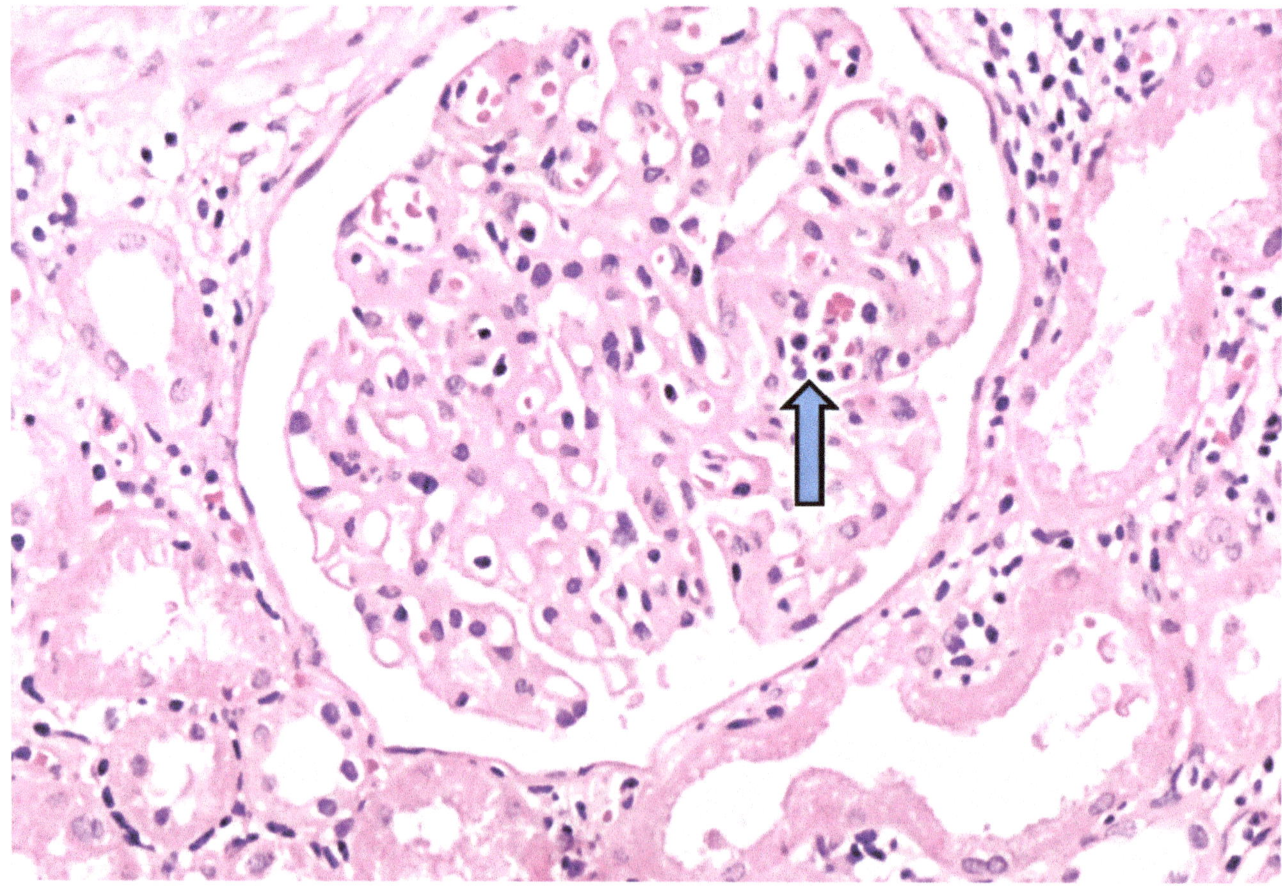

Figure 6:9.1: H& E Stain: 20x: Glomerulus: GBM thickening and segmental glomerulitis (blue arrow) with occasional neutrophils, surrounding moderate interstitial inflammation.

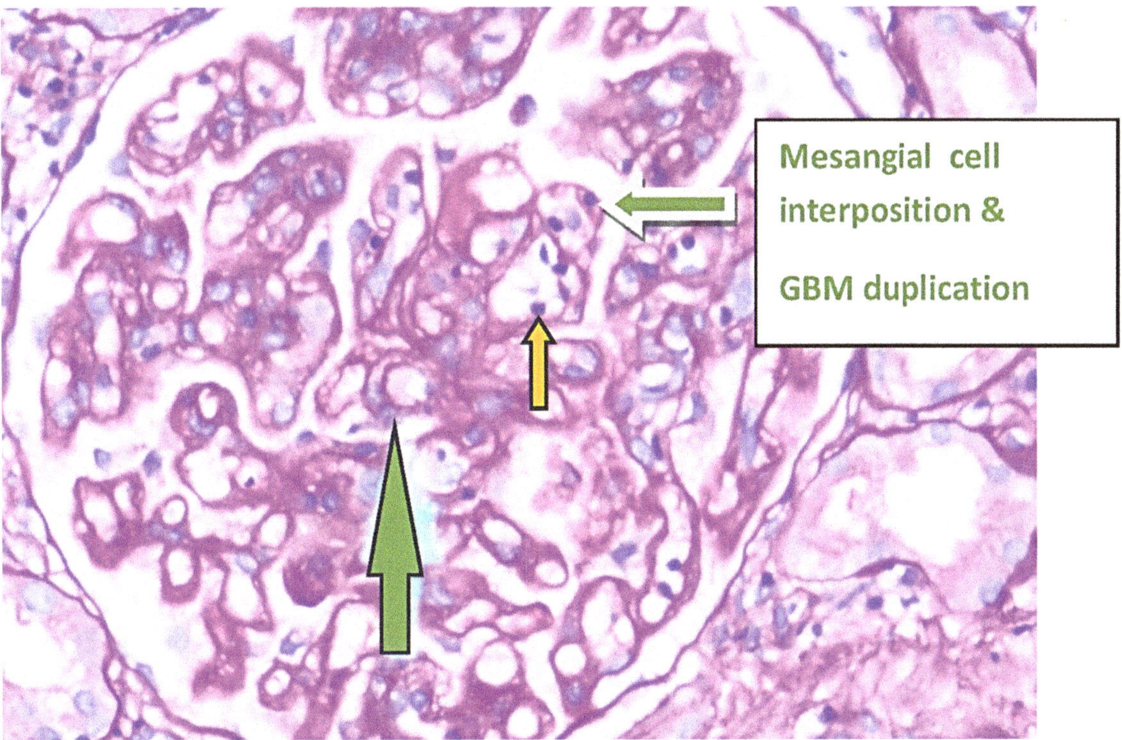

Figure 6:9.2: PAS Stain:20x:Glomerulus: GBM duplication (green arrows) and segmental glomerulitis (yellow arrow).

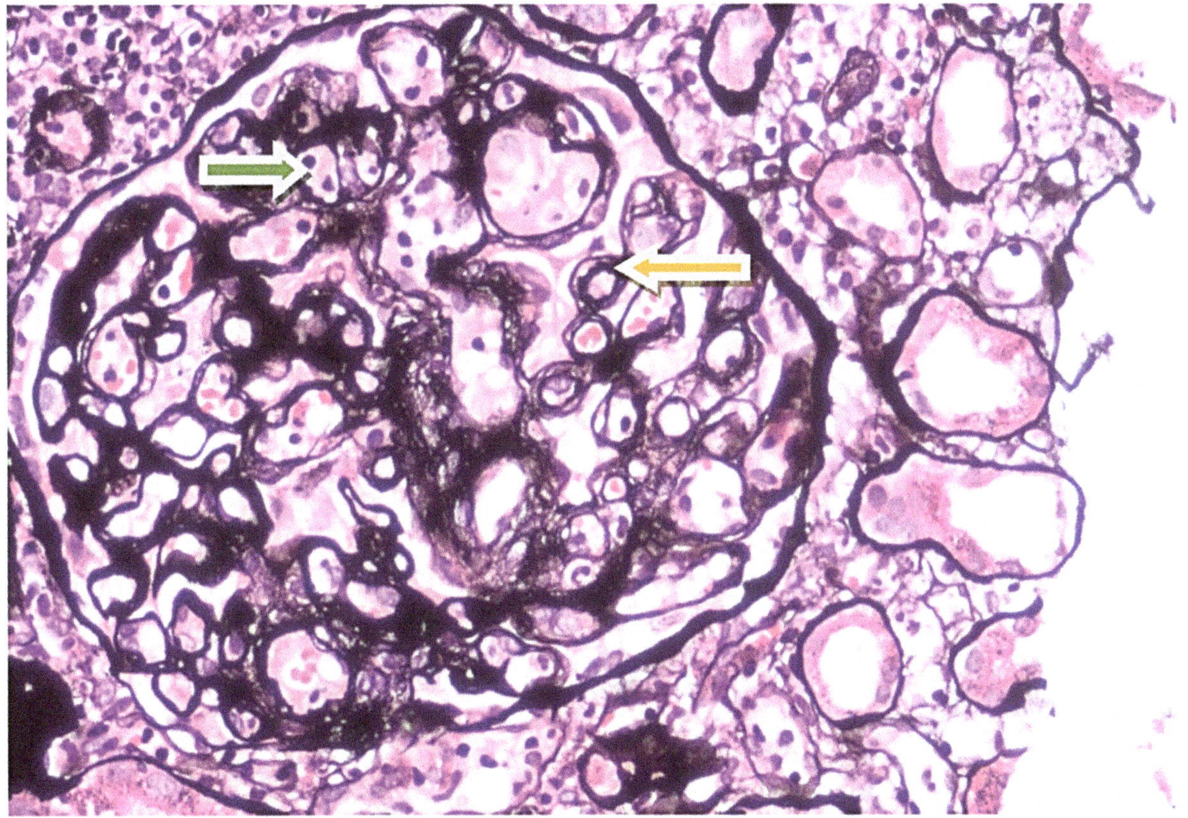

Figure 6:9.3: PASM Stain:20x: Glomerulus: GBM tram track appearance (yellow arrow) in about 50% of the GBM of the capillaries and segmental glomerulitis (green arrow).

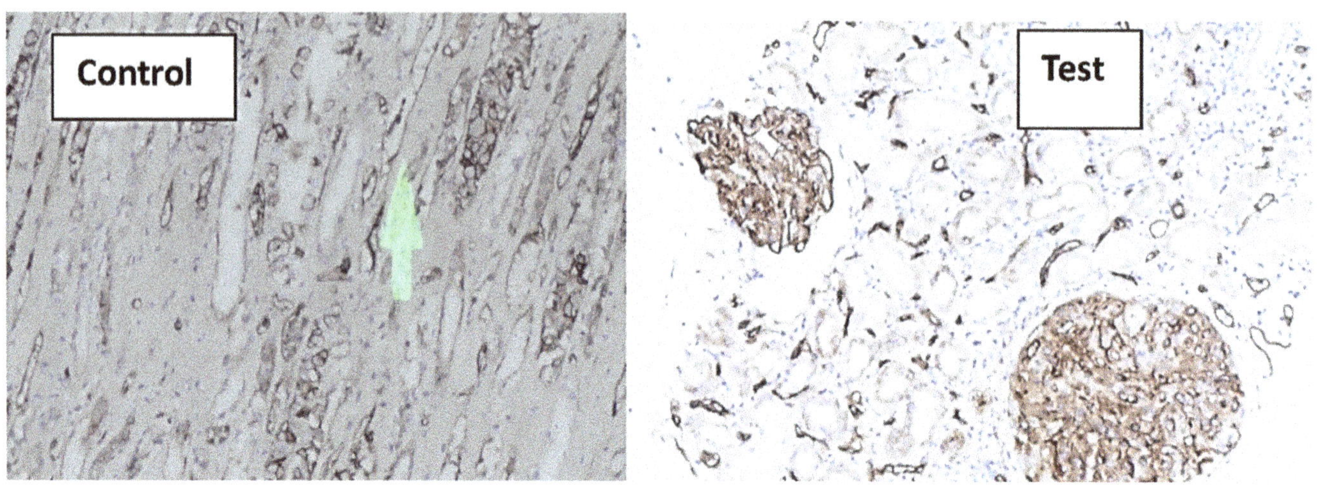

Figure 6:9.4: IHC :C4dStain:Test:10x: Diffuse strong linear circumferential positivity along the Glomerular basement membranes and peritubular capillaries.

Interpretation:

Features of transplant glomerulopathy, transplant glomerulitis, mild tubular injury, moderate peritubular capillaritis with diffuse C4d positivity is suggestive **of chronic active antibody mediated rejection**.

Banff score: g3, t0, i2, v0, cg2, ct1, ci1, cv1, aah1, mm0,C4d3, ptc2, ti2, i-IFTA1.

Additional investigation: Donor specific antibody test: positive.

Final Diagnosis: chronic active antibody mediated rejection.

CASE 10

History: 45 years old male, ESRD due to IgA Nephropathy, on MHD for 3years, underwent living donor renal transplant with wife as donor. HLA match: 2/6. Induction with ATG 3 mg/kg and Methyl prednisolone. Maintenance triple immunosuppression with Tacrolimus, MMF, steroid. CMV status D+/R+. Uneventful intraoperative and post operative course. Nadir creatinine = 0.9 mg/dl. Uneventful course for 2 years. 2 years post-transplant new onset hypertension with mild graft dysfunction.

Investigations: Serum Creatinine 1.6, Urine analysis: 1+ Protein, 10-12 RBC's, 4-5 Pus cells, Urine culture – Sterile. DSA: Negative. USG Graft: Normal perfusion, increased RI, Raised parenchymal echotexture. Tacrolimus drug level: 4 ng/ml.

Clinical DD: Allograft rejection/ Recurrence of IgA Nephropathy/ BKV Nephropathy.

Light microscopy:

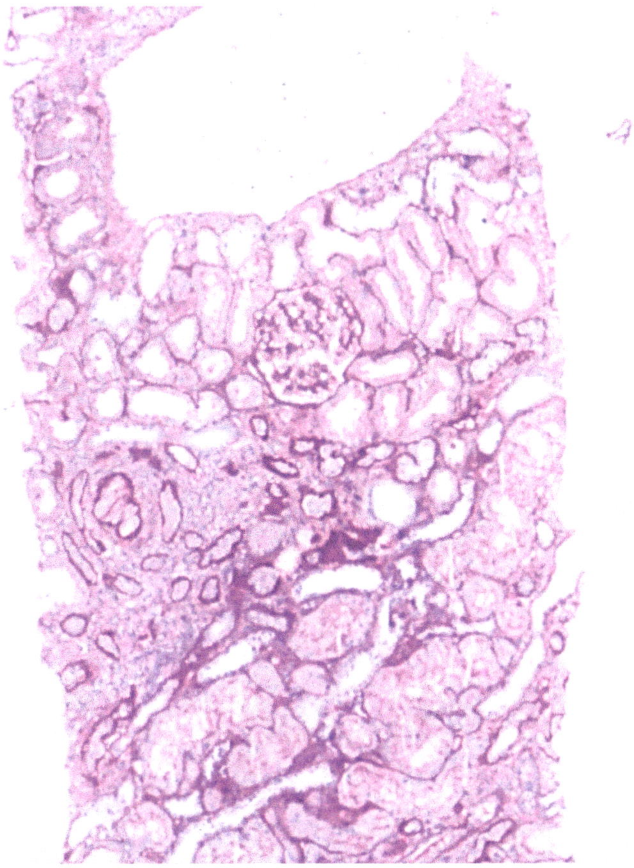

Figure 6:10.1: PAS Stain:10 x: Moderate tubulointerstitial changes of chronicity.

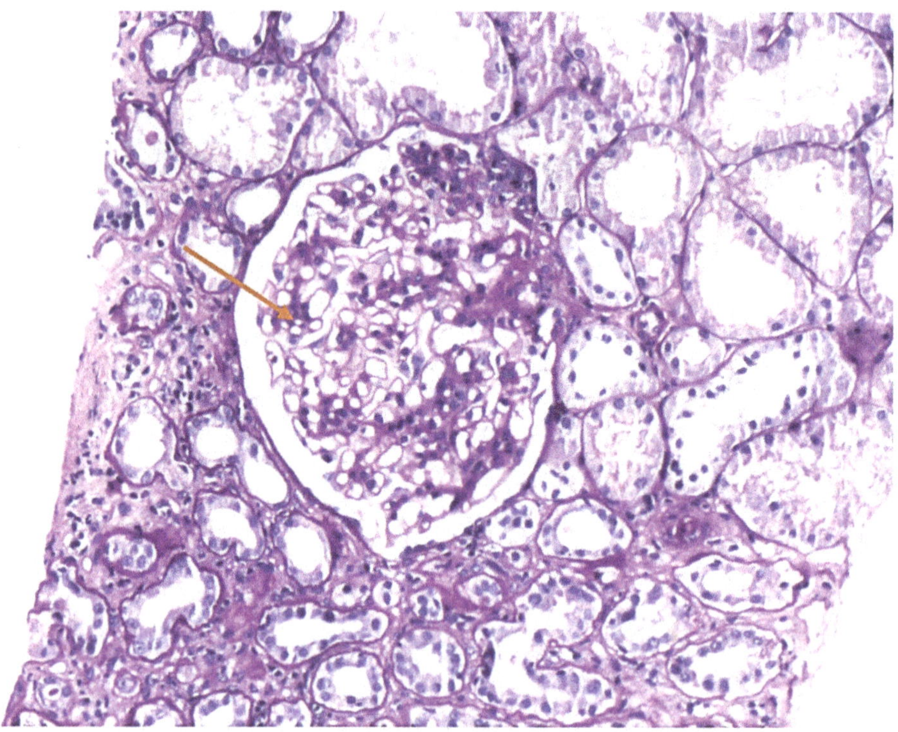

Figure 6:10.2: PAS Stain:20x: Glomeruli: Mild mesangial hypercellularity with mild PAS-positive mesangial widening in glomerulus.

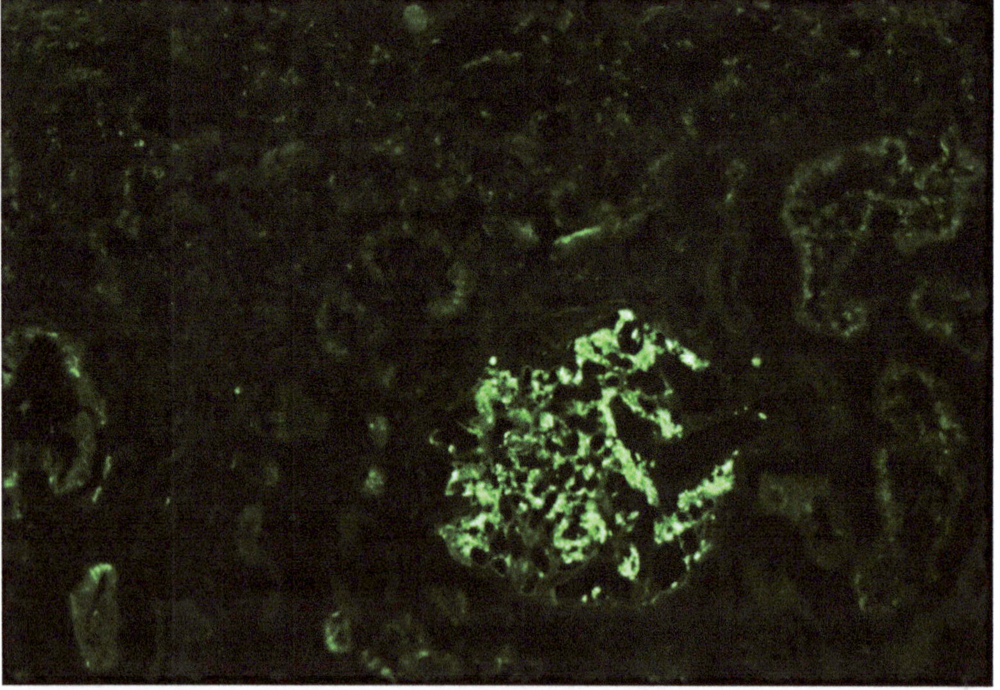

Figure 6:10.3: Immunofluorescence: IgA:10x:Glomeruli: Significant mesangial coarse granular immune deposits.

Interpretation: Features of recurrent IgA Nephropathy. (Oxford classification:M1E0S1T1-C0).

CASE 11

History: 42 years old male, ESRD due to biopsy proven Chronic interstitial nephritis of unknown aetiology, on MHD for one year, underwent living donor renal transplant with sister as donor. HLA match:4/6. Induction with Methyl prednisolone. Maintenance triple immunosuppression with Tacrolimus, MMF, steroid. CMV status D+/R+. Uneventful intraoperative and post operative course. Nadir creatinine: 1 mg/dl.5 years post-transplant came with progressive worsening pedal oedema and shortness of breath on evaluation found to have nephrotic range proteinuria. BP: 150/90 mm of Hg.

Investigations: Serum creatinine:1.41mg/dl, CUE: RBCs:4 to 6/HPF, WBCs:2 to 4/ HPF, 24 hours urine protein: 5gm/day.

Clinical DD: Post Transplant late onset Nephrotic range proteinuria with renal dysfunction – Denovo Glomerular disease / Recurrence of FSGS.

Light microscopy:

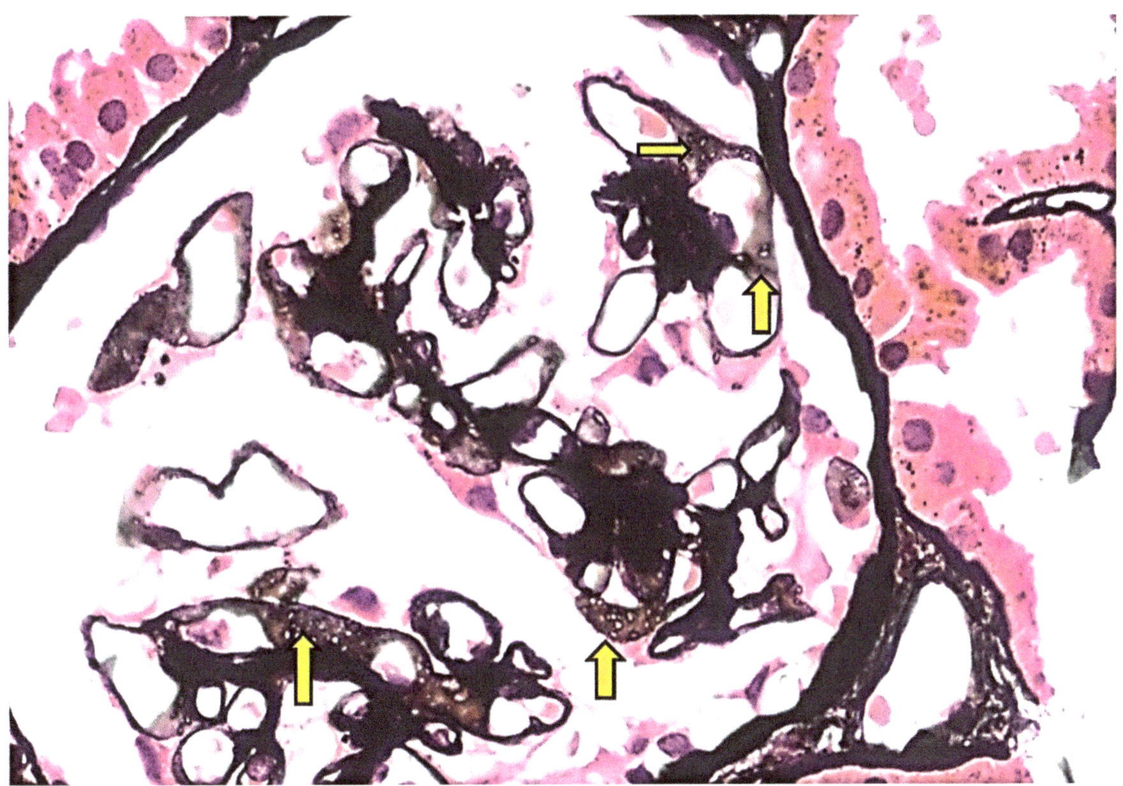

Figure 6:11.1: PASM Stain: 40x: Glomerulus: Non- argyrophilic (Silver negative) subepithelial holes (yellow arrows) with mild diffuse uniform thickening and rigidity of the basement membranes with no evidence of increase in cellularity/glomerulitis/fibrin thrombi/basement membrane duplication.

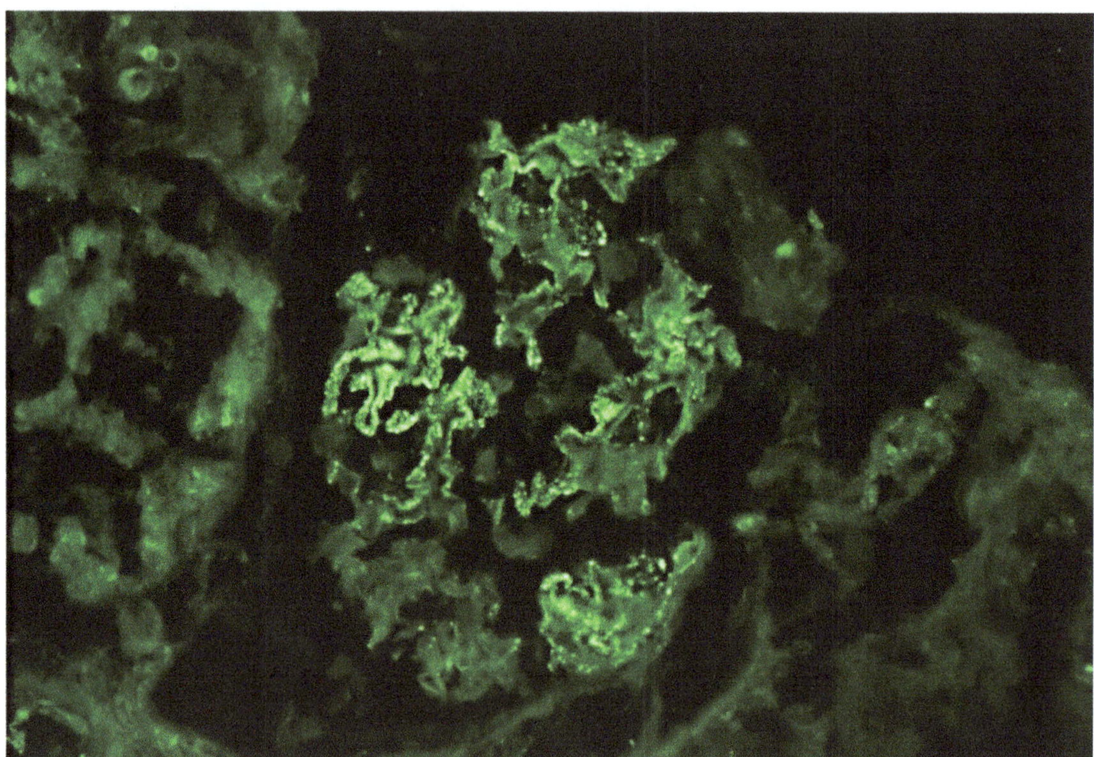

Figure 6:11.2: Immunofluorescence:20x: IgG: Glomerulus: Significant capillary wall fine granular immune deposits.

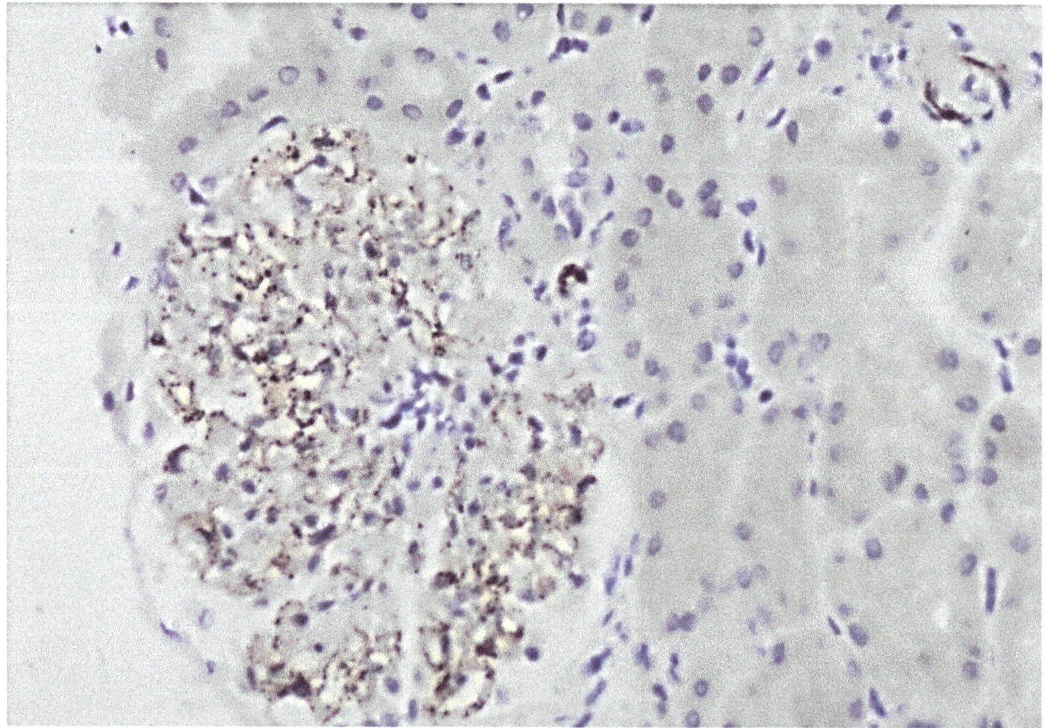

Figure 6:11.3: Immunohistochemistry:C4d Stain: 20x: Glomerular capillary wall granular positivity, negative in peritubular capillaries.

Interpretation: Features of a De novo Membranous Nephropathy with mild tubulointerstitial changes of chronicity (20%).

Additional investigations:

Serum PLA2Rantibody: Negative, ANA : Negative, Viral screen Negative, Malignancy screening: Xray chest , USG abdomen, Serum PSA level, Serum protein electrophoresis, Stool occult blood – were negative.

Pathology Pearls

Table 6:11.1: Difference between denovo and recurrent membranous nephropathy.

Sr. no	Features	Denovo Membranous	Recurrent Membranous
1	Onset	2 to 9 years	<2years
2	Mesangial hypercellularity	+/-	-
3	IgG subtype	Often IgG1	IgG4
4	Subepithelial spikes formation:	Inconspicuous often representing early stage of disease development	++
5	Electron microscopy: subepithelial deposits	Smaller and irregular in distribution	Larger and more regular in distribution
6	Serum anti- PLA2-R AB	-	Often +

CASE 12

History: 43 years old female, ESRD due to unknown aetiology, on MHD for one year, underwent ABO incompatible living donor renal transplant with brother as donor. HLA match:4/6. Immunosuppression: Received Rituximab as ABOi protocol. Induction with ATG 2 gm/kg and Methyl prednisolone. Maintenance triple immunosuppression with Tacrolimus, MMF, steroid. CMV status D+/R+. Uneventful intraoperative and post operative course. Nadir creatinine: 1.3 mg/dl. 3 months post-transplant mild graft dysfunction, serum creatinine 1.9 mg/dl. First graft biopsy showed CNI toxicity features and ATN. Tacrolimus level: 11 ng/ml. After Tacrolimus dose reduction and hydration serum creatinine decreased to 1.6 mg/dl. Now 8 months post-transplant, serum creatinine increased to 2.8 mg/dl. Tacrolimus drug level is 8 ng/ml. Urine analysis shows: Protein :1+, pus cells :7-8/HPF, RBCs: nil/HPF. Urine culture is sterile. USG graft: shows raised parenchymal echotexture and no obstruction.

Clinical DD: Tacrolimus toxicity / Rejection / CMV or BKV Nephropathy.

Light microscopy:

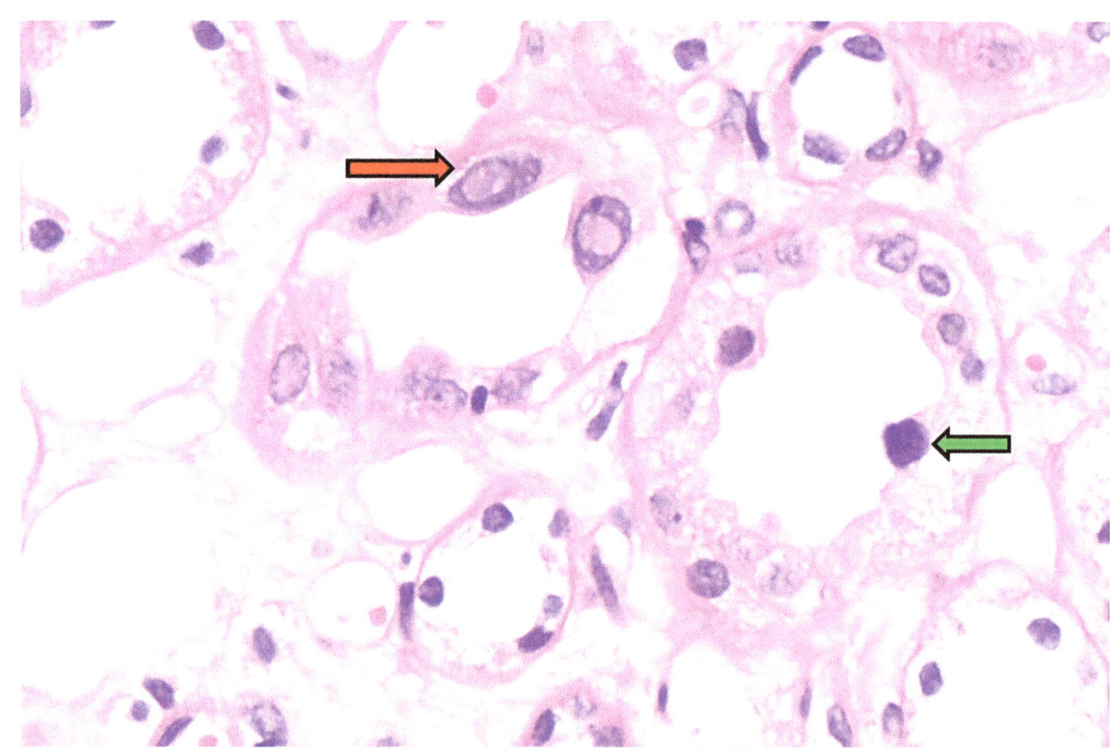

Figure 6:12.1: H&E Stain:40 x: Tubules: Type 1 (green arrow): intranuclear inclusion: ground glass -smudgy type 2 (red arrow): intranuclear granular inclusion body surrounded by mostly incomplete halo.

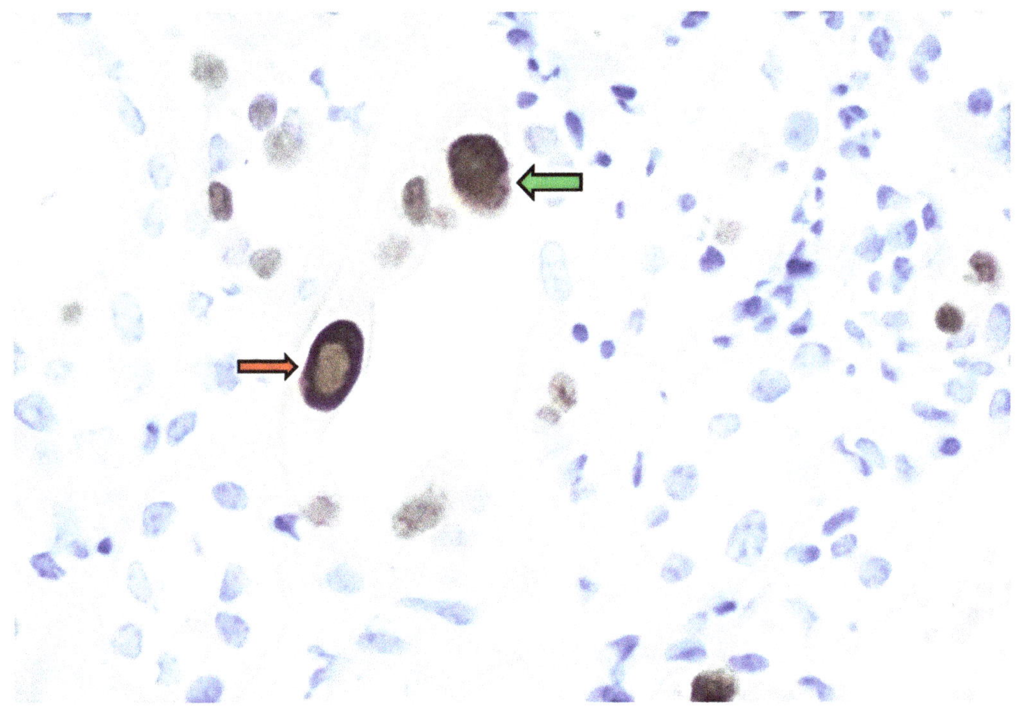

Figure 6 :12.2: IHC:SV 40 Stain: 40x:Tubules:positive for Polyoma virus: Type 1 (green arrow) &Type 2(red arrow).

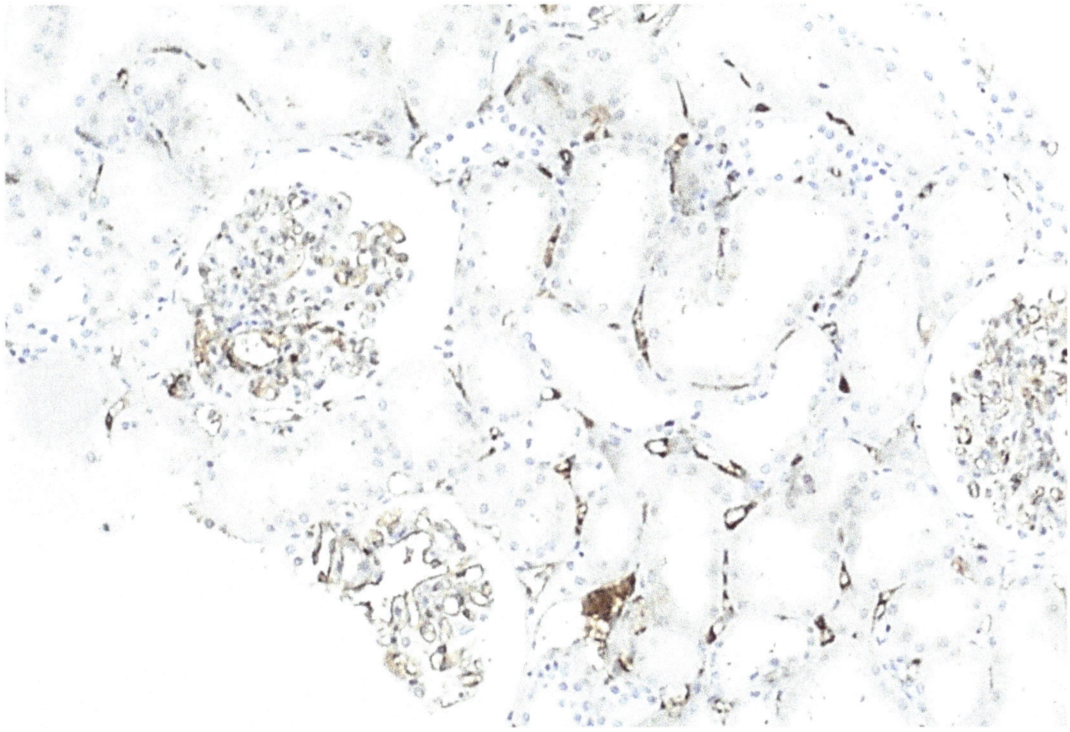

Figure 6 :12.3: C4d Stain:10x: Diffuse linear circumferential positivity around the GBM and Peritubular capillaries: Accommodation due to ABO Incompatibility IF/TA: 25% to 30%.

Interpretation: Polyomavirus Nephropathy: PVN Class 3.

*Suggested Reading:

Banff 2019: Category 5: polyomavirus nephropathy:

Specimen adequacy: two biopsy cores including portions of medulla in at least one of the two cores are required.

pvl scoring : is on the basis of the extent of virally induced tubular changes. A positive tubule: a tubule with intranuclear viral inclusion bodies (type 1 or 2) on the light microscopy and/or a positive IHC reaction for SV40-T antigen in one or more cells per tubular cross-section is considered and the overall percentage of positive tubular cross-sections is estimated in the entire biopsy sample (all available cores, cortex, and medulla).

pvl 1: ≤1% of all tubules/ducts with viral replication;

pvl 2: >1% to ≤10% of all tubules/ducts with viral replication;

pvl 3: >10% of all tubules/ducts with viral replication.

A Histologic class of definitive PVN:

morphologic degree of intrarenal pvl + Banff ci scores.

PVN Class 1 :

pvl 1 and ci 0-1

PVN Class 2 :

pvl 1 and ci 2-3 OR

pvl 2 and ci 0-3 OR

pvl 3 and ci 0-1

PVN Class 3:

pvl 3 and ci 2-3

.In PVN classes 1–3, interstitial inflammation and tubulitis can vary from Banff scores ti 0 to ti 3 /t 0 to t 3.

.PVN class 1 often lacks a significant inflammatory reaction. PVN and rejection (acute, chronic, cell mediated, and/or antibody mediated) can occur concomitantly.

Pathology Pearls

Parietal epithelial cells lining the Bowman capsule can show occasionally signs of viral replication, forming small **pseudocrescents***.

Nickeleit V. et.al:Polyomavirus of renal allograft recepients:from latent infection to manifest disease:J Am Soc Nephrol 1999;10(5):1080-1089.

Decoy cells*:

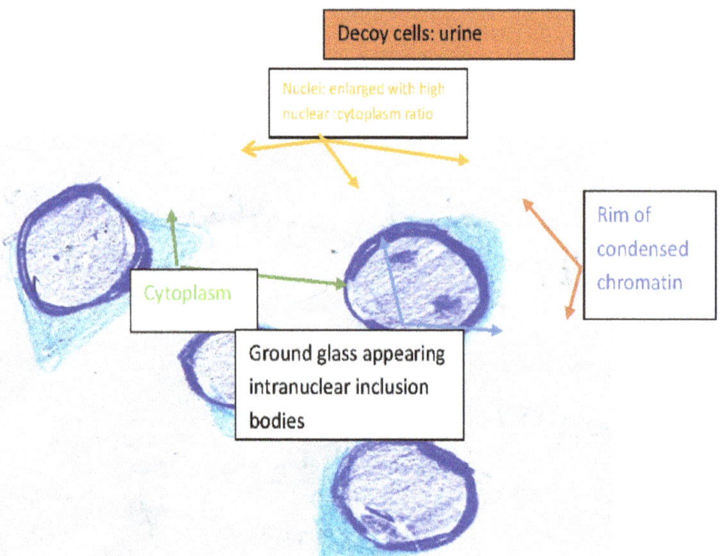

Figure 6:12.4: Diagrammatic representation of Decoy cells in urine :liquid based cytology: Papanicolaou Stain

Decoy cells*:

1. They are a morphologic sign of the activation of Polyomaviruses in the urinary tract, but not necessarily PVN.
2. Decoy cell analysis: threshold of ≥10 cells per liquid-based thin prep slide : excellent negative predictive value of greater than 99% but a positive predictive value of only 27%.
3. Quantitative urine PCR:
   Positive predictive value:27%
   Negative predictive value:99%
4. Quantitative plasma PCR:≥10,000copies per ml :74%probability of disease prediction .

Urine Polyomavirus-Haufen :

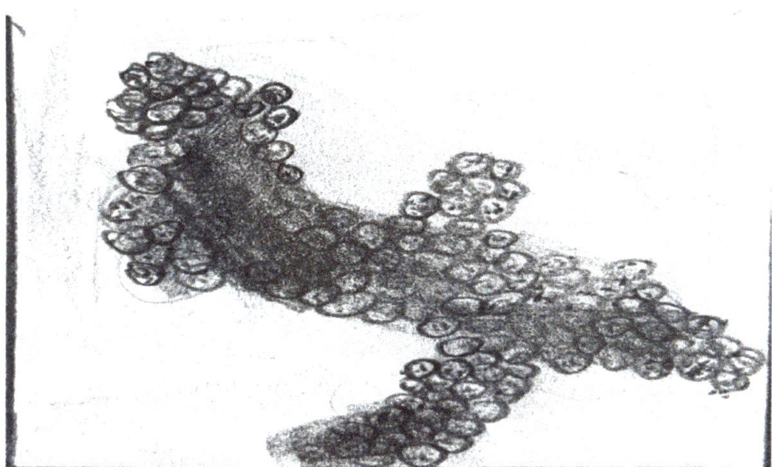

Figure 6:12.5: Diagrammatic representation of Polyomavirus-Haufen: Negative staining electron microscopy on a voided urine sample of a patient with Polyoma virus nephropathy.

Urine Polyomavirus-Haufen*:
These large three-dimensional cast-like viral aggregates, groups of virions, so called polyomavirus-Haufen are found in urine. Haufen (German for heap or stalk).
In PVN the viruses cluster and form cast-like structures in injured renal tubules containing high concentration of Tamm-Horsfall protein(THP). They are flushed into the bladder and can be detected in the voided urine as Polyomavirus-Haufen. These are pathognomic urinary biomarkers for PVN with positive and negative predictive values of >90%.

Cytomegalovirus (CMV) Inclusion:

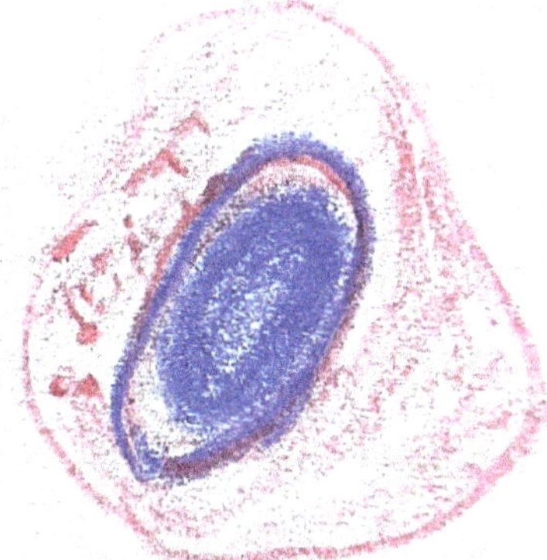

Owl-eye appearance of inclusion: CMV inclusions: central round inclusion body surrounded by a circumferential halo.

Figure 6:12.6: Diagrammatic representation of CMV inclusion: light microscopic view. These are seen in nuclei and cytoplasm of tubular epithelial cells(proximal tubules, collecting ducts), sometimes in endothelial cells and rarely in podocytes.

Table 6:12.1: *Histology of selected viral infections in allografts.

Sr.no.		Polyomavirus	Cytomegalovirus	Adenovirus	EBV-PTLD
A.	Virus inclusion type				
1.	Smudgy /ground-glass nuclear	common	Less common	common	-
2.	Central nuclear with halo	+	+++	+	-
3.	Cytoplasmic	-	+	±	-
B.	Sites of viral replication/staining				
1.	Tubular epithelial cells	+++	+++	+++	-
2.	Endothelial cells	-	++	-	-
3.	Inflammatory cells	-	±	++	+++
C.	Interstitial hemorrhage	-	-	+	May/not be
D.	Interstitial inflammation	Absent/present	±	Mild/moderate	-
E.	Granuloma formation	Often absent	±	++	-
F.	Acute tubular injury/necrosis	May/not be	Mild to moderate	Usually severe	May/not be
G.	Focal parenchymal necrosis	-	±	+-+++	±-++
H.	IHC stain	SV-40:+	CMV:+	Adenovirus:+	EBV:+

*Renal Transplant Pathology :Heptinstall's Pathology of the Kidney: volume II-seventh edition :page no.:1403.

CASE 13

History: 41 years old male, native kidney disease IgA Nephropathy treated with MMF and steroids for 2 years and progressed to ESRD. Underwent ABOi renal allograft transplant with sister as donor. Received PLEX and IVIG with Rituximab Pre-Transplant as per ABOi protocol. Received ATG 1g/kg as induction along with Methylprednisolone. Maintenance immunosuppression with CNI/MMF/Steroids. Serum creatinine 2mg/dl achieved at end of one week. Allograft biopsy done due to suboptimal decline in creatinine and persistent hypertension – it showed ATN. That time LDH :102 IU/L: Normal, Platelet count: normal, Urine analysis: Protein:1+, RBCs:8 to 10/HPF, Pus cells:10-12/HPF, Urine culture: sterile. So, Inj. Methylprednisolone 250 mg once daily given for 2 more days. DJ stent removed at 2 weeks. Serum creatinine decreased to 1.5 mg/dl. 3 weeks post-transplant, he presented with a serum creatinine of 2.9 mg/dl.

Other investigations: Urine analysis: Protein:2+, RBCs:8 -10/HPF, Pus cells:12-15/HPF. Urine culture: Sterile. USG findings: Enlarged and swollen graft, no fluid collection or features of obstruction, doppler: raised RI, no evidence of impaired perfusion. Serum DSA: Negative.

Second allograft biopsy done.

Clinical DD: Acute rejection/ CNI Toxicity / Thrombotic Microangiopathy / Acute tubular necrosis / Acute interstitial inflammation– Possibly due to Viral infections.

Light microscopy:

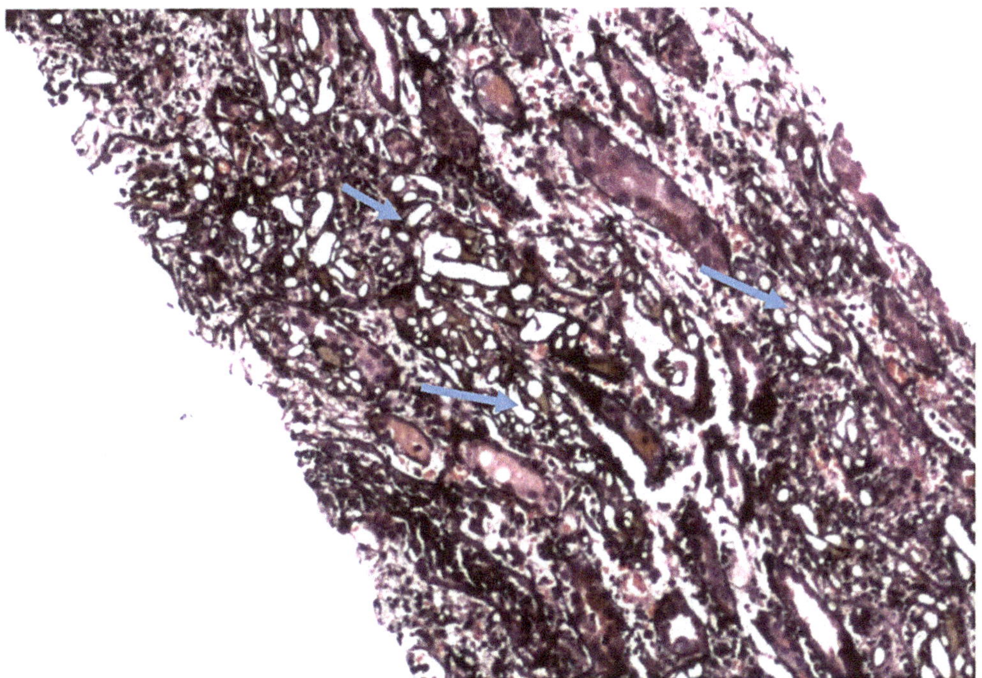

Figure 6:13.1: PASM stain:10x: Moderately dense patchy interstitial inflammation with mucormycosis hyphae mostly in tubules.

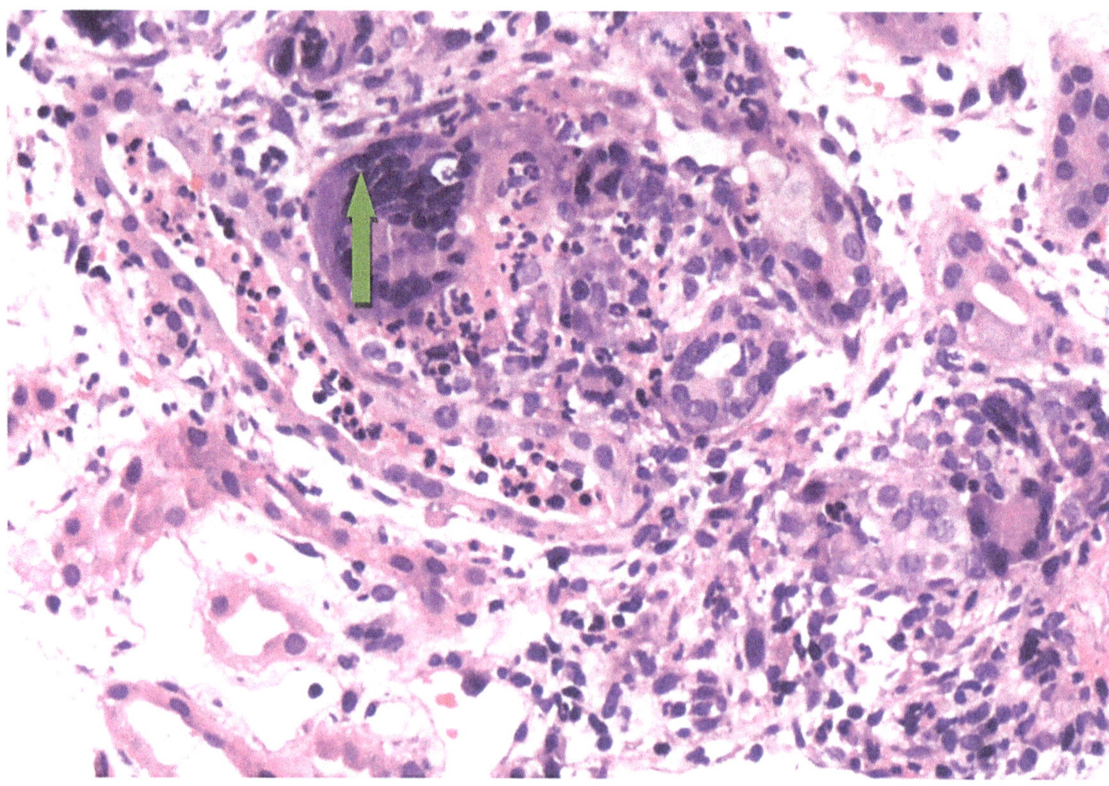

Figure 6:13.2: Haematoxylin and Eosin Stain:20x: interstitial inflammation forming ill-formed granuloma -multinucleated giant cells (green arrow).

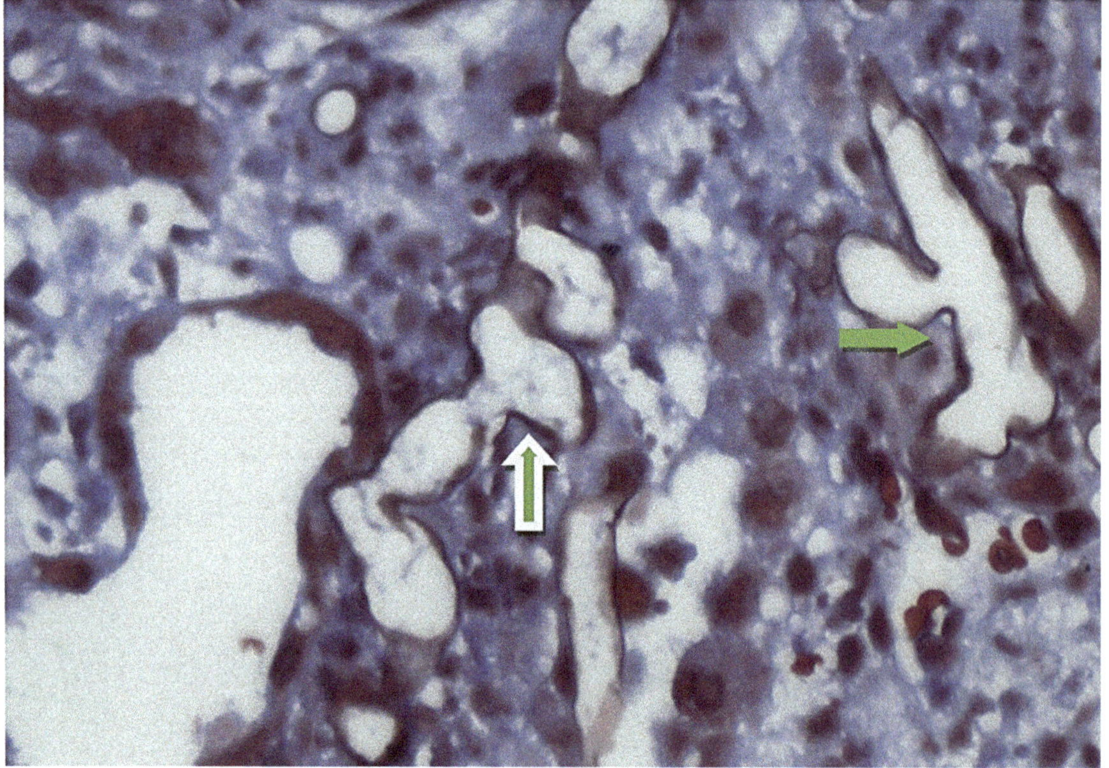

Figure 6:13.3: Masson Trichrome stain:40x: Mucor mycosis hyphae –right angle branching (green arrows).

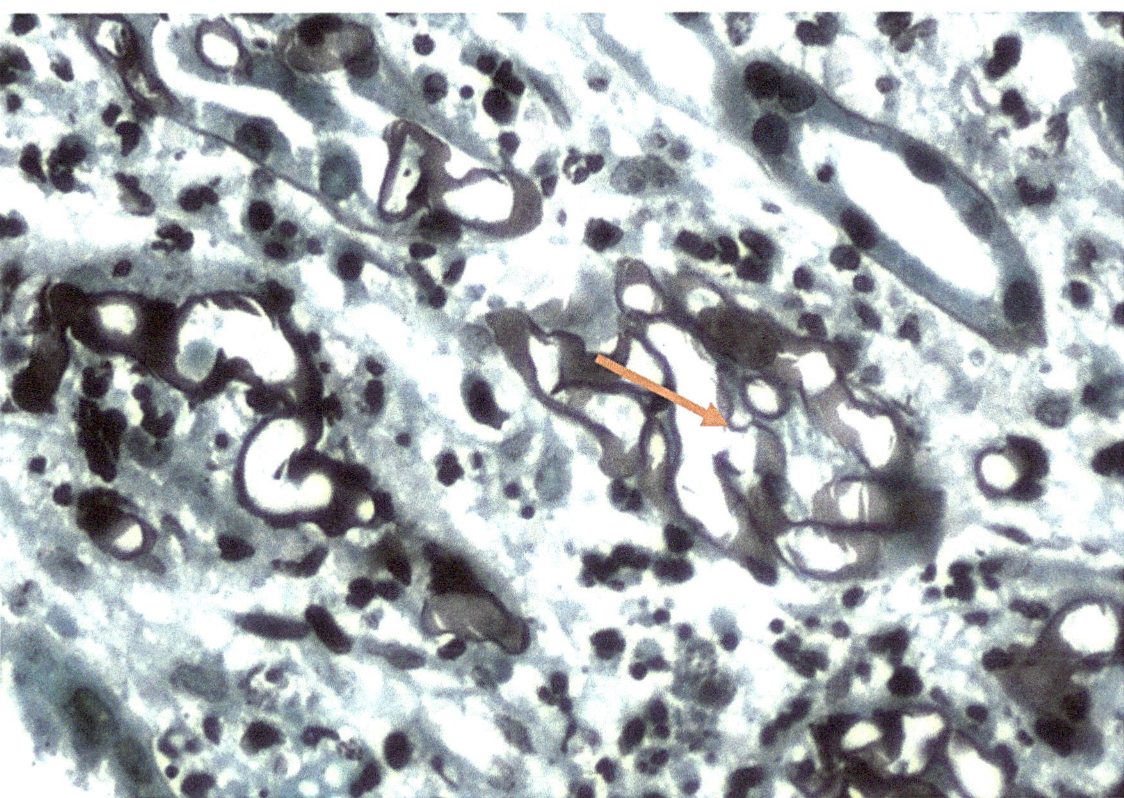

Figure 6:13.4: Grocott's Methenamine Silver stain:20x: Broad aseptate hyphae with right angle branching (orange arrow).

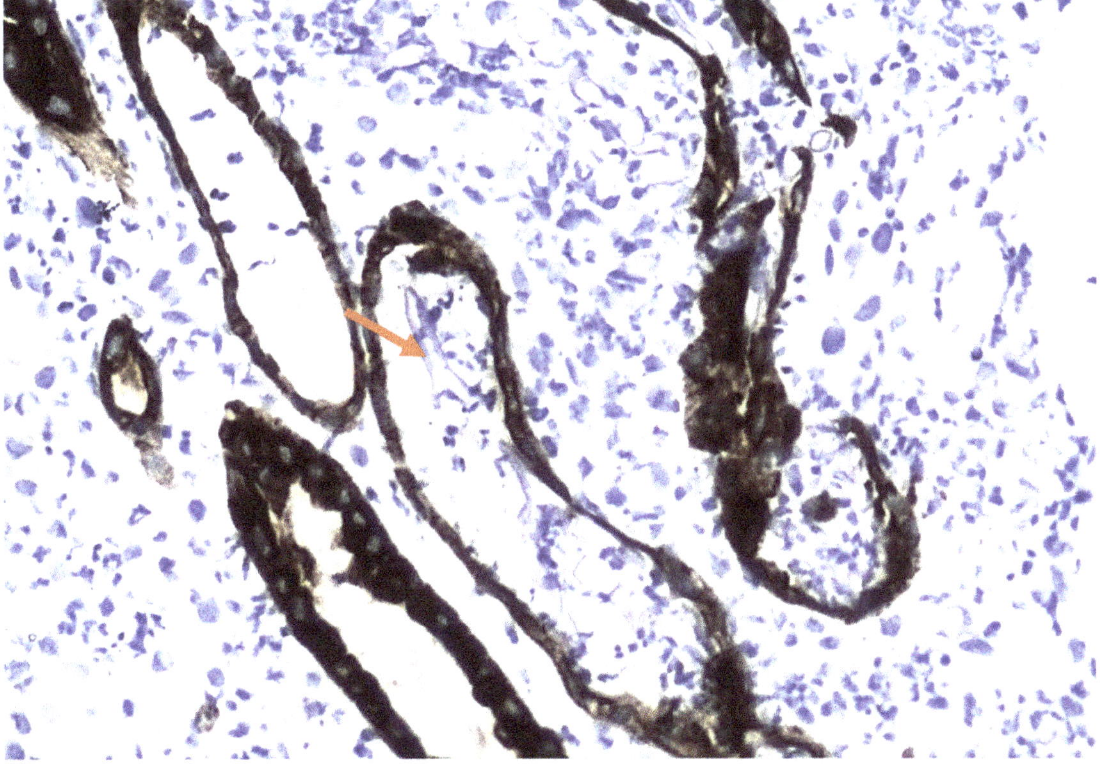

Figure 6:13.5: Immunohistochemistry:20x: Cytokeratin-7: Mucor (orange arrow) in distal convoluted tubules (DCTs)

Interpretation:

Allograft Kidney (needle) biopsy shows features of Mucormycosis. The C4d positivity is attributed to ABO incompatible status. There is no definite evidence of rejection seen in the biopsy studied.

Pathology Pearls

Mucormycosis: Mucormycosis is an angioinvasive fungal infection typically seen in vessels, peritubular capillaries and glomerular capillaries. In this case Mucormycosis is seen invading the tubules and not so much visible in vessels.

CASE 14

History: 45 years old male, ESRD due to unknown aetiology, on MHD for one year, underwent living donor renal transplant with mother as donor. Induction with Methyl prednisolone. Maintenance triple immunosuppression with Tacrolimus, MMF, steroid. CMV status D+/R+. Uneventful intraoperative and post operative course. Nadir creatinine:0.8 mg/dl. Last 10 days patient is having diarrhoea with 4-5 episodes of loose stools per day. Now one-month post-transplant he has graft dysfunction.

Investigations: Serum creatinine :3 mg/dl, Potassium :5.3mEq/L, Chloride :111mEq/L. Urine Protein: Nil, RBCs: 2-3/HPF, Pus cells :1-2/HPF. Tacrolimus trough level: 15 ng/ml.

Clinical diagnosis: AKI – Prerenal due to diarrhoea with CNI toxicity.

Light microscopy:

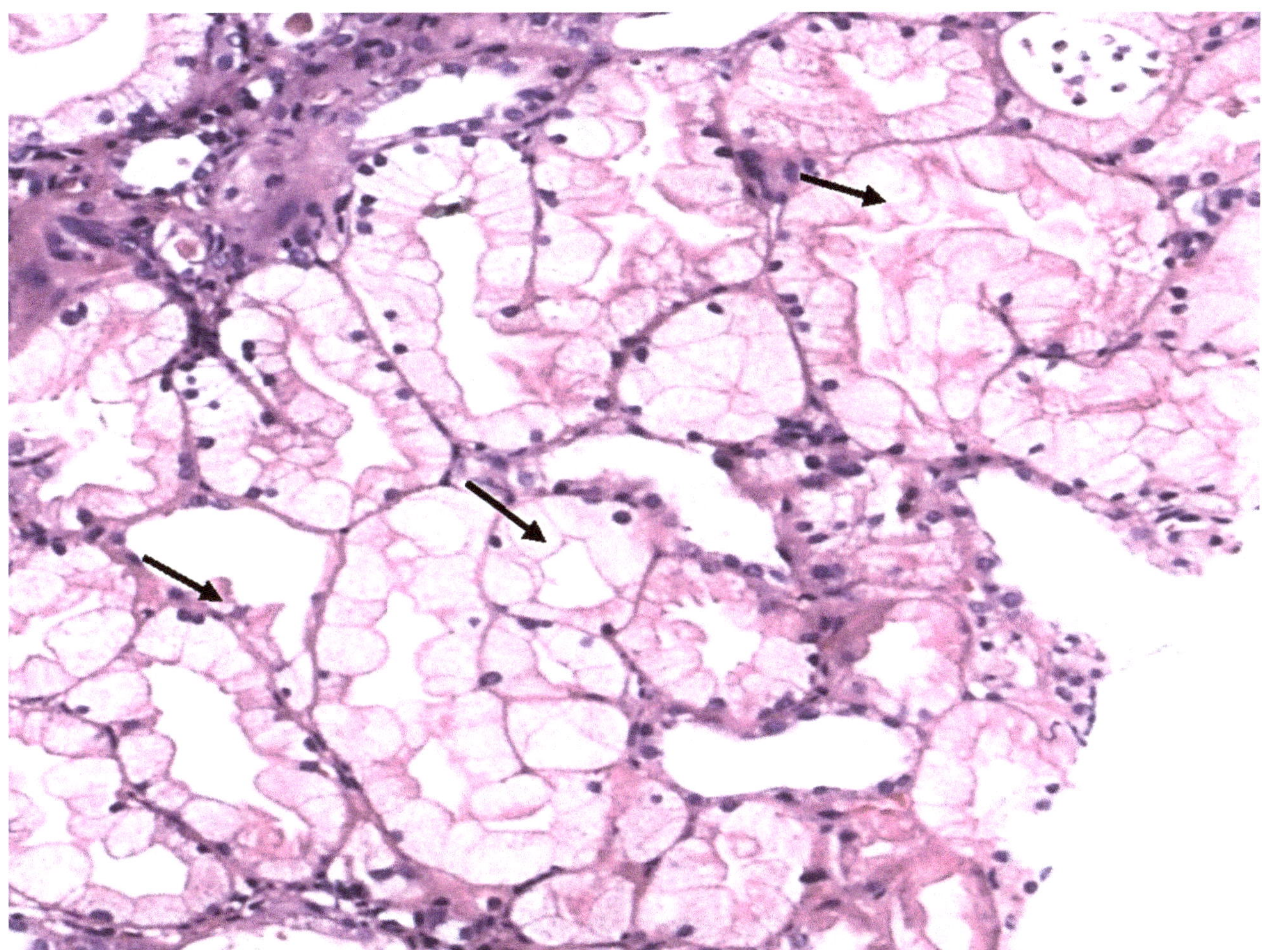

Figure 6:14.1: H&E Stain:20x: The tubular epithelial cell cytoplasmic vacuoles are isometric in nature (**black** arrows).

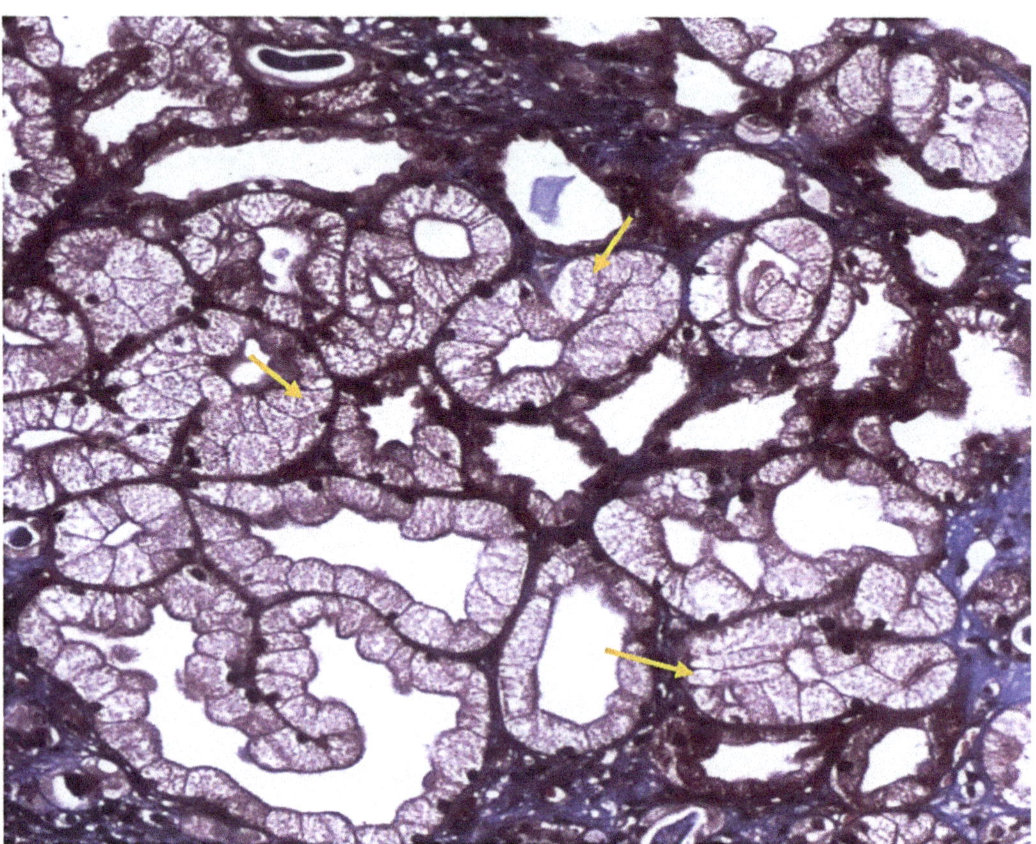

Figure 6:14.2: MT Stain:20x: CNI toxicity: Isometric cytoplasmic vacuolisations (yellow arrows).

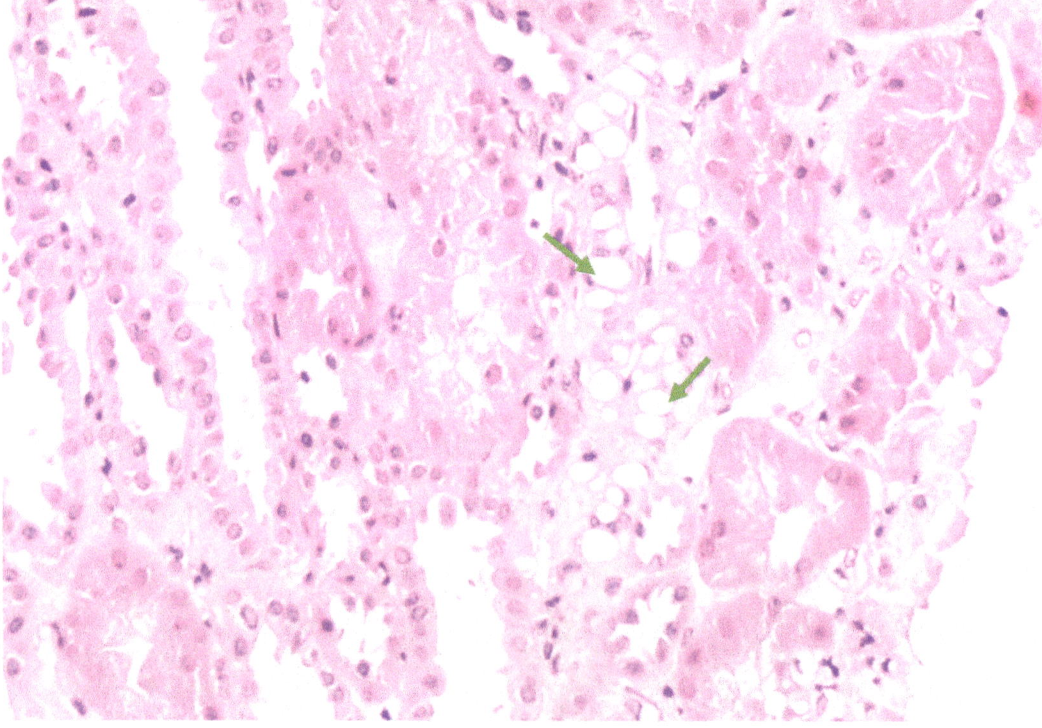

Figure 6:14.3: H&E Stain:20x:CNI arteriolopathy: Ballooning of smooth muscle cells of arterioles (green arrows).

Early Calcineurin Inhibitor (CNI) Toxicity

Pathology Pearls

Arteriolar ballooning in native kidneys:

1. Acute ischemic injury
2. Nephrotic syndrome with non-selective proteinuria.

*Heptinstall's Pathology of the kidney: seventh edition: Volume II: chapter 29: Renal Transplant Pathology: Page no.1395-1398.

CASE 15

History: 51 years old male, ESRD due to IgA Nephropathy, on MHD for 2 years, underwent living unrelated donor renal transplant. HLA match: 2/6. Induction with 3 g/kg ATG with Methyl prednisolone. Maintenance triple immunosuppression with Tacrolimus, MMF, steroid. CMV status D+/R+. Uneventful intraoperative and post operative course. Nadir creatinine = 1 mg/dl.4 months post-transplant patient had biopsy proven antibody mediated rejection treated with PLEX and IVIG. New baseline creatinine is 2.2 mg/dl. Tacrolimus trough level 8ng/ml. At end of one year serum creatinine is 2.6 mg/dl, repeat graft biopsy had no rejection or recurrence of IgA nephropathy but had 20% IFTA. BP is well controlled with 2 anti-hypertensives. Now he is 3 years post-transplant. Third biopsy is done.

Investigations: He has a serum creatinine of 3.8 mg/dl. Tacrolimus drug level of 8 ng/ml. Urine Protein: 2+, RBCs: 1-2/HPF, Pus cells :2-3/HPF, UPCR : 1.2 g/g.

Clinical diagnosis: CKD 4T – Chronic allograft Nephropathy.

Light microscopy:

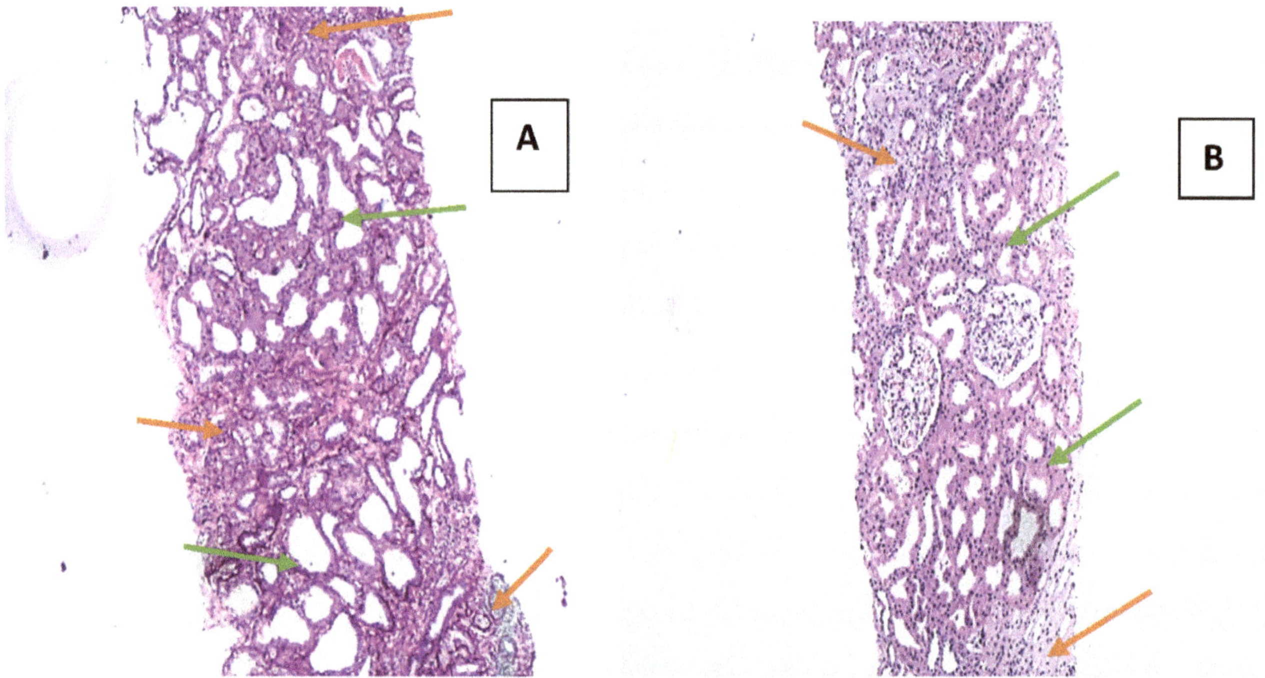

Figure 6:15.1: PAS Stain(A) and H&E Stain(b):10x: Moderate tubulointerstitial changes of chronicity: striped fibrosis: alternate viable (green arrows) and fibrosed areas (orange arrows).

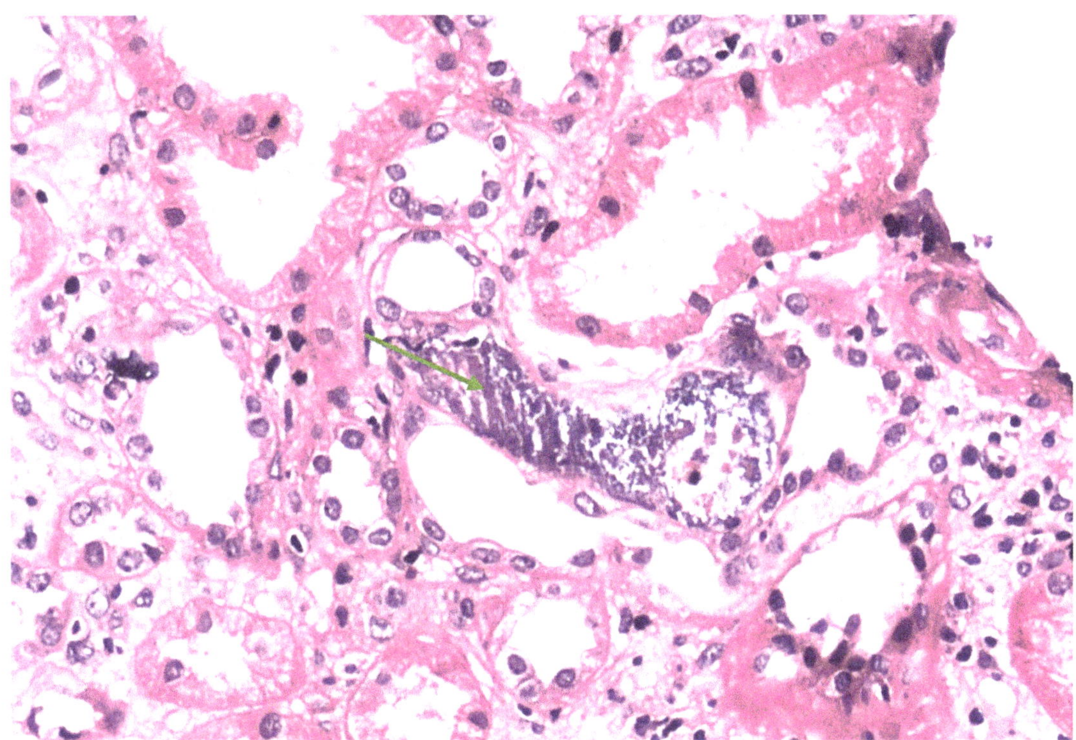

Figure 6:15.2: H&E Stain:20x: The tubule shows luminal calcification.

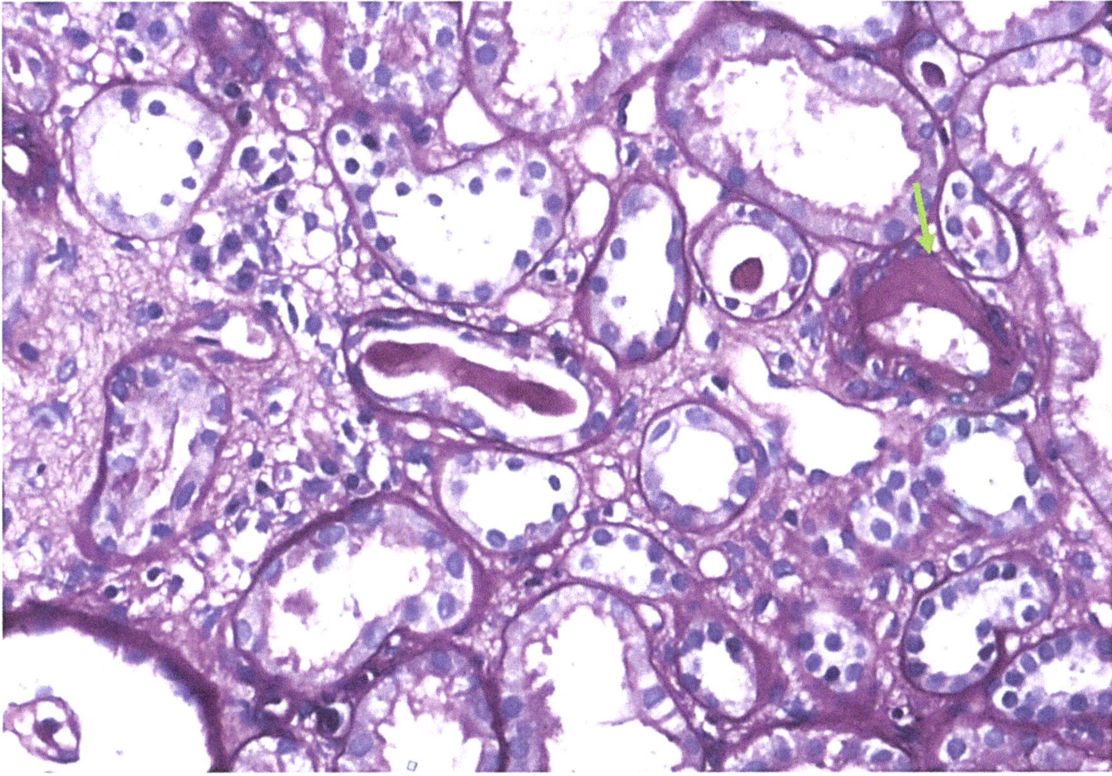

Figure 6:15.3: PAS Stain-20x: Arteriolar hyalinosis: intramural deposition: involving the muscle layer (green arrow): Hyaline is glassy smooth in appearance.

Interpretation: Late Calcineurin Inhibitor (CNI) Toxicity

Pathology Pearls

*The striped pattern of interstitial fibrosis seen in chronic tubular CNI toxicity is possibly a result of chronic ischemia in watershed zones of the medullary rays due to hyaline arteriosclerosis and direct tubular toxicity.

**Pearl-like pattern /beaded/nodular arteriolar hyalinosis: seen in late CNI arteriolopathy

*Diagnostic Pathology: Kidney Diseases, second edition; Colvin/Chang-page no.642.
**Heptinstall's Pathology of the Kidney: seventh edition: Volume II: chapter 29: Renal Transplant Pathology: Page no.1398.

Interpretation: Late Calcineurin Inhibitor (CNI) Toxicity

www.ingramcontent.com/pod-product-compliance
Lightning Source LLC
Chambersburg PA
CBHW040739150726
48196CB00011B/657